BDJ Clinician's Guides

This series enables clinicians at all stages of their careers to remain well informed and up to date on key topics across all fields of clinical dentistry. Each volume is superbly illustrated and provides concise, highly practical guidance and solutions. The authors are recognised experts in the subjects that they address. The *BDJ Clinician's Guides* are trusted companions, designed to meet the needs of a wide readership. Like the *British Dental Journal* itself, they offer support for undergraduates and newly qualified, while serving as refreshers for more experienced clinicians. In addition they are valued as excellent learning aids for postgraduate students.

The BDJ Clinicians' Guides are produced in collaboration with the British Dental Association, the UK's trade union and professional association for dentists.

Aws Alani • Mahul Patel

Adhesive Techniques in Restorative Dentistry

Springer

Aws Alani
Faculty of Oral Health,
University of Plymouth
Plymouth, London, UK

Faculty of Dentistry,
Oral and Craniofacial Sciences,
King's College London
London, UK

Mahul Patel
University College London
Faculty of Medical Sciences
Eastman Dental Institute
London, UK

Faculty of Dentistry,
Oral and Craniofacial Sciences
King's College London
London, UK

ISSN 2523-3327 ISSN 2523-3335 (electronic)
BDJ Clinician's Guides
ISBN 978-3-032-07345-7 ISBN 978-3-032-07346-4 (eBook)
https://doi.org/10.1007/978-3-032-07346-4

This Springer imprint is published by the registered company Springer Nature Switzerland AG
The registered company address is: Gewerbestrasse 11, 6330 Cham, Switzerland

Aws *would like to dedicate this book to his wife, Mimi, his parents Mustafa and Fatin, and his brother Faisal. He would like to thank his sons Zachary and Elias for their constant distraction during his writing.*

Mahul *would like to dedicate this book to his parents, Dilip and Kalpna; and to his children Nyla (his happiness) and Josh (his joy).*

Foreword

It is with great pleasure and privilege to write a foreword to this new book, *Adhesive Techniques in Restorative Dentistry*, by Drs Aws Alani and Mahul Patel. This book represents the paradigm shift in Restorative Dentistry, Prosthodontics and Operative Dentistry during the last 20 years. Contemporary adhesive approaches to tooth restoration provide a predictable and sensible option that is minimally invasive compared to the more traditional approaches of conventional tooth preparation and retention.

They have methodically delivered 10 chapters spanning various patient presentations, from tooth surface loss to tooth replacement, illustrating the text with step-by-step photographs. The sequential graphical presentation of procedures empowers and mentors the reader in understanding and appreciating how to deliver dentistry to the excellent standards presented. The text is an authoritative reference for undergraduates, postgraduates, specialist dentists and established practitioners in adhesive procedures, providing a comprehensive atlas for dentists to learn from or refer to when needed.

The authors, Drs Aws Alani and Mahul Patel, are diverse and different in their backgrounds and training, but are united by their expertise, knowledge and technical skill. Their meticulous attention to detail and clinical dexterity is captured masterfully through over 1000 clinical photographs, making this a standout addition to any dental library, bookshelf or learning resource collection.

It was a pleasure to read it!

Professor of Oral Function and Restorative Dentistry Bas Loomans
Radboud University Medical Centre
Nijmegen, The Netherlands

Preface

The purpose of this textbook is to highlight, describe and depict current adhesive techniques used to manage and treat common clinical conditions across the breadth of Restorative Dentistry. This book is an essential purchase for undergraduate and postgraduate students where modern operative techniques and contemporary restorative dentistry methods are taught. It is aimed to be used as an aide memoir instruction guide for both general and specialist practitioners working in primary and secondary care environments to develop and enhance existing clinical skill sets.

Achieving clinical outcomes whilst delivering minimally invasive techniques is supremely beneficial as teeth and their associated structures are irreplaceable. During our times opinions have swayed and new technology has replaced the old. Despite so much change one entity has remained true, adhesive dentistry applied optimally and with understanding, works. The delivery of treatment in this manner requires ingenuity and presence of mind through processing material science, dental anatomy and self-discipline. Clinical skills in Dentistry are won through the continual cycle of practicing, implementing and reflecting. The cases and knowledge captured in this text are the culmination of collective 40 years of experience and practice that have been incrementally built continually since our first phantom head sessions in the late 1990s as Dental Students at King's College London. Distinction is achieved through contemplating the last restoration, critiquing oneself, and saving those sentiments for the next. This notion was classically personified by Aristotle:

> **Excellence is an art won by training and habituation. We do not act rightly because we have virtue or excellence, rather we have those because we acted rightly. We are what we repeatedly do. Excellence is not an act but a habit.**

We would like to thank all our colleagues we have met through this great profession and more specifically those that trained and supported us through our journey to reach the level of knowledge and experience we enjoy today. We hope our debt is rewarded through the achievement of this book. We want to give a special acknowledgement to all the front-line National Health Service medical, dental, nursing and auxiliary healthcare workers who, during the global Corona virus (Covid-19) outbreak, worked with great spirit and bravery to ensure the comforts and care of our patients were met. We are forever grateful for your selfless courageous efforts during that turbulent time.

Plymouth, London, UK Aws Alani
London, UK Mahul Patel

Contents

About the Authors

Aws Alani, BDS, MFDS RCS (Eng), MSc, FDS RCS (Eng), LLM, FHEA, MFDT, FCGDent graduated from King's College London in 2003. He completed dental foundation training in Essex and held junior hospital positions at Guy's Hospital and King's College Hospital, before completing an MSc in Endodontics at the Eastman Dental Institute. He then moved to Morriston Hospital in South Wales to work in the maxillofacial unit where he spent four years as a trainee. He subsequently moved to Newcastle, where he completed his specialist training in restorative dentistry. During his training, he completed extensive relief work trips to Romania and Ghana with 'Young Smiles for Romania' and 'Global Brigades', respectively.

In 2013, Aws became the International Team for Implantology Scholar in Toronto, Canada, working at the Hospital for Sick Children and Bloorview Kids Rehabilitation Hospital. He returned to London in 2014 as an NHS consultant in restorative dentistry at King's College Hospital. His main remit is the management of congenital and acquired defects within a multidisciplinary team environment. In 2022, he was appointed Associate Professor in Restorative Dentistry at Peninsula Dental School. He is a UK registered specialist in Endodontics, Prosthodontics and Restorative Dentistry.

He has won numerous prizes and research grants from specialist societies and has lectured nationally and internationally. He has published over 50 peer-reviewed publications, book chapters and textbooks. He also holds a master's degree in medical law from Cardiff University. He is the course director for the Diploma in Operative Dentistry at Kings College London, which looks to upskill general dental practitioners in a multifaceted manner through seminars, hands-on simulated exercises and clinical treatment. He is also course director for the MSc in Endodontics at Peninsula Dental School, which is provided through blended learning with a focus on provision of root canal treatment minimally invasively with an emphasis on tooth tissue preservation and holistic restorative treatment planning. In 2025, he was invited onto the editorial board for the *British Dental Journal*.

Mahul Patel, BDS, MJDF RCS (Eng), MSc, MSc, MPros RCS (Ed). Mahul graduated from King's College London in 2002 and completed two master's degrees at the UCL Eastman Dental Institute in Restorative Dental Practice (2010) and Conservative Dentistry (2012). The latter was awarded with Distinction and the 3M ESPE post-graduate prize for excellence in clinical and academic achievement. He then gained Membership in Prosthodontics at the Royal College of Surgeons of Edinburgh in 2014.

He worked as a Specialty Dentist in Prosthodontics at King's College Dental Hospital for 9 years, in parallel with working in private referral practice in London. The remit of his clinical work is largely associated with the provision of Restorative Dentistry and Prosthodontics. In addition, he is a Senior Clinical Teacher at King's College London and a Senior Clinical Teaching Fellow at the UCL Eastman Dental Institute where he teaches on various post-graduate Restorative and Endodontic programmes. His research interests include the behaviour of restorative dental materials and novel methods of teaching practical hands-on prosthodontic techniques utilising digital media. He has lectured and presented nationally and internationally on a variety of clinical subjects and has published in peer-reviewed journals. He is a Key Opinion Leader and advisor for various multinational dental companies.

Rationale for Adhesive Techniques

1

Contents

Learning Outcomes

- Appreciate the ethos and advantages of minimally invasive adhesive techniques in the provision of restorative dentistry.
- Understand the differences between subtractive and additive techniques, where the latter results in reduced damage to natural tooth tissue.
- Realise that additive adhesive restorations are more likely to result in improved longevity of teeth when compared to more traditional conventional restorations.

1.1 Introduction

The perception of what may constitute a 'healthy' dentition is likely to be subjective and differ from patient to patient and dentist to dentist. At the very basic level, patients may expect, rather than aspire to, a dentition that is pain-free, functional and aesthetic. Meeting these expectations, despite their seemingly fundamental nature, may seem daunting to the clinician, depending upon the individual clinical challenges that present. The solutions to the clinician may be very apparent, but what may be more testing is the ideals and aspirations of the patient.

A. Alani, M. Patel, *Adhesive Techniques in Restorative Dentistry*, BDJ Clinician's Guides, https://doi.org/10.1007/978-3-032-07346-4_1

The paternalistic approach to oral care has progressively ebbed away from everyday practice due to the rapid increase in patient knowledge subsequent to the digital information revolution. Patients tend to question more readily, wanting to know the process, outcome and longevity of what we provide. Almost concurrently, the increase in dento-legal litigation has tempered clinicians to develop strategies to reach or even surpass patient expectations but achieving these utilising methods that minimise damage or reduce patient exposure to risk. The well-informed patient will be aware of technological advances and understand the positive repercussions of treatment. This 'knowledge' will not be to a professional level but to a degree that will result in an impetus to seek involvement in clinical decision-making, the outcome of which may be scrutinised by the patient to a greater level than ever before. This increased expectation, coupled with the potential legal repercussions, has resulted in the development of more innovative operative techniques to solve common clinical problems.

The philosophy of attaining successful clinical outcomes through 'maintaining health of what remains', as opposed to 'destroying to achieve a result', is likely to be the preferred aim of modern contemporary dentistry for both clinicians and patients.

1.2 Patterns of Need

The management of plaque-associated disease is the established core of the dental profession. Repercussions of caries or periodontal disease require comprehensive management from the optimisation of oral hygiene measures right up to the unfortunate need for tooth extraction. Patterns of need have changed due to the increased prevalence and reporting of non-plaque-associated disease processes and conditions such as tooth surface loss, congenital tooth malformations and dental trauma. Other emerging pathologies, such as cracked tooth syndrome, are challenging due to inconsistent signs and symptoms and the need to manage a sensitised vital pulpal complex with compromised dental structural integrity. If teeth lose pulp vitality, from cracks or caries, the planning for root canal treatment should embrace the need for an optimal coronal seal and cuspal coverage strategy at the outset of endodontic treatment. If teeth prove to be unrestorable, patients are less inclined to accept extraction as the remedy for their problem, however absolute a solution that may be, largely due to the social stigma as well as physical and mental co-morbidities associated with partial edentulism. Contemporary solutions for tooth replacement, such as dental implants, do carry significant morbidities during provision and have emerging biological and mechanical complications, the remedies for which are not forthcoming. Alternative tooth replacement methods must be explored.

The twenty-first-century patient is also more likely to suffer and report mental health issues. These can manifest in their opinions and requests for treatment. Patients with body dysmorphia may be convinced of the need for wholesale cosmetic changes to otherwise intact, healthy teeth. Managing these conditions whilst respecting the ideals of health and benefit, whilst reducing biological risk, can be a difficult task for the clinician. With this plethora of problems, plaque-associated or not, physical or mental, the 'value' in treatment should focus on how we can achieve patient satisfaction and health without undue damage. Patients may realise that treatment that preserves tooth health whilst improving function and aesthetics is more valuable than any other mode of provision.

1.3 The Need for Change

Traditional prosthodontic modes of indirect extra-coronal restorations focus on the attainment of resistance and retention form through a radial preparation that is near parallel or at least has a total occlusal convergence angle of 6°. This approach is 'subtractive' in its nature as it requires the removal of an increased volume of tooth tissue for the provision of the restoration. The genesis of these ideals occurred during a period where restorations were cemented to prepared abutment teeth with weak luting cements. This approach may result in a risk of pulp vitality loss. Heat generation or pulp exposure will compromise the pulp, making the need for root canal treatment more likely. It is known that loss of pulp vitality and the subsequent root canal treatment weaken teeth mechanically. Successful endodontics is also technique sensitive and brings co-morbidities to the patient, such as further pain and prolonged treatment. With the cervical extension of extra-coronal restorations, marginal fit becomes crucial to avoid positive or negative ledge creation, which aggregates plaque deposits and is a prelude to caries, gingivitis or periodontal defects. It would therefore seem a natural progression to reduce or even omit risks to patients by providing predictable restorations that do not compromise tooth tissue or threaten pulp or gingival health.

1.4 Survival—Tooth Versus Restoration

Research examining the longevity of restorations is popular as it provides clinicians with a tangible time period for the length of service of restorations. These research threads may focus on restoration survival as opposed to tooth survival, or the endpoint of restoration failure as opposed to tooth extraction. Tooth survival when linked to types of restoration would be more relevant to the patient and clinician.

These factors need to be considered more generally when considering the patient and the need for further treatment. The placement of a restoration for a patient of 20 years of age is likely to require replacement at least, at a conservative estimate, six times during the lifetime of the patient if it is assumed that the tooth is retained and not extracted. This is on the assumption that by the sixth replacement, there is adequate tooth tissue available to seal the remaining structure and manage occlusal loads without catastrophically failing. If the initial preparations remove significant tooth tissue or the disease process, such as extensive caries, leaves minimal volume remaining, the tooth may not be retained in the long term. The 'subtractive' approach, by definition, removes tooth tissue at every point that the restoration requires replacement. This then progressively increases the risk of tooth loss as less and less tissue remains. Fundamentally, plaque-associated disease threatens tooth retention, as can overtly aggressive dental intervention.

1.5 The 3 A's of Adhesive Dentistry

Traditional prosthodontic approaches to the assessment of teeth prior to restoration may consider the volume and height of the tooth to deliver either an intra-coronal or extra-coronal restoration, depending on clinical case presentation. This is also true of the adhesive approach to treatment, which wholly depends on the bonding surface area. The key to successful adhesion is the presence of an optimal bonding substrate, its subsequent isolation and observing an adhesive bonding protocol. This largely translates to the presence of enamel, ideally, throughout the prospective margin of the restoration, the ability to isolate the tooth and proficiency in a bonding sequence.

Tooth tissue is physiologically responsive to its environment. At the higher level, this may involve the utilisation of growth factors present within the pulp or dentine to respond to bacterial invasion. More routinely, teeth can adapt to occlusal loading through bending and deforming largely due to the elasticity of dentine and the ability of the periodontal ligament to manage applied forces. Unfortunately, dental materials are yet to be able to mimic natural tooth tissues in this way without the combined use of dental adhesives. In addition, minimising tooth tissue removal during restoration is likely to retain many biomechanical advantages.

The key advantage of adhesive dentistry is that it can be provided on both a 'subtractive' and on an 'additive' basis, nullifying the need to remove tooth tissue and the co-morbidities that may bring. Without a significant volume of tooth tissue removal, treatment is provided 'atraumatically'; any initial pulp insult through caries or tooth surface loss is not worsened or amplified by treatment. Gingival health is also maintained where restoration margins are kept equi- or supragingival, or the gingiva is retracted during the procedure without the creation of a positive ledge profile.

'Additive' as opposed to 'subtractive' restorative dentistry is more technique sensitive and requires improved operator skill and a greater appreciation of restorative material science, knowledge of occlusion and the physiology of tooth movement. Where indirect restorations are essentially designed and constructed by technical colleagues through information provided to them, the direct adhesive additive approach puts more onus onto the clinician to formulate restoration design and manage its delivery through various chairside clinical stages. In essence, the dental surgeon can now interplay the roles of both technician and clinician.

The digital age has increased the visual scrutiny of dental restorations. Patients may analyse the treatment we provide through photographs of themselves, putting greater pressure on clinicians to deliver aesthetic outcomes. Recreating tooth tissue, the small nuances, from surface texture to colour and shape, can be challenging and humbling. Conventional restorations, provided in a wholesale manner for multiple adjacent anterior units, remove the onus of reproducing natural tooth appearance from the clinician onto technical colleagues. In comparison, the techniques and cases showcased in this book have been wholly designed and delivered through the hands of the clinician who can better appreciate the features of the natural dentition as they reside during the clinical appointment. The breadth of resin materials available to clinicians, and treatment adjuncts such as gingival recontouring and tooth bleaching, needs to be fully utilised to produce an optimal 'aesthetic' outcome.

The 3 A's of adhesive dentistry; 'additive', 'atraumatic' and 'aesthetic' (Fig. 1.1), all combine with good clinician motivation and a self-critical approach, resulting in consistent outcomes that are predictable and reduce patient morbidity. When putting this into perspective, it may seem a daunting change in mindset, but with a wider remit of role, there comes greater adaptability, variety of skills that can be applied to different clinical situations and potentially greater job satisfaction.

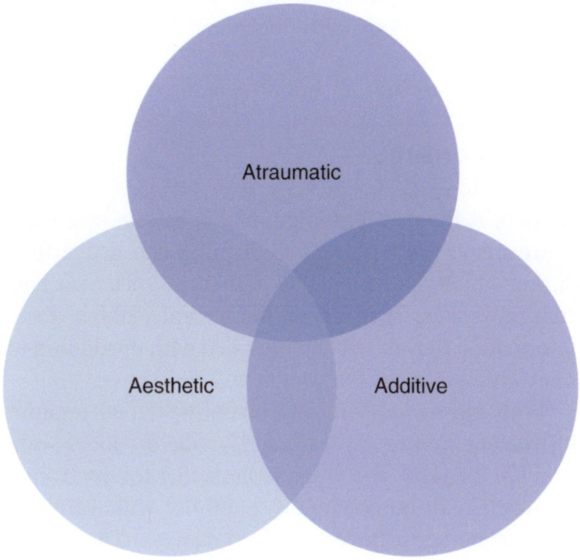

Fig. 1.1 The 3 A's of adhesive dentistry

1.6 Business Model

One of the main keys to business is customer satisfaction, the ability to satisfy patients to a degree that they return to your clinic rather than to another office and attract their family and friends to attend for your clinical service. This is a key determinant of business growth and profitability. What could be more convincing to family and friends than an improved smile, 'whiter' and more uniform without gaps, that did not require local anaesthetic or 'drilling'? These positive aspects of ethical minimally invasive aesthetic dentistry are huge selling points over other modes. This provides the satisfaction to the patient or 'value' attached to the treatment they are being provided with. 'Value' may not only be provided when comparing the ratio between the monetary outlay to the treatment provided. With healthcare and more often invasive procedures, the biological cost of treatment triangulates the inter-relationship. The patient is not simply purchasing a direct adhesive restoration or a tooth bleaching treatment; they are choosing self-preservation and self-maintenance. The business advantages for the clinician are apparent in more ways than one.

Through the additive adhesive approach, restoration renewal can be relatively predictable and consistent, provided the highly biologically 'valuable' enamel is maintained. However, the latter cannot be said with any guarantee for the provision of replacement conventional restorations. Hence, the business model is based on the selling points of minimal invasive treatment provision from the outset, but also the predictability in inevitably replacing the restoration and the future treatment fees attached to this.

1.7 Consent

Consent is the permission granted in full knowledge of the possible consequences of treatment. This process is ongoing and active throughout treatment provision, during which the patient can withdraw consent at any time. The robustness of the consent process is based on the patient making decisions about their care on the information they have been provided with in addition to the benefits of treatment but more crucially risks the patient will be exposed to.

With the majority of any operative dental treatments, the physical process of instrumentation removal of tooth tissue produces some form of morbidity or damage. For example, the repercussions that follow from the provision of a subtractive approach may be potentially multiple, with varying consequences and levels of tooth-related or soft tissue-related damage. These risks need to be balanced against the biological, functional and aesthetic improvements the patient may gain from the restorative procedure. In comparison, adhesive additive techniques are significantly less likely to result in pulpal issues but are open to the increased risk of soft tissue inflammation and thus marginal breakdown of the restoration as the margin of the new restoration is positively veneered onto the natural emergence profile of the tooth. Open and frank discussions about such factors need to be recorded in the patient's clinical notes and referred to at future appointments during subsequent treatment.

Further Reading

1. Alani A, Kelleher M, Hemmings K, Saunders M, Hunter M, Barclay S, Ashley M, Djemal S, Bishop K, Darbar U, Briggs P, Fearne J. Balancing the risks and benefits associated with cosmetic dentistry - a joint statement by UK specialist dental societies. Br Dent J. 2015;218(9):543–8.
2. Chadwick B, Treasure E, Dummer P, Dunstan F, Gilmour A, Jones R, Phillips C, Stevens J, Rees J, Richmond S. Challenges with studies investigating longevity of dental restorations - a critique of a systematic review. J Dent. 2001;29(3):155–61.
3. Langeland K, Langeland BK. Pulp reaction to crown preparation, impression, temporary crown fixation and permanent cementation. J Prosthet Dent. 1965;15:129–42.
4. Mjör IA. Repair versus replacement of failed restorations. Int Dent J. 1993;43:466–72.
5. Saunders WP, Saunders EM. Prevalence of periradicular periodontitis associated with crowned teeth in an adult Scottish population. Br Dent J. 1998;185:137–40.

Optimising Adhesion

2

Contents

Learning Outcomes

- Understand the 'bonding stack' factors considered to optimise adhesive outcomes for restoration success.
- Outline the basics of composite resin material constituents and classification.
- Appreciate composite resin material selection and handling for clinical success.
- Outline the required clinical steps for bonding agent application.
- Understand surface treatment stages required to prepare indirect restorative materials for adhesive bonding.

A. Alani, M. Patel, *Adhesive Techniques in Restorative Dentistry*, BDJ Clinician's Guides, https://doi.org/10.1007/978-3-032-07346-4_2

2.1 Introduction

The success of any adhesive dentistry technique is built upon a good foundation understanding of restorative dentistry and how this relates to the manipulation of dental materials and their adhesive adjuncts, coupled with the management of the residual tooth bonding substrate. Any adhesive restoration, be it a direct composite resin restoration or the replacement of missing teeth with indirect resin-bonded bridges, can only be as good as the procedural technique and optimisation of the materials utilised to retain it. A nonchalant attitude to adhesive bonding protocols, from lack of moisture control, not following manufacturers' recommendations on how to manage adhesive materials or the assessment and control of the occlusion, cannot be excused when the treatment outcomes are poor. The development of adhesive technology and understanding of factors required to gain predictable clinical outcomes should be observed by clinicians to establish greater predictability and result in increased confidence in the treatment modality provided. The foundation of good adhesive practice is based upon following recommended evidence-based treatment protocols and applying them to the presenting clinical case as best as possible.

2.1.1 The 'Bonding Stack' Concept

The success of any adhesive bonding process is reliant on every step being delivered as optimally as possible. Any weak or sub-standard steps in the process are likely to result in a deficient restoration or one that is more likely to fail in an undefined shorter time period. The hydrolytic stability of the bond at the interfacial layer is subject to degradation over time by the process of ageing; therefore, care must be taken from the outset to carry out this procedure in dry conditions to eliminate moisture contamination. The 'bonding stack', from management of the operative environment, optimising substrate treatment up to and including the adhesive techniques and occlusal control can 'collapse' if one stage or process is compromised. The onus for clinicians should be that of instilling good adhesive bonding protocols for the treatment they provide and ensuring that this is integral to the provision of the restoration.

2.2 Soft Tissue Manipulation

The larger the dental hard tissue surface area available for adhesive bonding, the improved retention of the restoration. The opportunity to increase the surface area of enamel or dentine availability for bonding can take the form of soft tissue manipulation or removal prior to the adhesive procedure.

Soft tissue gingivectomy in clinical situations where there is residual periodontal pocketing can be achieved by various different instruments and techniques. These include a surgical scalpel blade, dry gingival curettage with a diamond bur or a soft tissue removal bur or the use of an electrosurgery unit. These methods aim to sculpt gingival soft tissues and reposition the gingival margin to reveal the underlying tooth structure without encroaching upon or invading the periodontal attachment complex that may otherwise result in chronic gingival inflammation or recession from the restoration margin.

The exposure of tooth tissue through gingivectomy can optimise various adhesive techniques. It may allow exposure of deep preparation margins for impression taking and adhesive cementation of indirect restorations (Fig. 2.1). Palatal tissue removal can accommodate greater adhesive bonding potential for both the management of tooth surface loss and the wing retainer for resin-bonded bridges (Fig. 2.2). In contrast, the sculpting of buccal soft tissue can increase surface area for bonding but can also result in aesthetic improvement via tooth form and soft tissue modification (Fig. 2.3). Gingival contour is significant when considering its role in the overall shape of the tooth, especially in the aesthetic zone. The shape and position of the gingival zenith, where the gingival apex is offset in either mesial or distal directions, can result in improvement in symmetry. An 'excess' of healthy gingiva resulting in the absence of the gingival zenith arc shape can result in teeth looking too 'square' or 'rectangular'.

Where these soft tissue procedures are required, it may be prudent to delay the adhesive stages of the treatment to another clinical appointment to allow healing and gingival maturity if haemorrhage of the tissues is anticipated. A controlled operating environment is key to success.

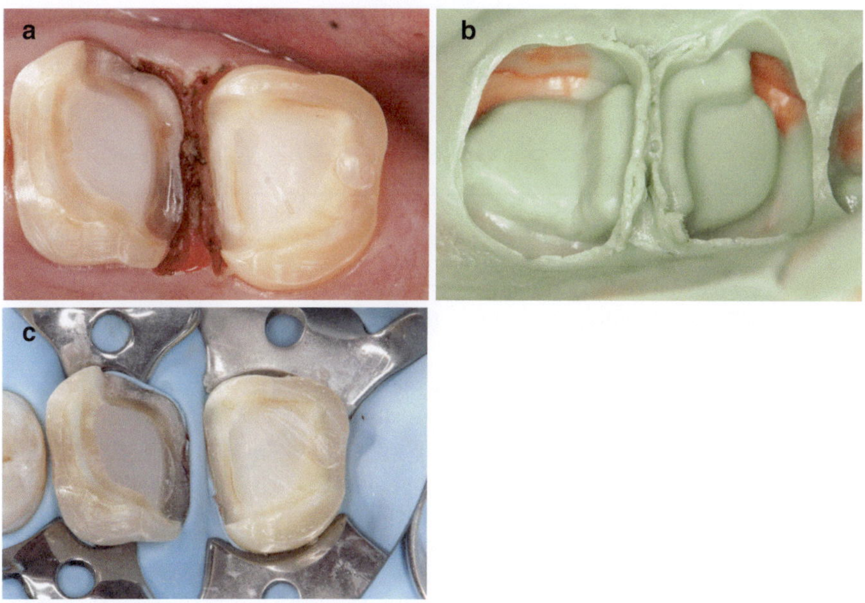

Fig. 2.1 (**a**) Teeth 17 & 16 with electrosurgery exposure of the deep preparation margins to aid (**b**) impression taking and (**c**) rubber dam isolation for the adhesive cementation of the indirect glass-ceramic restorations

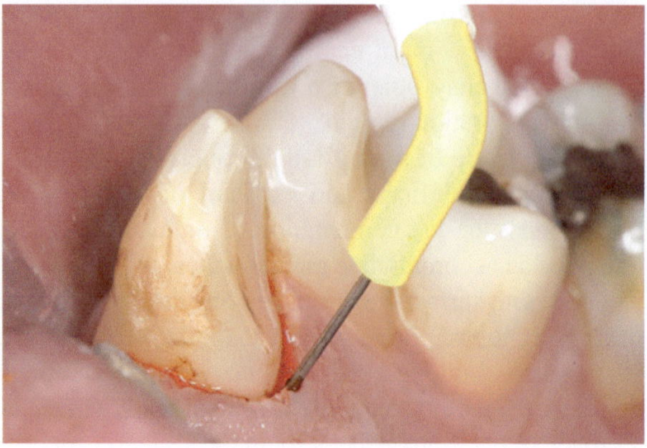

Fig. 2.2 Tooth 22 palatal tissue removal with electrosurgery unit to increase the bonding surface area and expose the palatal cingulum for the provision of resin-bonded bridge wing retainer

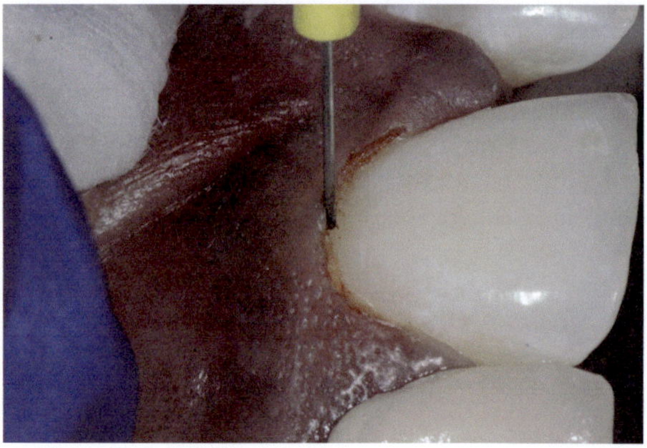

Fig. 2.3 Tooth 11 sculpting of buccal soft tissue with electrosurgery unit to increase surface area for the provision of composite resin restoration and aesthetic improvement

2.3 Environment Control

The need for a clean and dry isolated operating field provides assurances when carrying out adhesive bonding procedures to prevent contamination of the substrate and adhesive materials being utilised.

Isolation with a rubber dam provides a means to ensure consistent moisture and contamination control throughout most restorative operative procedures. Time invested appropriately isolating the oral environment restricted to the area of clinical interest enhances soft tissue retraction and improved access. This pays dividends through improved visibility and allows the dental team to focus efforts on the bonding protocol rather than the potential distraction that constant moisture control can bring (Fig. 2.4). Further to this, patient airway and soft tissue protection is vital, especially when using caustic materials required for adhesive procedures (Fig. 2.5). The advantages of rubber dam isolation are listed in Table 2.1.

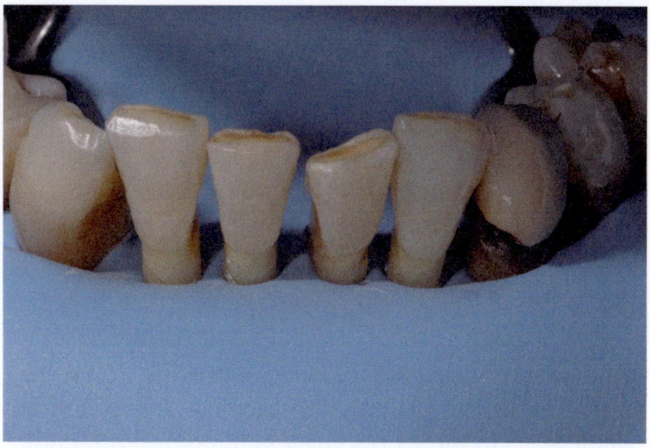

Fig. 2.4 Lower arch rubber dam isolation allows a clean and dry isolated operating field, enhancing soft tissue retraction and improved access and visibility of the operating field

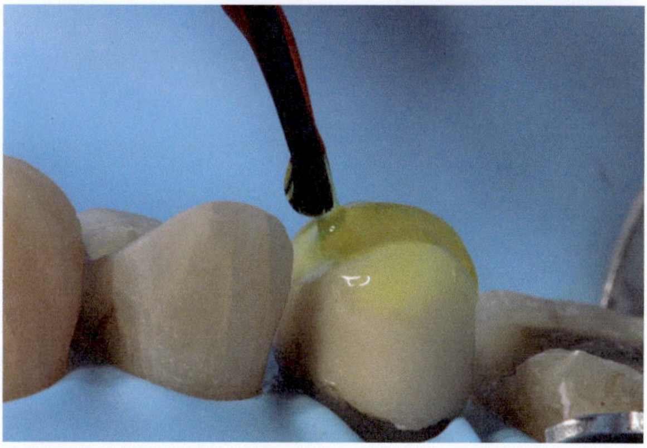

Fig. 2.5 Rubber dam isolation allowing protection of soft tissues during adhesive procedures requiring intra-oral use of caustic substances (e.g. 9.5% hydrofluoric acid etching a ceramic crown restoration)

Table 2.1 Advantages of rubber dam isolation

Rubber dam isolation advantages
Patient protection—airway and soft tissues
Reduced aerosol generation
Improved access to the operating area—retraction of soft tissues
Improved operative efficiency
Controlled operative field—moisture and contamination

The key to successful rubber dam application is the exposure of the maximum amount of tooth tissue without compromising the tooth/teeth seal, resulting in fluid seepage exchange between the operative area and the oral cavity. This may seem straightforward, but it is essentially an art form. Rubber dam sheet materials (latex and non-latex) and thickness gauges differ (Fig. 2.6), consequently they have varying handling characteristics to aid inverted isolation of single or multiple teeth (quadrant or full arch isolation). Common adjuncts to achieve isolation with a rubber dam include a hole punch, frame (metal or plastic), forceps (Stokes or Brewer), stabilisation clamps, rubber wedges and floss ligatures. The combination of these components can provide isolation for all adhesive procedure applications where the patient allows. An awareness of the number of teeth that require isolation and how the isolation achieved can impact the procedure of restoration provision needs to be borne in mind from the outset.

Optimal tension-free isolation can be difficult to achieve consistently and may impact the ease of the adhesive bonding procedure. If the rubber dam sheet is slipping up the tooth in a coronal direction, it could interfere with the bonding procedure (Figs. 2.7, 2.8 and 2.9). Where direct or indirect adhesive restorations are planned extending to, or are in close proximity to the gingival margin, retraction and stabilisation of the rubber dam can provide access beyond these areas. Methods of stabilising the rubber dam sheet include the utilisation of floss ligatures or clamps, which serve to retract the sheet in a gingival direction away from the proposed restoration margin (Figs. 2.7, 2.8 and 2.9). Other common issues that can arise are the difficulty in the engagement of sectional matrix band components, complete seating of silicone matrices/stents or passive seating of resin-bonded bridges due to the taut

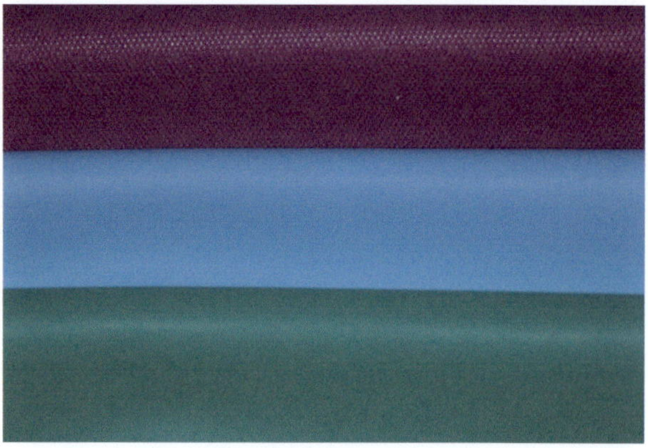

Fig. 2.6 Rubber dam sheet, latex and non-latex material options

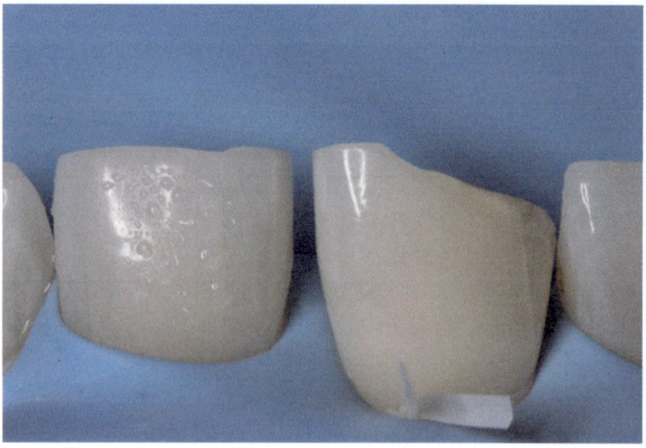

Fig. 2.7 Coronal slipping of rubber dam on tooth 21. Floss ligature placement on tooth 11, providing rubber dam retraction in a gingival direction, exposing the buccal surface

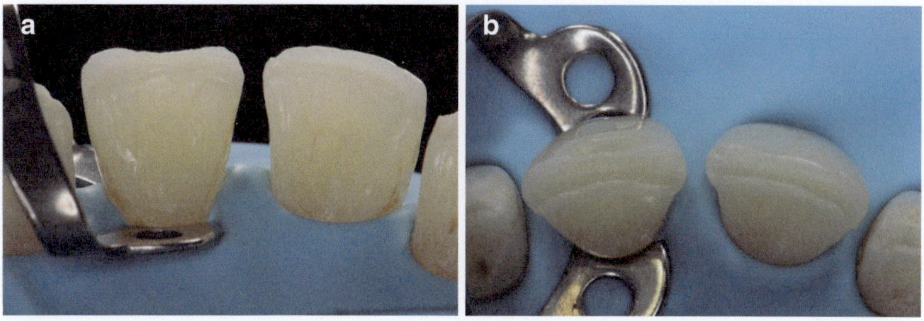

Fig. 2.8 (**a**) Coronal slipping of the rubber dam on tooth 21. (**b**) Clamp placement on tooth 11, providing rubber dam retraction in a gingival direction, exposing the palatal surface

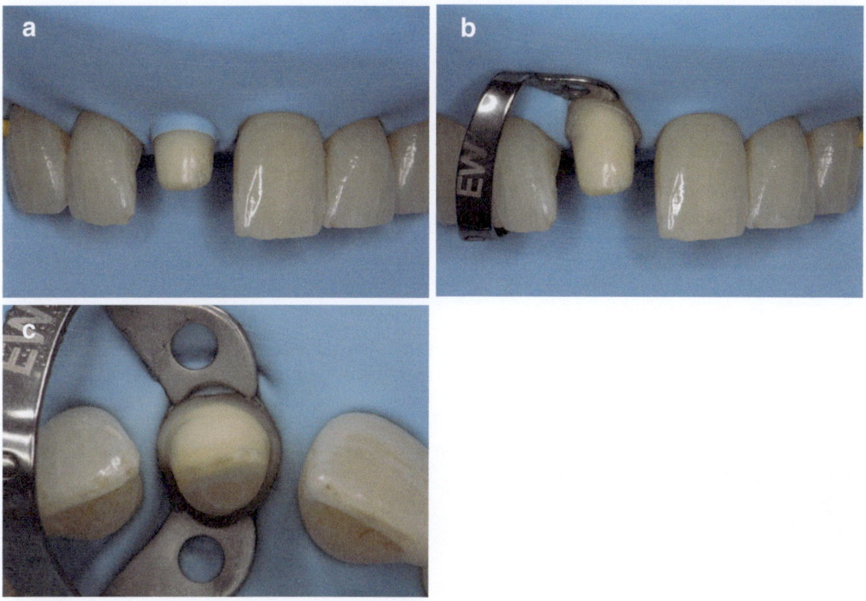

Fig. 2.9 (**a**) Coronal slipping of the rubber dam on tooth preparation 11. (**b**, **c**) Clamp placement on tooth 11, providing rubber dam retraction in a gingival direction, exposing tooth preparation finish lines

area of the rubber dam sheet extending over the edentulous span area (Figs. 2.10, 2.11 and 2.12).

The awareness, dexterity and motor skills of the dental assistant are also tested, due to the various stages required for bonding different restorations. Prolonged bonding of single or multiple restorations may lend itself to investing the time and effort into rubber dam equipment training and practice of subsequent clinical application.

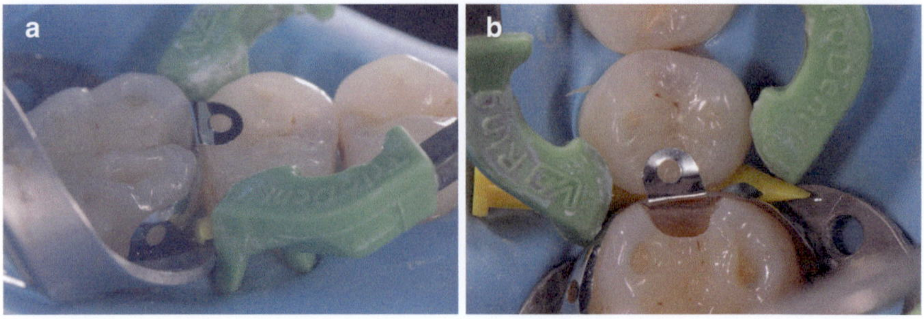

Fig. 2.10 (**a**, **b**) Rubber dam clamp on tooth 16 interfering with palatal embrasure engagement of the sectional matrix ring tine. This will lead to a composite resin restoration with inadequate interdental contact

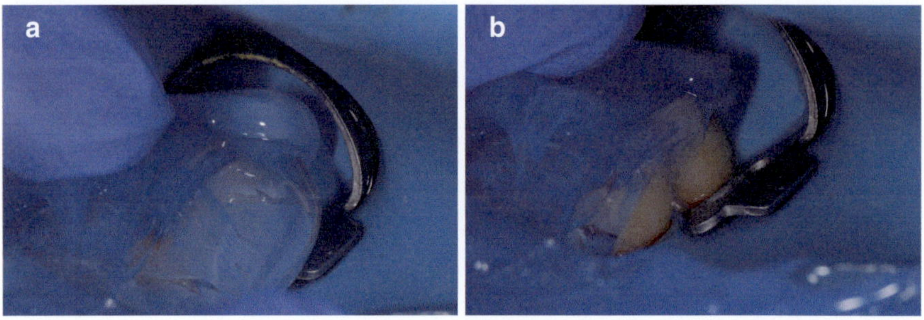

Fig. 2.11 (**a**) Rubber dam clamp interfering with the positioning of a transparent silicone stent. (**b**) Silicone stent trimmed away from the clamp to allow its complete seating

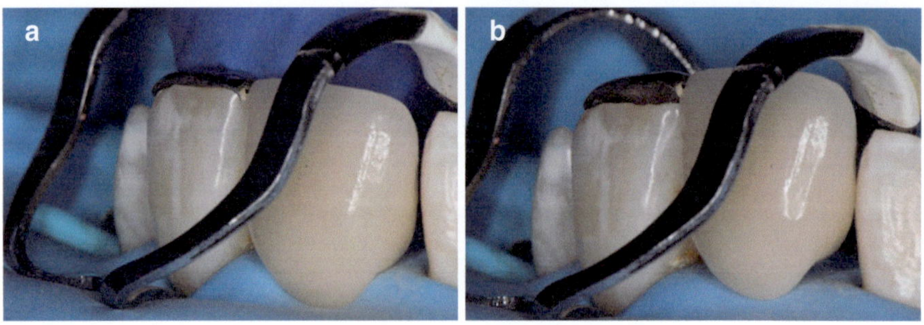

Fig. 2.12 (**a**) Try-in of resin-bonded bridge prosthesis pushing against the taught area of the rubber dam sheet extending over the edentulous span, which can prevent passive restoration seating. (**b**) When digital pressure is removed, the bridge pontic (tooth 11) is lifted in a coronal direction, causing the bridge retainer to separate away from the abutment tooth 21

The well-isolated environment, in which direct or indirect restorations are adhesively bonded, will change the clinician's mindset by improving their confidence through improved restoration performance.

2.4 Substrate Management

The key to optimising adhesion is managing and conditioning the substrate in conjunction with the paired crucial steps in applying the adhesive bonding agent and composite resin material.

2.4.1 Barrier Removal

Any intervening layer (e.g. oral fluids, pellicle, plaque, calculus, restorative material) that compromises the contact between the resin and tooth structure will reduce adhesive bonding efficacy. Poor surface adhesive bonding could manifest as marginal discolouration, gingival inflammation, caries development and restoration loss/failure.

Contamination of the pre-etched proposed bonding surface will prevent appropriate acid etch conditioning and infiltration with the resin bonding agent. Hence, it is good practice to first clean the tooth surface with an ultrasonic scaler and oil-free prophy paste (using a prophy brush or cup) or pumice powder to reduce any barrier remnants that could compromise the adhesive bond. Alumina blasting tooth surfaces in addition will aid the further removal of stubborn surface stains and any remnant restorative material (Fig. 2.13).

Matrix metalloproteinases (MMPs) produced by odontoblasts are inherently present in dentine and can be reactivated in acidic environments (during the caries process or acid etching). Their presence can cause degradation of the hybrid layer within the adhesive–dentine bond interface. MMP inhibitors, e.g. chlorhexidine, may be scrubbed onto the dentine surfaces to negate this prior to acid etching.

Ideally, a patient's self-maintenance of plaque control provides the best outcome as prophylaxis just before bonding procedures can result in unwanted haemorrhage and contamination. If plaque is present on smooth surfaces with associated gingival inflammation, it may be prudent to reconsider the provision of the restorations until such time that the patient's self-maintenance improves. The cervical and palatal/lingual surfaces of teeth may be more commonly implicated as areas with biofilm. This represents a key issue for the clinician. If areas of plaque are identified (via disclosing solution or test etching), the clinician must decide whether to provide oral hygiene instruction and abort bonding provision or provide tooth surface cleaning and prophylaxis and continue treatment.

The intaglio surfaces of indirect restorations may be contaminated before and during try-in procedures by inappropriate handling, oral fluids, try-in oil-based paste mediums and oil/water droplets from the 3:1 syringe (Fig. 2.14). There is a requirement to identify potential sources of this barrier contamination, to remove

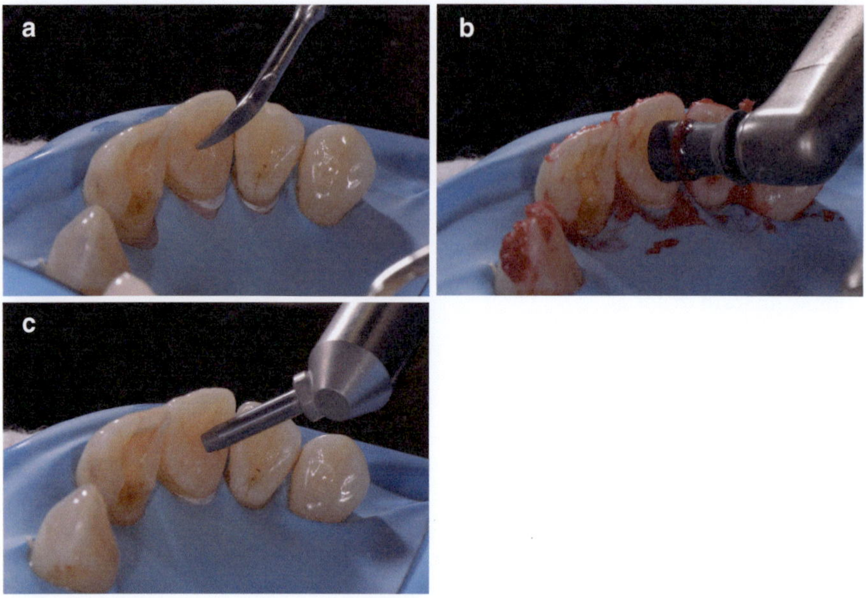

Fig. 2.13 Palatal tooth surface cleaning with an (**a**) ultrasonic scaler, (**b**) prophy paste and (**c**) sandblasting

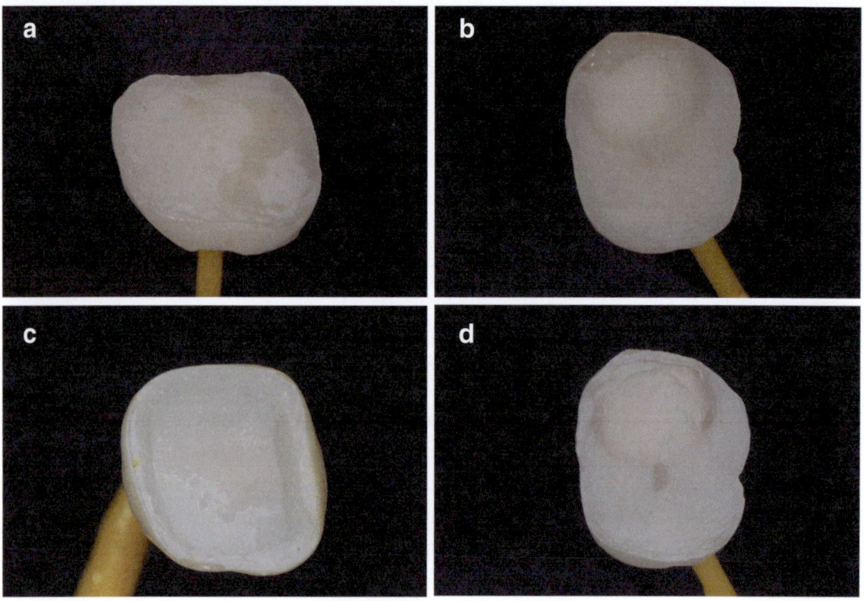

Fig. 2.14 Examples of glass-ceramic indirect restoration surface contamination by; (**a**) inappropriate handling (incomplete laboratory hydrofluoric acid etch conditioning and die spacer remnant particles) prior to restoration try-in; (**b**) oral fluids (saliva leakage through rubber dam isolation) during restoration try-in; (**c**) oil-based try-in paste (preventing continuous hydrofluoric acid etch conditioning of surface); (**d**) oil/water droplets from the 3:1 syringe (during drying stage after hydrofluoric acid etch conditioning and rinsing)

and eliminate them, such that the efficacy of surface treatments to condition and prepare the restoration for adhesive bonding is not affected. Cleaning restoration surfaces after try-in procedures should involve the use of steam cleaning in conjunction with alcohol cleaning. Alcohol solutions that may be used are 99% isopropyl alcohol, which may also be ultrasonically activated.

2.4.2 Finish Lines

Teeth to be restored may require minor preparation to augment adhesive bonding procedures. The shape of the tooth may be modified at the proposed restoration junction by the placement of a finish line.

Bevel finish lines prepared on the facial surface of a tooth allow an increased surface area of the composite resin restoration to be bonded to. The oblique bevel opens the enamel prisms in cross-section to allow for improved resin infiltration and micromechanical adhesion. The bevel will also aid blending the transition of the composite resin restoration into the tooth seamlessly allowing optimal aesthetic integration. The bevel (short or long) may be continuous or interrupted (feathered) in its shape and along its length to allow scattering of light to help permit restoration aesthetic transition to tooth (Figs. 2.15 and 2.16).

Chamfer finish lines prepared on the palatal/lingual surface of a tooth allow for a thicker placement of restorative material, improving restoration durability and functional performance over the long term. In these non-visible areas, the demarcation line that may show at the restoration margin is of no aesthetic concern. The finish line must be placed away from areas of occlusal static and dynamic contact such that the restoration margin is not placed in high mechanical stress that would allow premature breakdown and failure of the adhesive bond (Fig. 2.16).

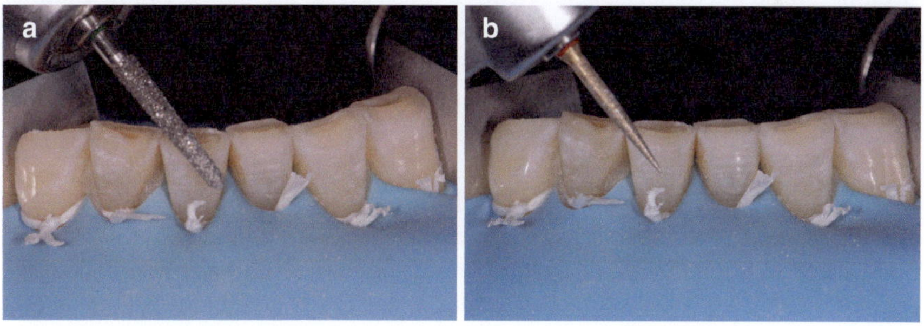

Fig. 2.15 Preparation of bevel finish lines with (**a**) coarse and (**b**) fine grit diamond burs

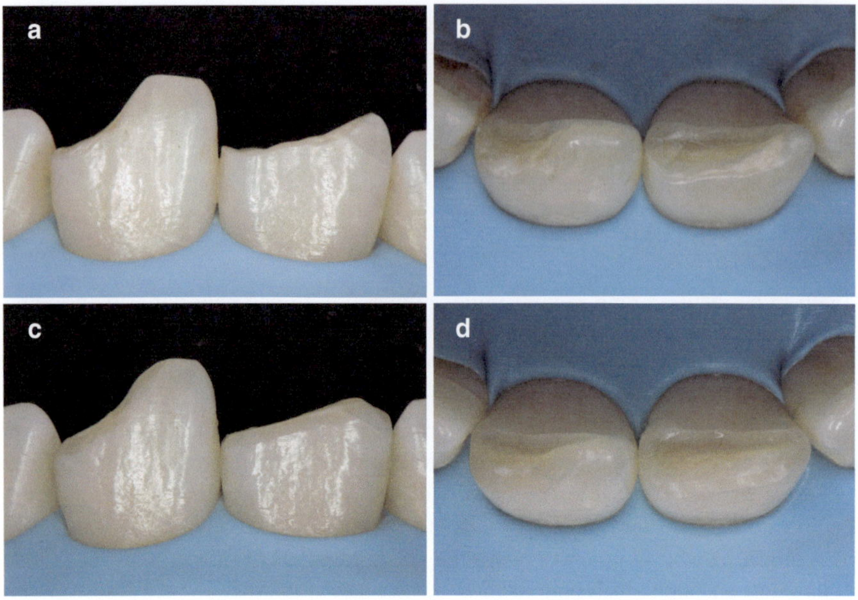

Fig. 2.16 (**a**, **b**) Class IV fractures of teeth 11 & 21. (**c**, **d**) Aesthetic bevel finish lines prepared on facial and interdental surfaces and functional chamfer finish lines prepared on the palatal surfaces

2.4.3 Sand (Alumina) Blasting

A further method to prepare the bonding surface of teeth is the utilisation of sandblasting (alumina blasting) with alumina particles (Al_2O_3). Sandblasting tooth surfaces will aid the removal of surface stains, remnant restorative materials (temporary or definitive) and imparts a rough surface topography to create a reactive surface for 'wetting' to aid micromechanical retention (Figs. 2.13c, 2.17 and 2.18). In a similar fashion, restoration surfaces (metal alloys and resin-based materials) should also be prepared for adhesive bonding by sandblasting treatment, which cleans and abrades the restoration surface prior to adhesive bonding treatment. This produces a rough surface topography to aid micromechanical retention of the resin (Figs. 2.19 and 2.20).

The blasting process occurs ahead of the handpiece, involving the propulsion of alumina particles (20–50 microns diameter size) under high pressure (30–45 PSI) that collide with the surface of the tooth or restoration, resulting in abrasion cleaning and roughening. This can be carried out in wet or dry conditions in conjunction with high volume aspiration (Fig. 2.21). The further the handpiece sits from the instrumented site, the wider the area of abrasion treatment. The converse is true if the handpiece is closer to the site, resulting in a more focused area of action. The efficiency of sandblasting abrasion is inherently multifactorial. Particle size plays a role, where larger particles result in greater aggressiveness of the blasting. The greater the pressure applied, the increased efficacy of abrasion, which also concurrently raises the risk of patient discomfort during the procedure.

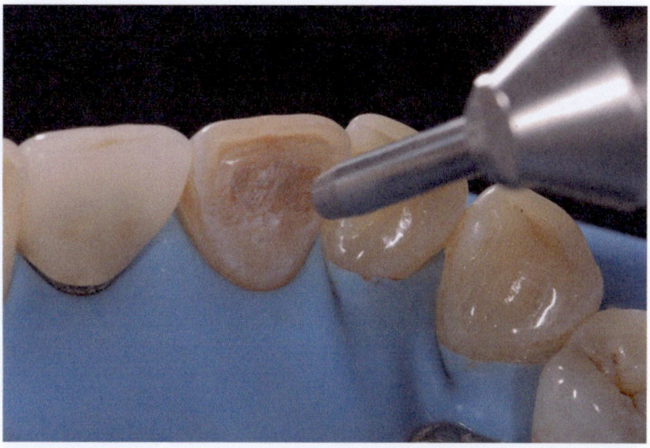

Fig. 2.17 Sandblasting tooth 21 palatal surface with stubborn surface stains

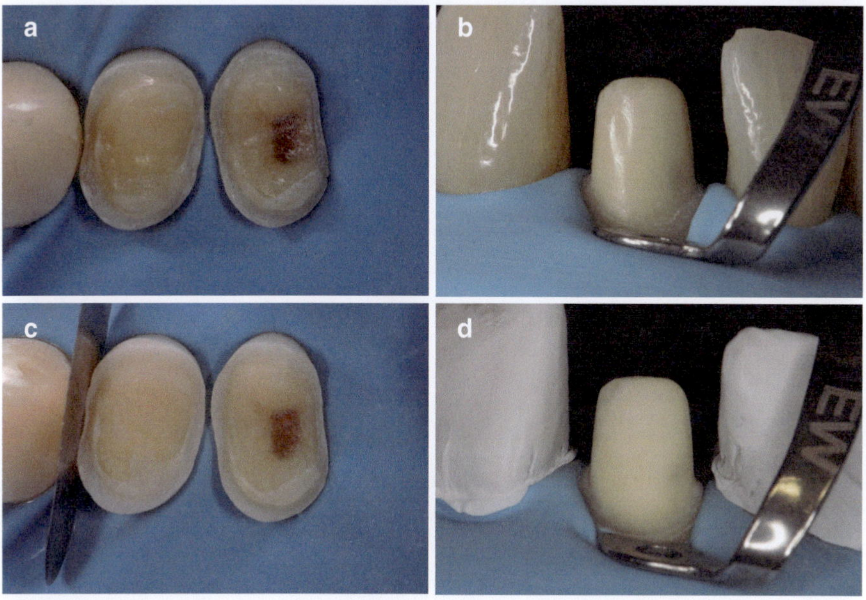

Fig. 2.18 (**a**, **b**) Teeth 24, 25 onlay and tooth 11 crown preparations. (**c**, **d**) Preparations were sandblasted to remove temporary cement material and roughen surfaces for adhesive treatment. Metal strip and PTFE tape barriers are used to protect adjacent teeth 23, 21 & 12

Some precautions are advised when using alumina blasting. Eye protection should be worn by the clinical team and the patient. The authors would recommend the application of rubber dam isolation prior to the process and the use of high-volume aspiration during the process. This will reduce pooling or ingestion of the alumina particles. The rubber dam will also protect the soft tissues from epithelial abrasion and laceration. Adjacent teeth and restorations not intended to be alumina blasted should be protected by way of barrier materials. The barrier materials that could be used include Polytetrafluoroethylene (PTFE) tape, acetate or metal strips (Fig. 2.22).

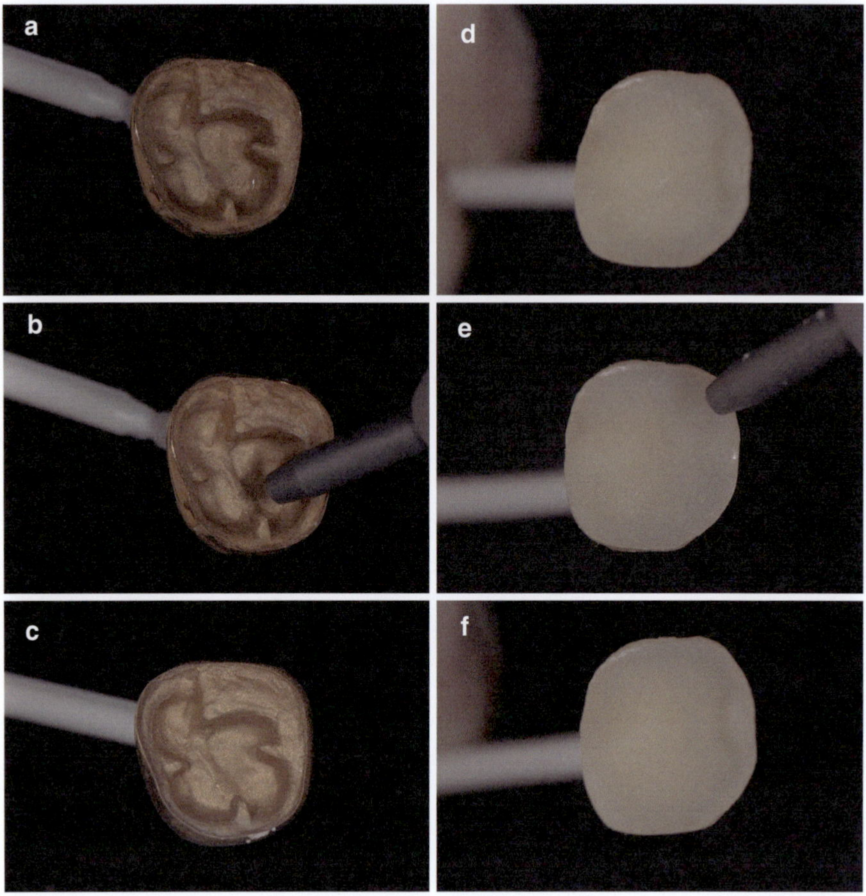

Fig. 2.19 Sandblasting intaglio surfaces of onlay restorations, before and after. (**a**, **b**, **c**) Type III gold alloy and (**d**, **e**, **f**) resin-based materials

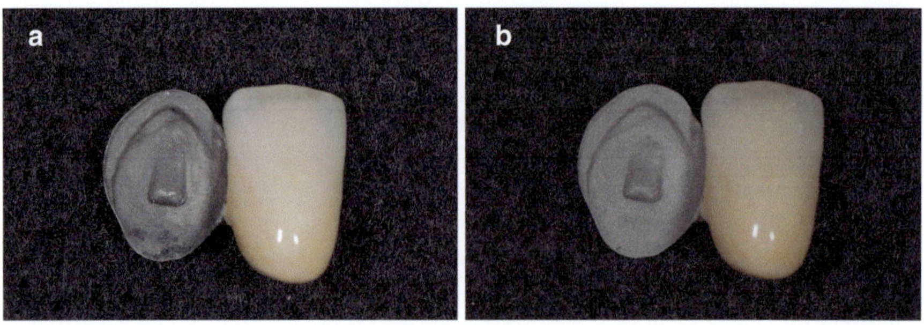

Fig. 2.20 Resin-bonded bridge wing retainer intaglio surface sand blasted (**a**) before and (**b**) after

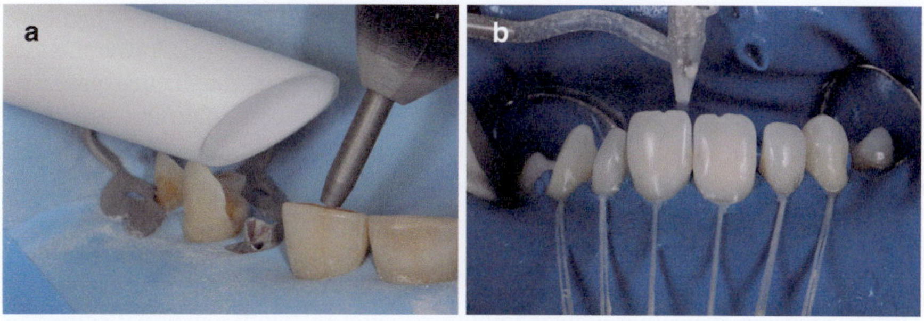

Fig. 2.21 Sandblasting with high-volume aspiration in (**a**) dry and (**b**) wet conditions. (Image 2.21(b) courtesy of Dr Monik Vasant)

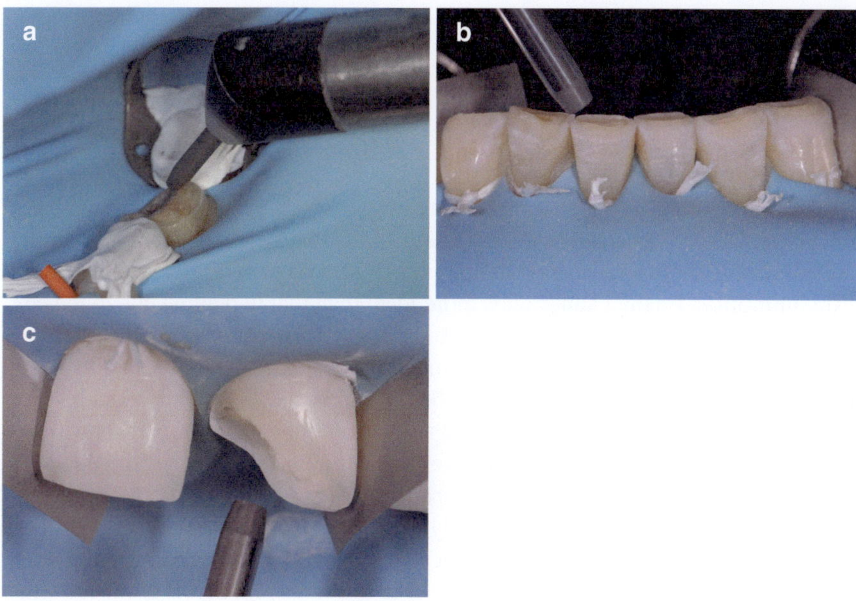

Fig. 2.22 Protection of teeth not intended to be sandblasted with (**a**) PTFE tape and (**b**, **c**) metal strip barriers

Sandblasting differs in tactile sensation when compared to handpiece feedback and needs to be compensated for in the clinician's mindset. Without awareness of the settings during the abrasion process and monitoring of roughening progress, sandblasted sites can be overtreated quickly without the appropriate care and attention. Maintaining a gentle motion of the handpiece will help minimise this.

2.5 Adhesion

Dental adhesion typically involves joining a dental restorative material (direct or indirect restoration) to tooth structure resulting in two adhesive interfaces; one between the tooth structure and the adhesive resin, and the other between the adhesive resin and the restorative material. It is a complex physico-chemical process that occurs at the interface of the two intimately contacting materials, which results in the formation of an attractive force. The strength of the adhesive bond is chemo-mechanical, and failure can occur either adhesively (failure at the adhesive interface, i.e. substrate separation) or cohesively (failure within the adhesive layer).

2.5.1 Tooth Substrate

Adhesion to enamel tooth structure is the key to success for any adhesive-based procedure. In 1955, Michael Buonocore, at the Eastman Dental Centre in Rochester, United States, discovered enamel bonding through a process of enamel etching and resin infiltration. Enamel adhesion is more ideal than that to dentine due to the consistency of the bond, its strength and durability. This marries with the minimally invasive approach as conservation of as much of the tooth as possible and results in the more ideal bond interface. As such, bonding procedures that are more invasive and purposefully remove the full enamel surface are inherently less efficient.

Dentine, due to its significantly different structural characteristics, organic composition and moisture content, has a reduced bonding potential. The organic component of dentine, which is approximately 30%, and the presence of odontoblasts means there is fluid present in its surface further complicating adhesive bonding potential when compared to enamel. Further to this, adherent debris produced when instrumenting the tooth surface known as the smear layer also compromises the adhesive bond. The smear layer is a 1–2μm thick layer of with plugs that block the dentinal tubules and so reduce their porosity.

Adhesive bonding to enamel and dentine structures produces bond strengths of between 10 and 30 MPa, which may be carried out by etch and rinse methods (Fig. 2.23), or self-etch methods utilising either fourth-, fifth-, sixth-, seventh- or eighth-generation bonding agents with the option of both light-cure and dual-cure capabilities (Fig. 2.24). Both methods will aim to fully or partially remove the smear layer that is left on the tooth tissue after instrumentation. The smear layer is an aggregate of mainly fragmented and compacted tooth material and debris (Figs. 2.25 & 2.26).

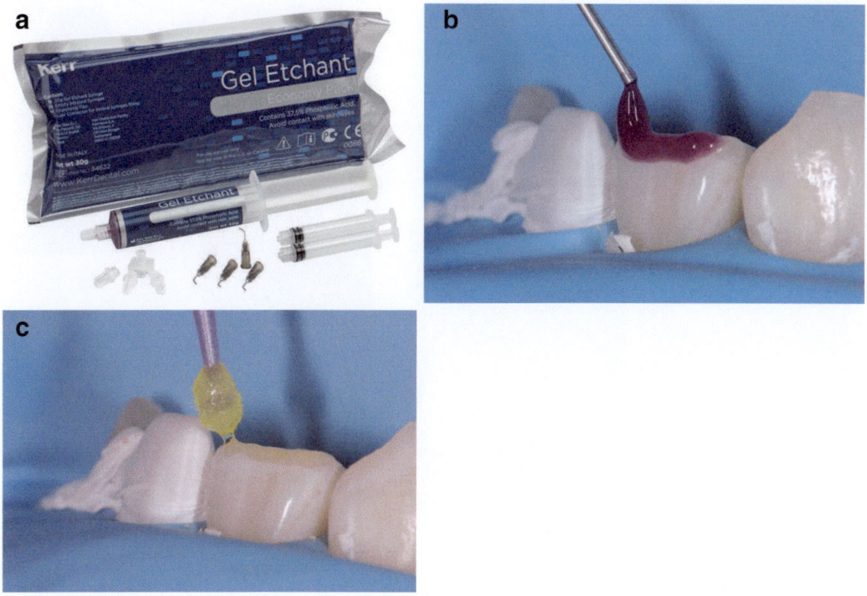

Fig. 2.23 Etch and rinse method. (**a**, **b**) Placement of 37.5% phosphoric acid. (**c**) After rinsing and drying, the application of eighth-generation 'Universal' adhesive for the provision of direct Class IV composite resin restoration

Fourth-generation (two-bottle system) agents yield the highest values in laboratory testing for microtensile bond strengths to tooth tissue and require the full etch and rinse protocol with separate etch conditioning, primer and adhesive application steps. Fifth-generation (one-bottle system) agents are most commonly used by clinicians requiring separate etch conditioning and combined primer/adhesive application steps. Eighth-generation (one-bottle system) agents termed the 'Universals' can be used in one of three modes: total-etch, selective-etch or self-etch. The differences are in the method of use of the 37% phosphoric acid conditioner, which is left to operator preference (Table 2.6). Self-etching occurs by way of the phosphoric acid-modified acrylate resin acidic primer within the bonding solution. Solvents (acetone, ethanol or water) are often present to carry the primers and aid primer penetration into the tooth structure. They must be evaporated before the primer is light polymerised

The basis of enamel bonding is the ability of 37% phosphoric acid conditioner to remove the smear layer (thereby increasing surface energy and wettability) and selectively dissolve the interprismatic tissue surface, creating a combination of Types I–III etching patterns of micro-porosities which are approximately 20 microns in depth (Figs. 2.27 & 2.28). The use of phosphoric acid etching is always advised by the authors for the adhesive treatment of any enamel tissue irrespective of the bonding agent system used. If contamination of the highly reactive freshly etched surface occurs by contaminating fluids (of any kind), it is prudent to re-etch the

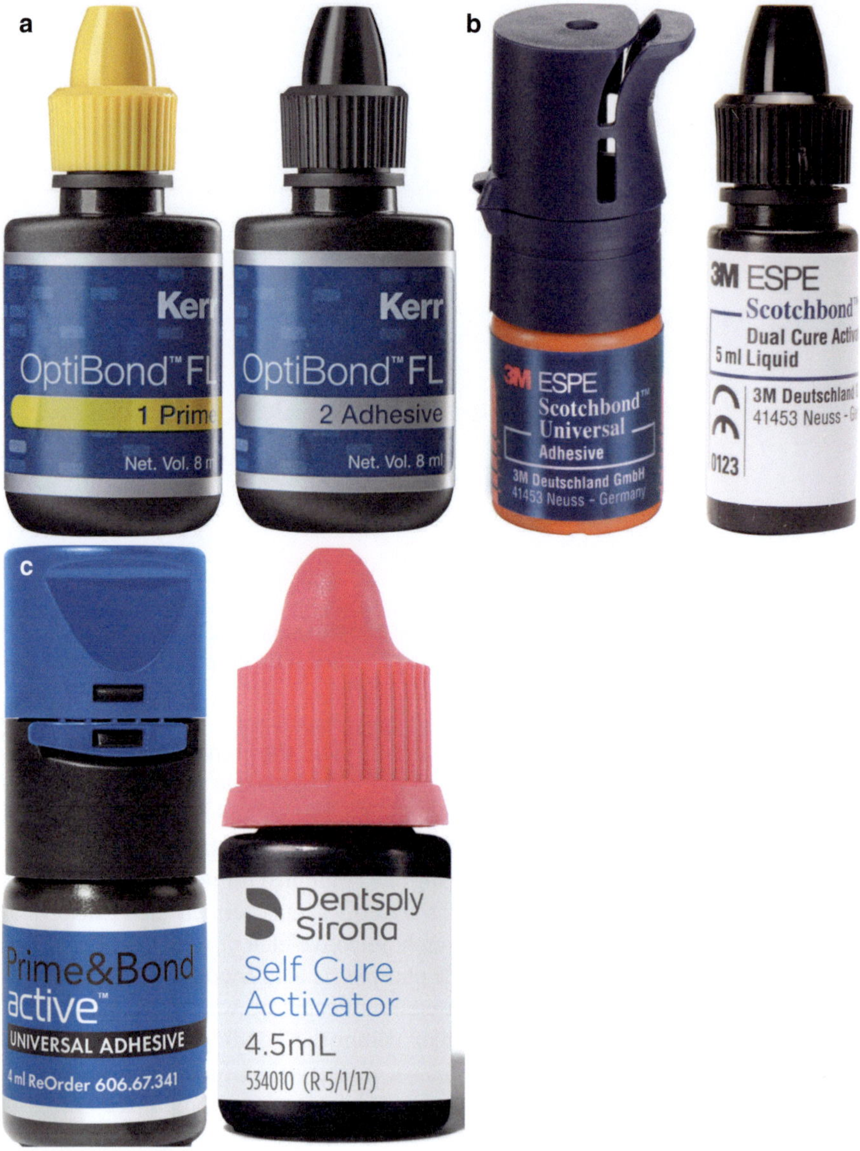

Fig. 2.24 Examples of light-cure adhesive bonding agents; (**a**) fourth generation (two bottle system) and (**b**, **c**) eighth generation 'Universal' (one bottle system) with paired match activator product for dual-cure capability. (Images courtesy of Kerr, 3M ESPE & Dentsply Sirona)

affected surface for a further 5–10 s, followed by appropriate rinsing and drying stages) (Fig. 2.29). The creation of micro-porosities provides a highly energised surface with voids to increase the surface area and an exposed organic matrix protein into which a low viscosity resin can flow via capillary action, resulting in adequate wetting of the etched enamel surface. The unfilled adhesive resin locks into these areas and once light polymerised are otherwise known as resin tags (Fig. 2.30).

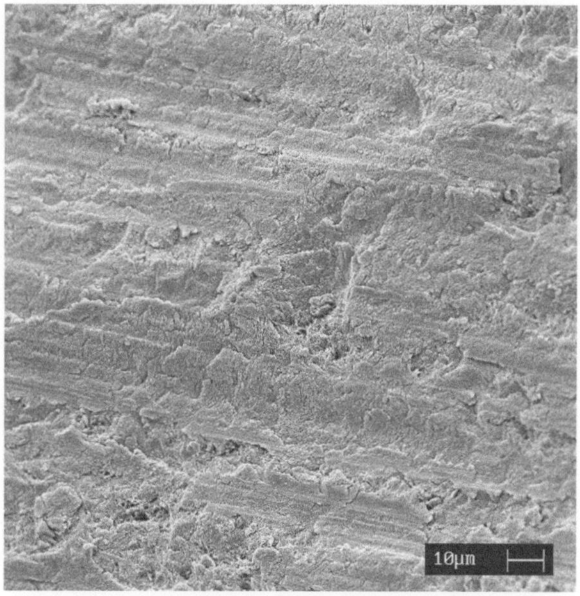

Fig. 2.25 Scanning electron microscopy (SEM) image of the enamel smear layer after cutting with a diamond bur. (Image with permission from Springer Nature)

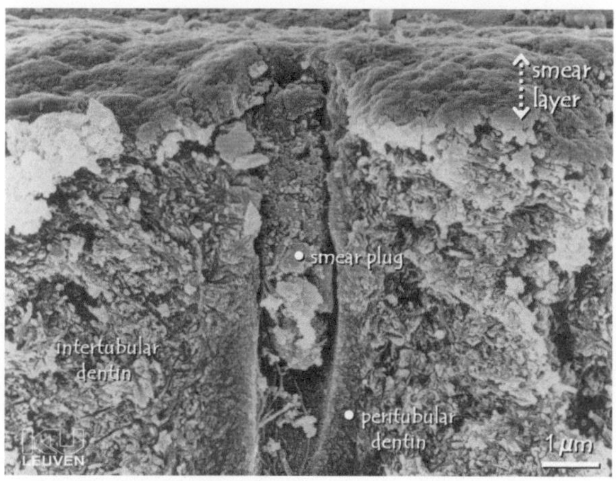

Fig. 2.26 Dentin surface prepared by wet grinding showing a smear layer covering the entire dentin surface and a smear plug extending several micrometres into the dentin tubule, occluding the tubule's orifice. (Image with permission from Springer Nature)

This process forms 'micro-mechanical retention' from which the main body of the restorative composite resin material is anchored to this surface layer of adhesive resin.

Adhesive bonding to dentine requires the use of 37% phosphoric acid conditioner for smear layer removal, or use of an acidic primer that penetrates the smear layer and dentinal tubules forming hybridisation with the dentine collagens. Independent dentine etching completely removes the smear layer and demineralises the hydroxyapatite in the peritubular dentine up to 5–8 microns in depth, leaving exposed collagen fibrils (Figs. 2.31 & 2.32). This permeable layer allows resin tag infiltration of hydrophilic adhesives into and around the tubules and collagen fibrils. This collagen fibril reinforced resin layer is known as the 'hybrid layer' (Fig. 2.33).

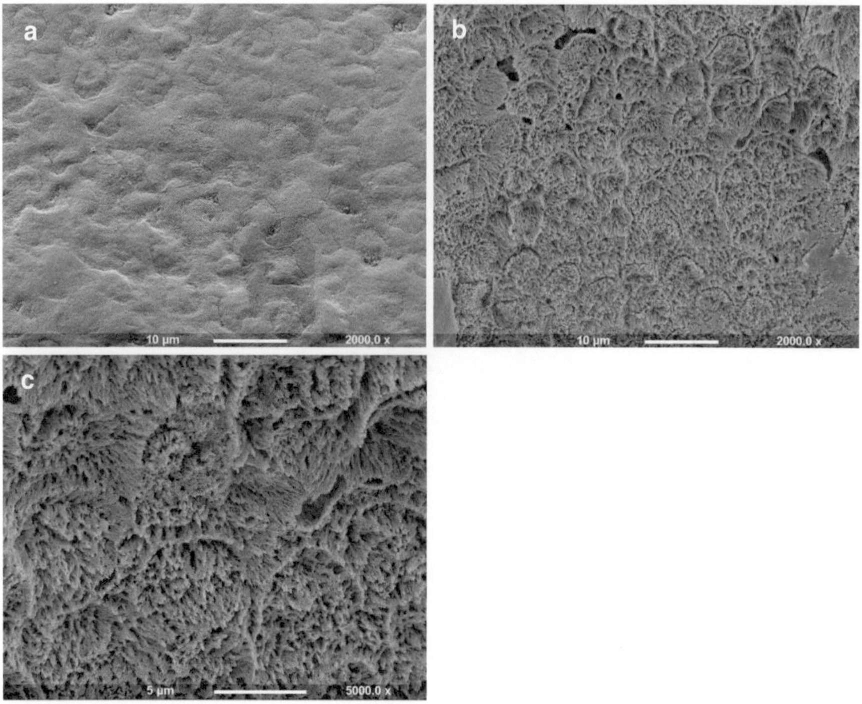

Fig. 2.27 SEM images of enamel surfaces, (**a**) unetched (x2000 magnification) and (**b**, **c**) etched (x2000 & x5000 magnification). (Images courtesy of Dr Nicky Mordan, Eastman Dental Institute, London, UK)

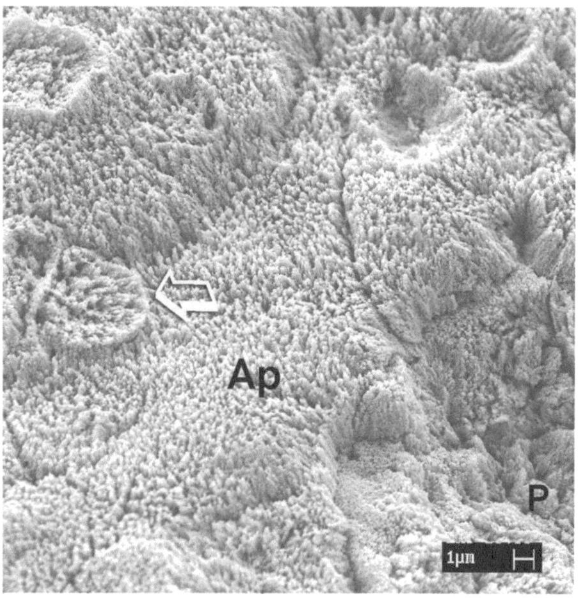

Fig. 2.28 SEM image of uncut enamel after application of phosphoric acid. The aprismatic enamel (*Ap*) is almost completely dissolved, with partial exposure of the rod heads of the prismatic enamel (*arrow*). Complete dissolution of the aprismatic enamel on the right side reveals differentially etched enamel prisms (*P*). (Image with permission from Springer Nature)

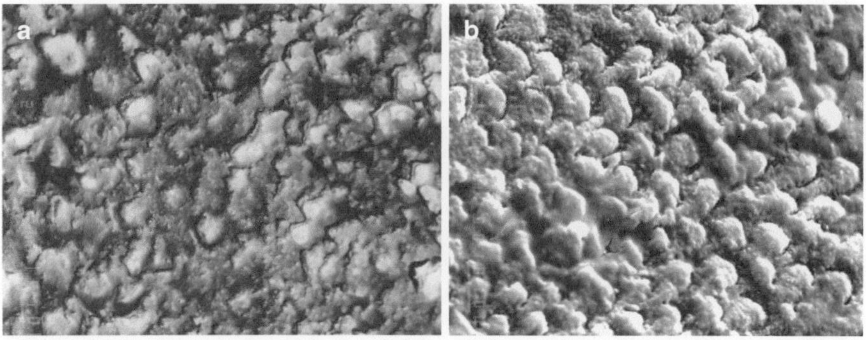

Fig. 2.29 (**a**) Saliva covers the microporosity of an etched (36% solution of phosphoric acid, 30 s) enamel surface. (**b**) Re-etching (15 s) of the surface recovered partially the initial etching pattern. (Images with permission from Springer Nature)

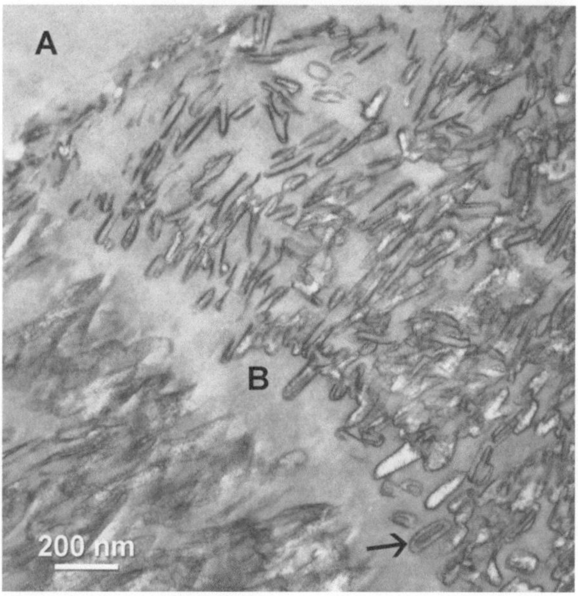

Fig. 2.30 Adhesive (**a**) infiltration into interprismatic boundaries (**b**) within enamel hybrid layer. *Arrow* indicates central hole region of a partially dissolved crystallite (stained, demineralised TEM). (Image with permission from Springer Nature)

Collagen is hydrophilic in nature, and composite resin materials are hydrophobic. Hydrophilic monomers (e.g. 2-hydroxyethyl methacrylate, HEMA, or tri-ethylene glycol dimethacrylate, TEGDMA) are contained in the primer to permeate the demineralised collagen matrix. Hydrophobic monomers (e.g. bis-phenol-A-glycidyl dimethacrylate bis-GMA or urethane dimethacrylate, UDMA) are contained in the resin adhesive bonding agent, facilitating adhesion of the restorative composite resin material to the conditioned hydrophobic dentin surface.

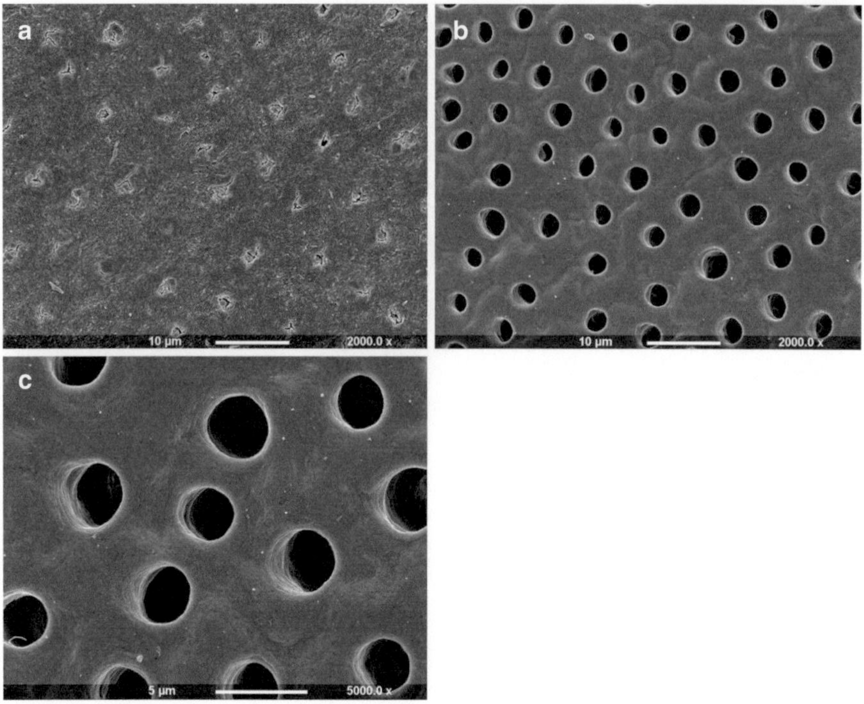

Fig. 2.31 SEM images of dentine surfaces, (**a**) unetched (x2000 magnification) and (**b**, **c**) etched (x2000 & x5000 magnification) showing removal of the smear layer and smear plugs, the dentin tubules are widened and a porous network of collagen fibrils is exposed. (Images courtesy of Dr Nicky Mordan, Eastman Dental Institute, London, UK)

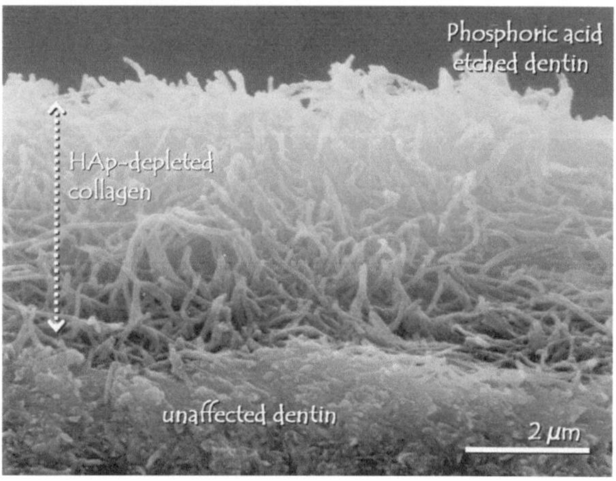

Fig. 2.32 Field-emission scanning electron microscopy photomicrograph of demineralised dentin after 15 s etch treatment with 35% phosphoric acid for 15 s. A scaffold of collagen fibrils that is nearly totally depleted of hydroxyapatite is exposed, creating a retentive network with interfibrillar spaces. (Image with permission from Springer Nature)

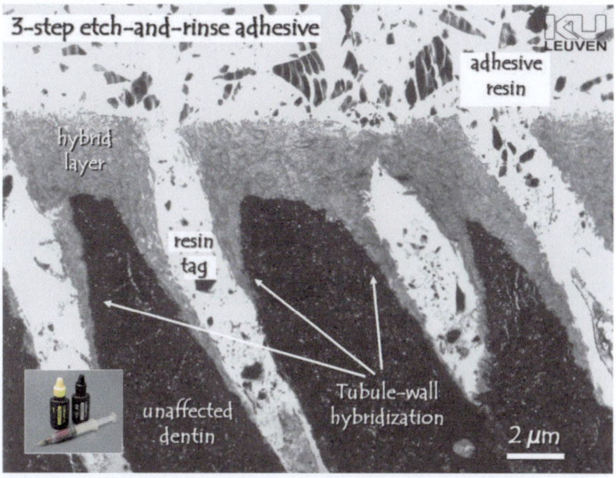

Fig. 2.33 Transmission electron microscopy photomicrograph of the interface produced by Optibond (Kerr) showing the hybrid layer extending into the dentinal tubules, attaching the resin tags to the tubules walls producing hermetic sealing to act against microleakage. (Image with permission from Springer Nature)

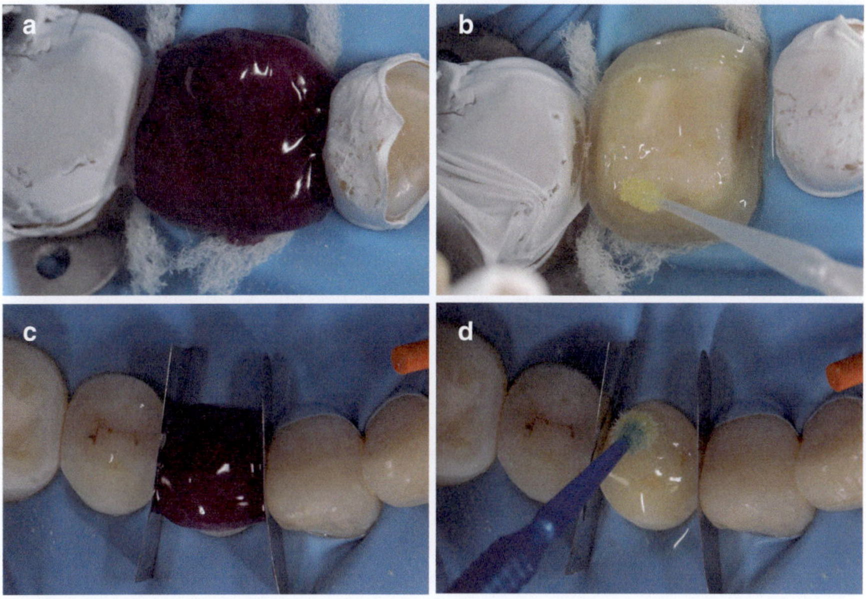

Fig. 2.34 Adhesive treatment (acid etch and bonding agent application) of (**a**, **b**) tooth 16 and (**c**, **d**) tooth 34. PTFE tape and metal strip barriers are used to protect the adjacent teeth not intended to be adhesively treated. (**b**, **d**) Different-sized microbrushes are used for optimum application of the bonding agent in all the required areas

In all cases, adjacent teeth and restorations not intended to be adhesively treated should be protected by way of barrier materials. Barrier materials of selection are polytetrafluoroethylene (PTFE) tape, acetate or metal strips (Fig. 2.34). Different sized and shaped microbrushes will aid the scrub application of the adhesive agent to all the required surfaces of the cavity or tooth preparations (Figs. 2.34 & 2.35).

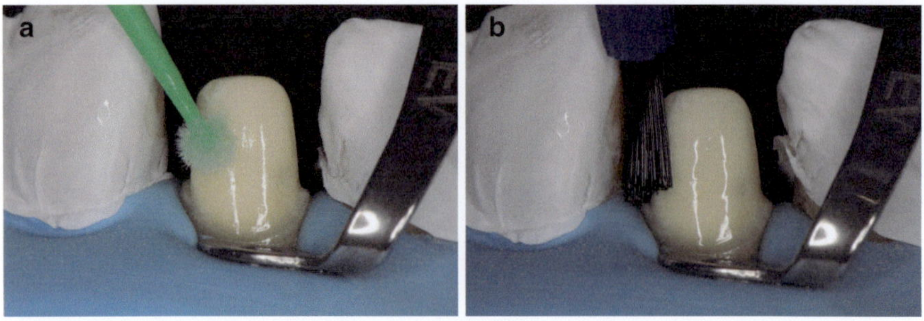

Fig. 2.35 (**a**, **b**) Tooth 11 preparation adhesive treatment (bonding agent application) using different-shaped microbrushes for optimum application of bonding agent in all the required areas. PTFE tape barriers are used to protect adjacent teeth not intended to be adhesively treated

The use of these barrier adjuncts will prevent bonded restorations and adjacent units being adhesively fused and will also aid the removal of excess resin material in interproximal areas.

2.5.2 Replacing, Refurbishing or Repairing Composite Resin Restorations

The task of optimising the adhesive bond becomes more crucial where restorations require replacement and the enamel substrate has already been bonded to once before. The clinician is faced with the challenge of removing the residual restoration in its entirety whilst also avoiding damage to the precious enamel substrate, which is key for the achievement of the remedial treatment. Utilisation of magnification in combination with LED lighting can aid the process and remove the guesswork in whether the defective restoration has been removed and if the enamel is clean and intact, ready for the new restoration (Fig. 2.36).

When refurbishing or repairing composite resin restorations where the defect lies within the restoration and not on tooth structure, the surface to be repaired should be roughened with a diamond bur or sandblasting; cleaned with acid etch and water, primed with an unfilled resin primer and then repaired with a similar composite resin material. Where defects lie on both restoration and tooth substrate, a traditional approach to the adhesive strategy should be utilised.

2.5.3 Restorative Material Substrates

Indirect restorative materials such as metal alloys, resin-based materials and ceramics may be conditioned and bonded to using similar concepts to that of tooth tissue substrates. Creating a roughened surface topography on the intaglio surface of the restoration allows infiltration of resin primers to micromechanically and chemically

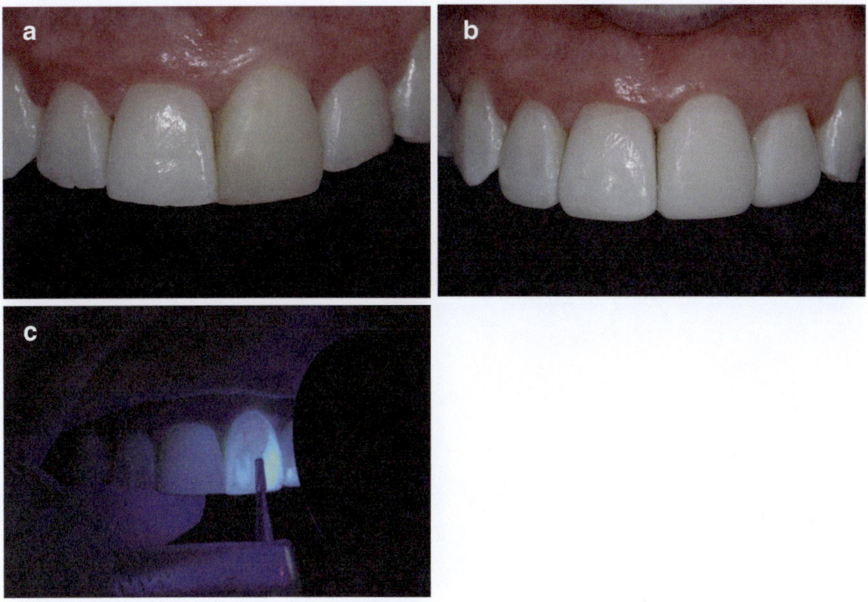

Fig. 2.36 (**a**) Defective and poorly contoured composite restoration on tooth 21 with an underlying discoloured tooth substrate subsequent to trauma. (**b**) The completed case with a new composite resin restoration placed on tooth 21 and additional edge bonding on teeth 12 and 22. (**c**) Utilisation of the LED light to identify existing composite resin material to be replaced and avoid the removal of sound enamel substrate

adhere. Micromechanical adhesion may be achieved by alumina blasting or by acid etch conditioning with 5–9.5% hydrofluoric (HF) acid (Figs. 2.19, 2.20 & 2.37). Chemical adhesion is achieved by the application of bifunctional coupling agents to cross-link the primer components (e.g. 10-methacryloxydecrydihydrgenphosphate, MDP) to the bonding resin cement at one adhesive interface (Fig. 2.38), whilst the other interface, the composite resin, is adhered to the tooth structure. This double-bonding adhesive mechanism to restorative materials allows for a strong and durable bond producing bond strengths of between 20 and 30 MPa irrespective of restoration material type. The added advantage to adhesively bonding specific to ceramic restorations is that where flaws and tensile stresses are highest at their internal surfaces, restoration failure may occur at lower functional mechanical loads. Therefore, adhesive bonding provides strengthening of the tooth-restoration interface via physico-chemical interaction between the ceramic restoration surface, the adhesive and the adhesive cement and allows greater transmission of these forces into the abutment tooth.

An example of an intra-oral adhesive bonding procedure to a ceramic restorative material is shown (Fig. 2.39). The required clinical steps of restorative material intaglio surface treatments are listed in Sect. 2.7.2 in Table 2.10.

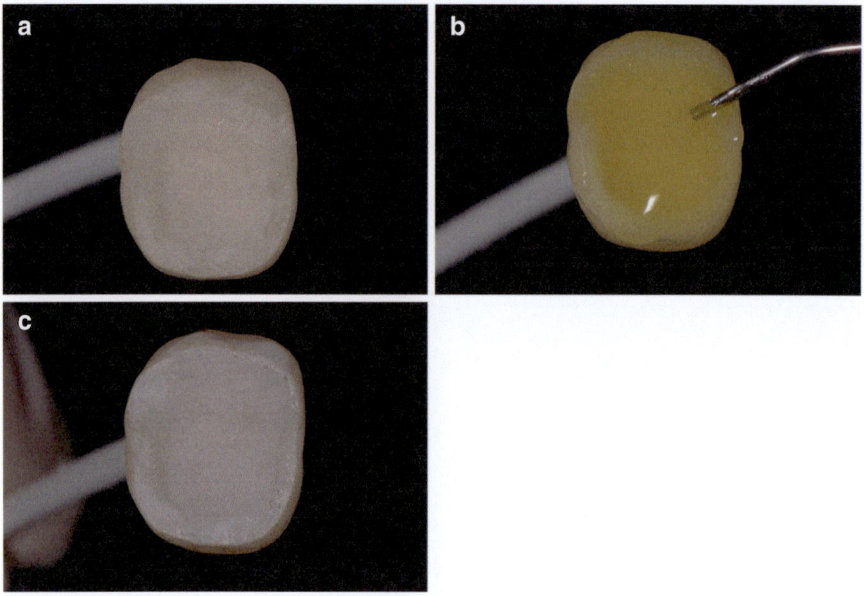

Fig. 2.37 (**a**, **b**, **c**) Acid etch surface treatment of glass-ceramic restoration with 9.5% hydrofluoric acid to impart a roughened surface topography upon the intaglio surface of the restoration to allow infiltration of resin primers to micromechanically adhere

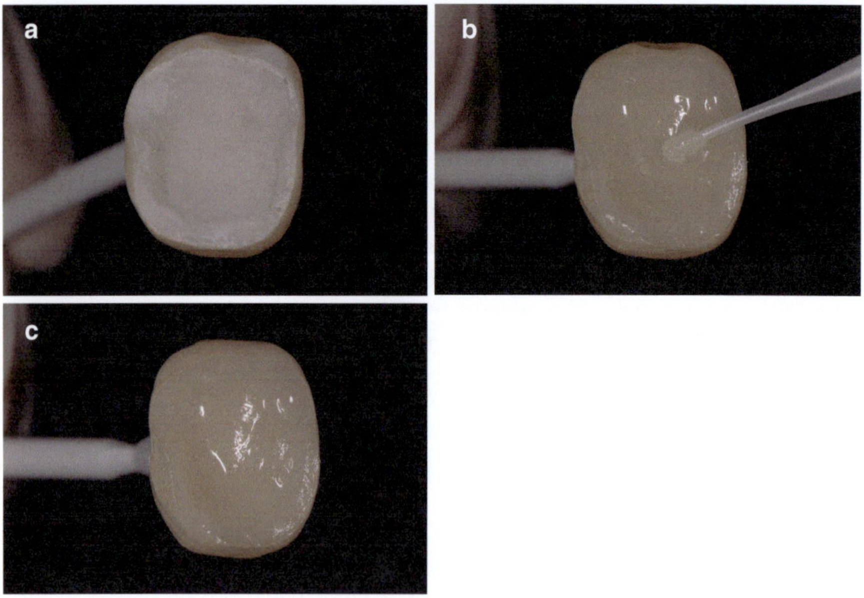

Fig. 2.38 (**a**, **b**, **c**) Infiltration surface treatment of the glass-ceramic restoration with a siliane coupling agent to infiltrate the etched micromechanically roughened ceramic intaglio surface

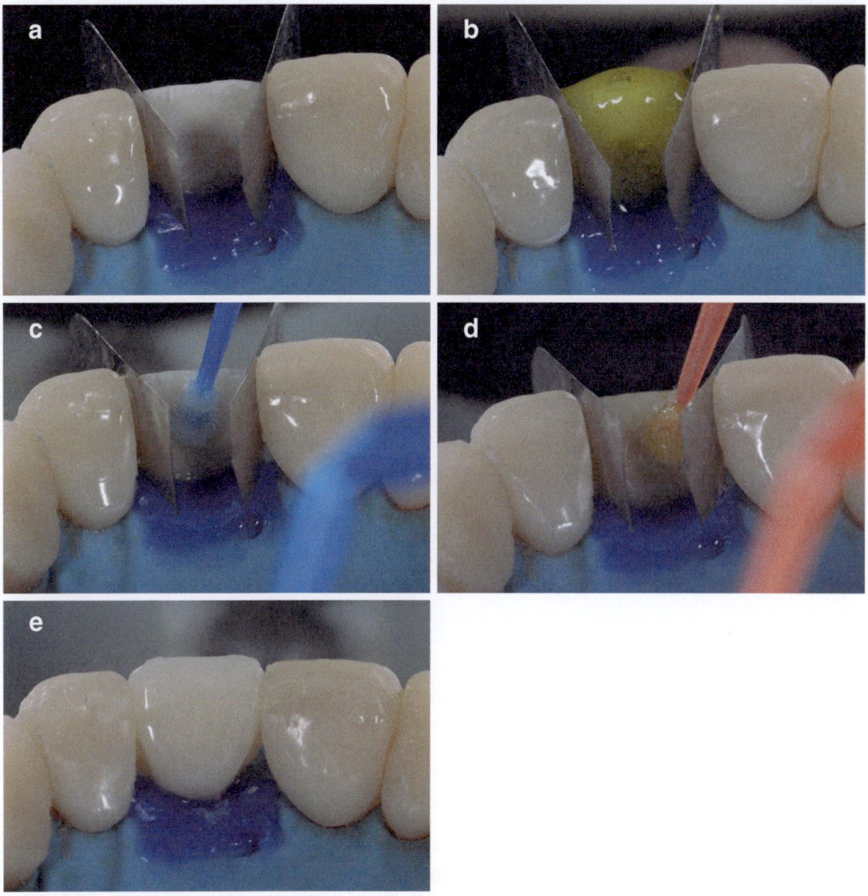

Fig. 2.39 (**a**) Tooth 11 metal-ceramic restoration palatal surface treatment (**b**) with 9.5% hydrofluoric acid and (**c**) application of silane and (**d**) eighth-generation bonding agent for (**e**) cementation of a composite resin indirect palatal veneer restoration

2.6 Composite Resin Materials

The advantages and the disadvantages of utilising composite resin materials are listed in Table 2.2.

Composite resin restorative material is composed of numerous components, which allow it to successfully adhesively bond to tooth tissue and restorative material interfaces. Bis-phenol-A-glycidyl dimethacrylate (Bis-GMA) forms the organic resin matrix into which other components can reside. Urethane dimethacrylate (UDMA) is a commonly used alternative monomer. Inorganic inert filler components such as quartz, silica, glass and ceramic (zirconia) particles regulate material translucency, control polymerisation shrinkage and influence physical properties,

Table 2.2 Composite resin material advantages and disadvantages

Advantages	Disadvantages
1. Cost—economical to the patient 2. Application versatility—chemical, light and dual cure modes 3. Aesthetic—various shades and translucencies 4. Adhesive bonding to tooth structure 5. Conservative to tooth structure 6. Reinforcement of tooth structure 7. Additive technique 8. No corrosion products 9. Ability to easily refurbish and repair	1. Cost—expensive to the clinician 2. Technique sensitive 3. Polymerisation shrinkage 4. Dentine sensitivity 5. Higher coefficient of thermal expansion 6. Low modulus of elasticity 7. Lack of anti-cariogenic properties 8. Water sorption 9. Surface wear—attrition and abrasion 10. Poor long-term aesthetics—staining (loss of filler content)

Table 2.3 Composite resin material classification and clinical uses

Classification type	Filler diameter size (μm microns)	Polymerisation shrinkage (vol%)	Clinical uses
Nanofill	0.005–0.01μm	4+ vol%	Non-stress bearing areas Class III, V
Microfill	0.01–0.4 μm	3–4 vol%	Non-stress bearing areas Classes III, V
Hybrid	0.6–1μm	2–3 vol%	Classes I–V
Small particle	1–5μm	2–3 vol%	Stress-bearing areas & abrasion-prone Classes I, II, IV
Macrofill	8–12+μm	0.5–1 vol%	Stress-bearing areas Class II, IV

e.g. viscosity, strength and hardness of the material. Highly filled composite resin materials will exhibit less polymerisation shrinkage. The filler size will also help to classify the composite resin materials (Table 2.3).

A silane-coupling bifunctional-binding agent is required to allow the inorganic filler and the organic filler to successfully connect. The inorganic filler is treated by the silane-coupling agent to facilitate this connection. A photo-initiator is required to initiate the polymerisation process, activated by a visible wavelength of blue light (465 nm wavelength). An example of this photosensitizer is Camphorquinone, which generates a free radical catalysed by organic aliphatic amines required for material polymerisation. To control the shade of the composite resin material, pigments and opacifiers are added, which are usually metal oxide molecules. One further component is the addition of ultraviolet light stabilisers to reduce discolouration on sun exposure.

Handling characteristics of the composite resin material are affected by the composition of the material itself and the manner with which it is managed prior to and during clinical placement. Other than Bis-GMA or UDMA, matrix dilutent components such as 2-hydroxyethyl methacrylate (HEMA) or tri-ethylene glycol dimethacrylate (TEGDMA) can reduce viscosity and increase the depth of cure of the composite resin material, making it more favourable to handle.

Composite resin undergoes a process of volumetric shrinkage when polymerising. This is caused by largely dispersed monomer components linking tightly together, resulting in a net reduction in volume proportional to the degree of monomer to polymer conversion. The amount of polymerisation shrinkage (1–4+ vol%) varies upon the classification of the composing resin material used and light polymerisation conditions (Table 2.3). Resin-based cements show similar or higher shrinkage values. Some unwanted effects can result from this process; namely, debonding between the restoration/tooth interface or at restoration margins, leading to internal or marginal spaces. This may be a prelude to post-operative sensitivity, marginal staining or caries. Where tooth tissue is undermined, or craze lines exist, cracks or cuspal fractures can also develop. There are some recognised methods for minimising polymerisation shrinkage. Shrinkage occurs towards the light source, with most stress occurring at the bonding interface. Bearing this in mind is crucial during composite resin restoration placement as it can reduce the amount of unfavourable shrinkage. Incremental composite resin material placement and slowing the rate of polymerisation also reduce the amount of shrinkage stresses developing (Table 2.4).

A 1–2 mm material thickness incremental layered placement approach for deep posterior cavities will allow reduced shrinkage stress to develop by reducing the C-factor. This, however, is time-consuming and technique sensitive. Low-shrinkage, filler and viscosity bulk-fill flowable composite resin materials may be used as the base layer in deep cavities. These materials adapt well to the cavity floor, reduce void potential and allow single-step placement and light polymerisation of up to 4 mm material thickness depth in order to decrease technique sensitivity and increase efficiency of the clinical procedure. They will also reduce the incidence of cuspal deflection.

Where the cavity configuration C-factor and aesthetics allow, the authors favour the use of large dispensing tubes of composite resin material as opposed to injection delivery compules applied through the use of an injecting dispensing gun. The advantages of larger storage mediums, especially when considering the techniques illustrated in this book where multiple units are restored, means that there is inherently less intervening layers of air or folds within the composite resin material as it is applied to the tooth surface. As a result, the delivery through a seamless block

Table 2.4 Stress development factors and clinical considerations for the provision of composite resin restorations

Stress development factors	Clinical Considerations
Material—modulus of elasticity	Classification of material—filler content
Cavity configuration (ratio)	Configuration C-factor = Bonded walls/Unbonded walls
Restoration application technique	Incremental layering technique Bulk fill technique with flowable material
Polymerisation rate (kinetics)	Continuous activation Discontinuous activation

volume of material results in a stronger restoration without areas of weakness that may arise due to interruptions in the material mass.

The light polymerisation activation of composite resin materials is a key stage in the provision of adhesive restorations. Light polymerisation activation methods are listed in (Table 2.5).

Reducing the rate (kinetics/speed) of the initial polymerisation shrinkage will benefit the restoration bond integrity. This may be achieved by step, ramp or pulse light polymerisation activations. Without adequate polymerisation, the restoration provision is compromised as the optimum physical characteristics of the material are not achieved. This is not only important for the main body of the restoration but essential for the bonding interface junction between the resin material and the tooth structure.

Final light polymerisation of any composite resin material may be carried out through a water-based oxygen-blocking translucent barrier material, e.g. glycerine (Fig. 2.40) to order to eliminate the oxygen inhibition unreacted resin layer (approximately 10 microns thick). Any factor that reduces the intensity of light transmission compromises the proficiency and completeness of resin material polymerisation and, therefore, adhesive restoration success. Resin materials can be light polymerised through tooth structure, translucent restorations or oxygen-blocking barrier mediums, but this reduces the intensity of the light (Figs. 2.40, 2.41 & 2.42). One crucial factor for adequate material polymerisation is the position and distance of the light source from the restoration surface. Placing the curing light tip at multiple positions around the restoration can aide the totality of cure. This is especially relevant where there are areas blocked to light penetration as a result of access issues or adjacent teeth or restorations. The position of the light cure tip should be approximated close to the surface of the restoration at a 90° angulation (Figs. 2.40 & 2.41). The further the distance of the light cure tip, the light intensity diminishes (Fig. 2.42). The depth and thickness of the restoration also require consideration, perhaps the need for incremental light polymerisation where possible. The darker the shade is of the composite resin material, the more light absorbent the material is and less likely the efficiency of light polymerisation, and so the more likely the need to cure from multiple angles. Where filler content results in a more opaque mass, the ability to cure diminishes much in the same way as the darkness of the material. For all factors, light polymerisation activation durations extended over the recommended timings suggested by the manufacturers will not improve upon polymer conversion. The light output intensity should be optimised, and the light-cure unit meter tested on a regular basis. The output of the light cure unit is specified in the manufacturer's guide, and meter testing methods for light output efficiency should be adhered to.

Table 2.5 Light polymerisation activation methods

Light polymerisation activation methods	
Continuous activation	Uniform
	Step
	Ramp
Discontinuous activation	Pulse

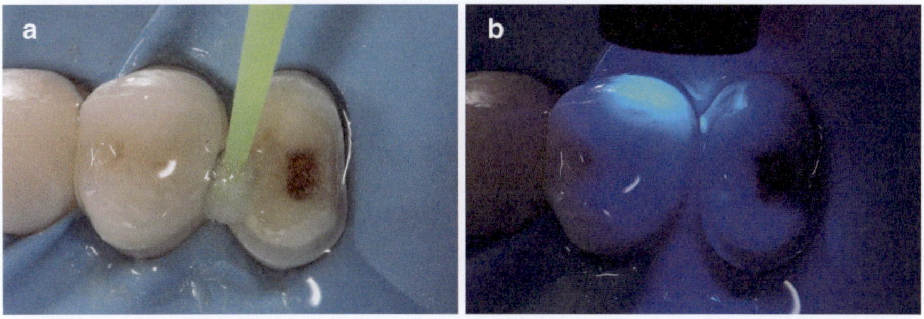

Fig. 2.40 Tooth 24 indirect glass ceramic onlay restoration (**a**) oxygen-blocking glycerine application and (**b**) final light curing of resin cement to eliminate the oxygen inhibition layer of unreacted resin

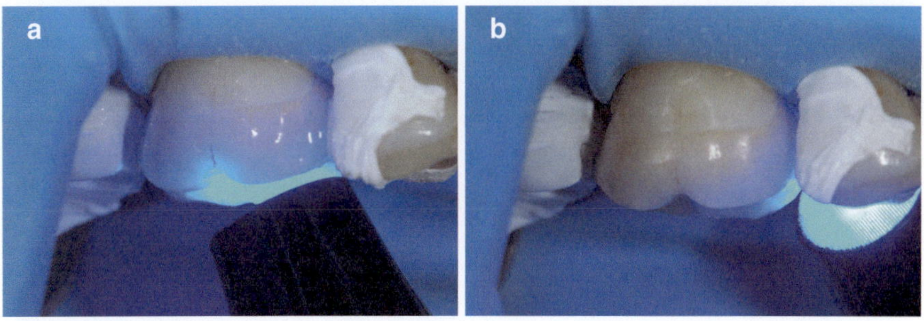

Fig. 2.41 (**a**, **b**) Light curing of composite resin cement through indirect glass ceramic onlay restorations on tooth 26. Note the close proximity and angulation of the light cure tip for optimum penetration of light for improved efficacy of resin cement polymerisation

Fig. 2.42 Light curing of composite resin cement through indirect glass ceramic onlay restorations on tooth 36. In this case, the light-cure tip should be approximated closer to the restoration for better penetration of light for improved efficacy of resin cement polymerisation

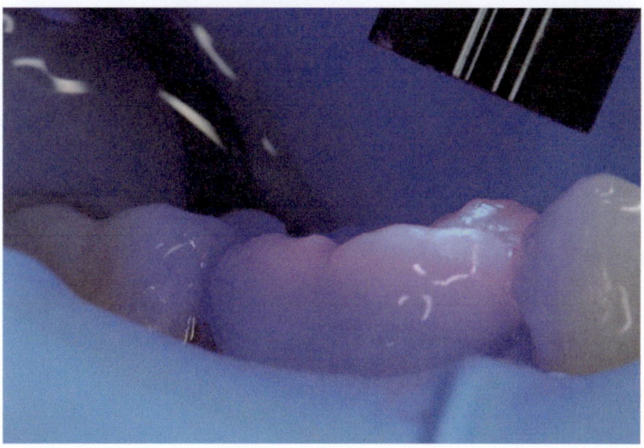

With regard to the cementation of indirect adhesive restorations, dedicated composite resin cement systems are available that offer dual-cure and light-cure versions of the cement; however, composite resin restorative paste materials may also be used (Fig. 2.43). This may be advantageous in that the higher filler load in the composite resin restorative paste will provide a 'stronger cement' and that excess expressed cement material removal is made easier due to its viscous nature. This 'cement' material may be heated in a hot water bath or with a dedicated composite resin material heater (Fig. 2.44) to allow a decrease in material viscosity for improved flow during the cementation process. Another advantage is that the working time of the cement is extended in that it is command cured by light. If there is concern over the depth of cure to activate polymerisation of the resin cement, a dual-cure resin cement may be used. This may be beneficial in the provision of posterior adhesive restorations, where the restoration thickness and limited access for the light-cure tip may reduce light transmission and prevent complete resin cement polymerisation.

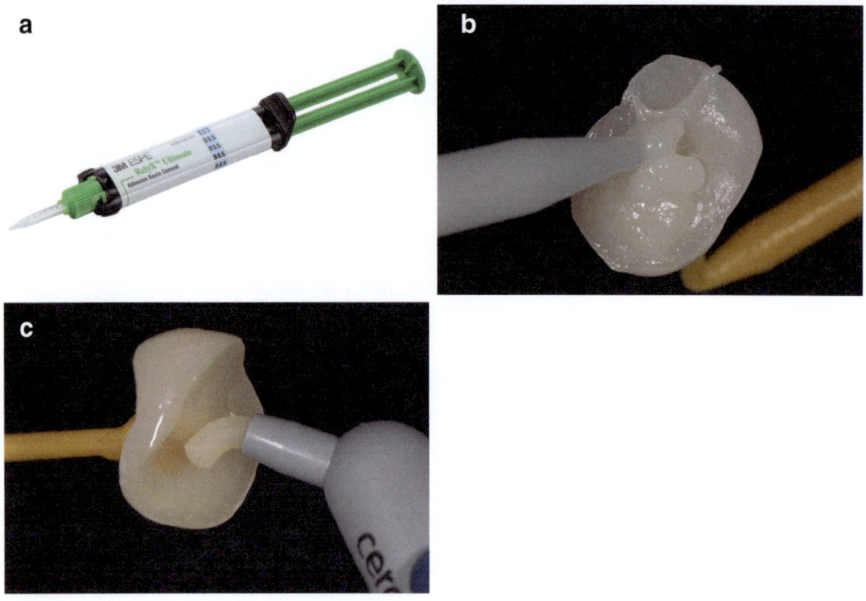

Fig. 2.43 Loading of glass ceramic restorations with (**a**, **b**) light-cure or dual-cure composite resin cement and (**c**) composite resin restorative paste materials. (Image (a) courtesy of 3M ESPE)

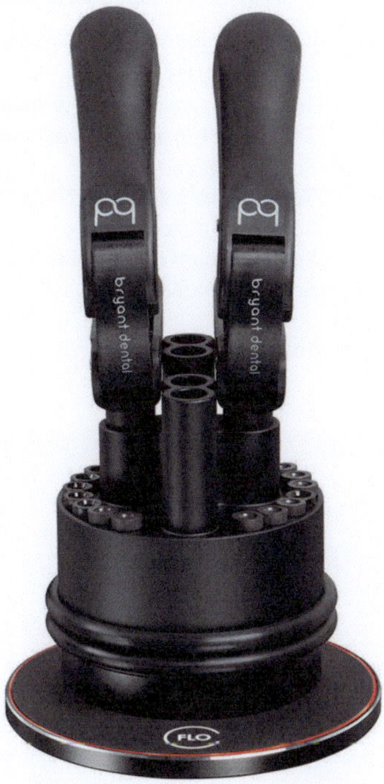

Fig. 2.44 C-Flo composite resin heater. (Image courtesy of Bryant Dental)

2.7 Adhesive Technique

The clinical procedures highlighted in this book have been performed utilising the adhesive techniques described and depicted below.

2.7.1 Bonding Agents

A summary of the bonding agent generations and their methods of use is listed in Table 2.6.

The required clinical steps for fourth-generation bonding agents are shown (Fig. 2.45) and listed in Table 2.7.

The required clinical steps for fifth-generation bonding agents are shown (Fig. 2.46) and listed in Table 2.8.

The required clinical steps for eighth-generation bonding agents are shown (Figs. 2.46, 2.47 & 2.48) and listed in Table 2.9.

Table 2.6 Summary of bonding agent generations and methods of use

Bonding agent generation	37% Phosphoric acid etch (Substrate) & rinse	Primer (bottle 1)	Adhesive (bottle 2)
Fourth	Total-etch (enamel 30 s & dentine 15 s)	+	+
Fifth	Total-etch (enamel 30 s & dentine 15 s)	+	
Sixth	Self-etch (none)	+	+
	Selective-etch (enamel 30 s)		
Seventh	Self-etch (none)	+	
	Selective-etch (enamel 30 s)		
Eighth UNIVERSAL	Self-etch (none)	+	
	Selective-etch (enamel 30 s)		
	Total-etch (enamel 30 s & dentine 15 s)		

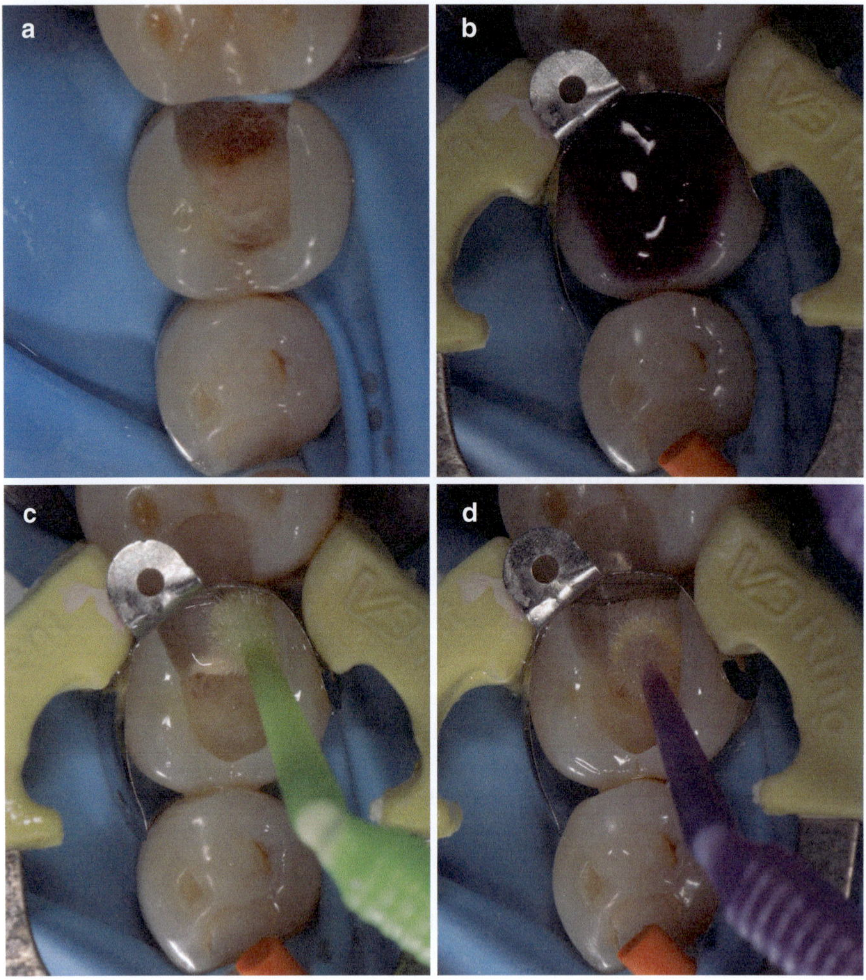

Fig. 2.45 (**a**, **b**) Total-etch technique (fourth-generation bonding agent), enamel and dentine surface acid etch. (**c**, **d**) Application of bonding agent (primer & adhesive, two bottles)

Table 2.7 Adhesive technique for fourth-generation bonding agents

Etch technique	Enamel	Dentine
Total-etch	37% Phosphoric acid etch (30 s) Rinse & air dry Primer scrub (15 s) Air dry Adhesive scrub (15 s) Air dry Light polymerise (20 s)	37% Phosphoric acid etch (15 s) Rinse & air dry (do not desiccate) Primer scrub (15 s) Air dry Adhesive scrub (15 s) Air dry Light polymerise (20 s)

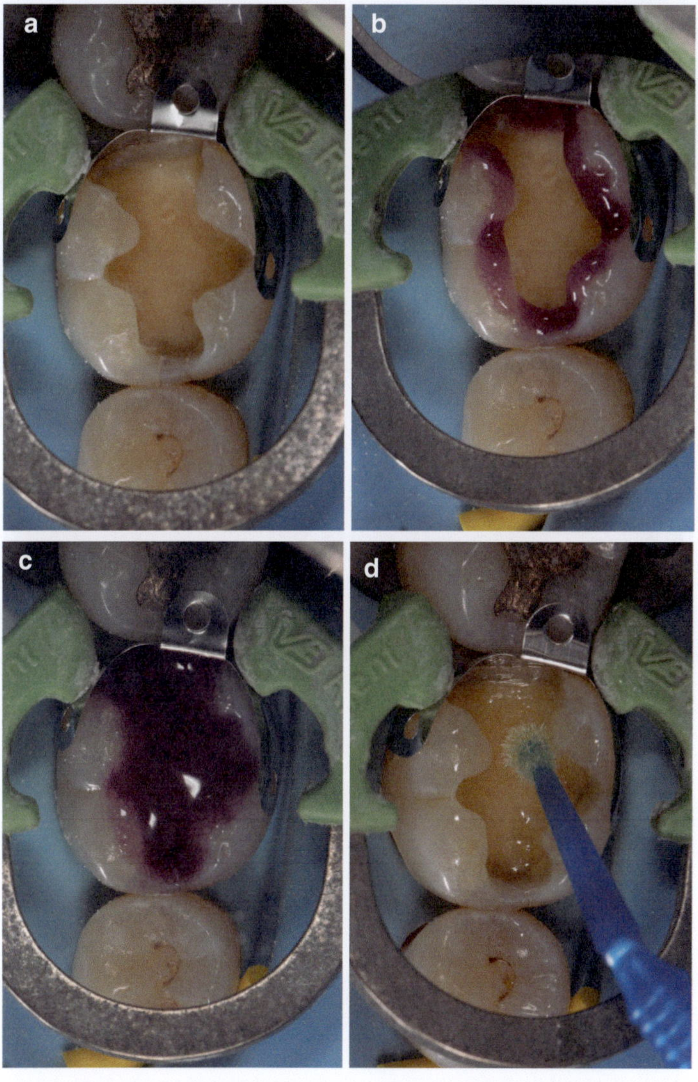

Fig. 2.46 (**a**, **b**, **c**) Total-etch technique (fifth- and eighth-generation bonding agent), enamel and dentine surface acid etch. (**d**) Application of bonding agent (one bottle)

Table 2.8 Adhesive technique for fifth-generation bonding agents

Etch technique	Enamel	Dentine
Total etch	37% Phosphoric acid etch (30 s) Rinse & air dry Bonding agent scrub (20 s) Air dry Light polymerise (20 s)	37% Phosphoric acid etch (15 s) Rinse & air dry (do not desiccate) Bonding agent scrub (20 s) Air dry Light polymerise (20 s)

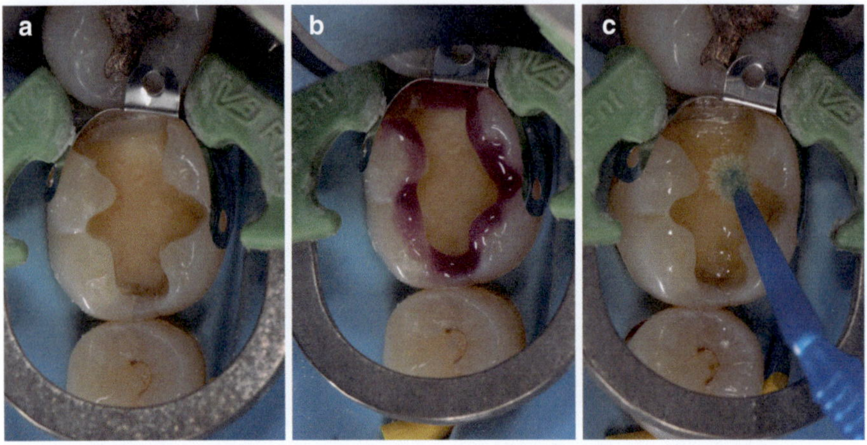

Fig. 2.47 (**a**, **b**) Selective-etch technique (eighth-generation bonding agent), enamel surface acid etch. (**c**) Enamel and dentine surface application of bonding agent (one bottle)

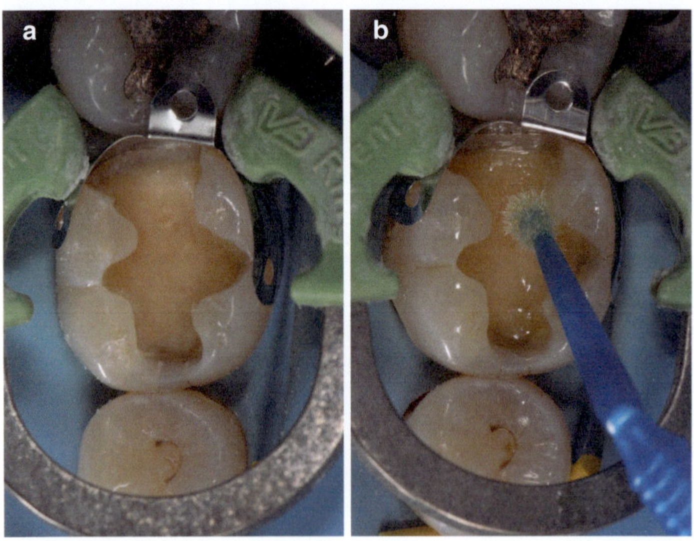

Fig. 2.48 (**a**, **b**) Self-etch technique (eighth-generation bonding agent), enamel and dentine surface application of bonding agent (one bottle)

Table 2.9 Adhesive techniques for eighth-generation bonding agents

Etch technique	Enamel	Dentine
Total-etch	37% Phosphoric acid etch (30 s) Rinse & air dry Bonding agent scrub (20 s) Air dry Light polymerise (20 s)	37% Phosphoric acid etch (15 s) Rinse & air dry (do not desiccate) Bonding agent scrub (20 s) Air dry Light polymerise (20 s)
Selective-etch	37% Phosphoric acid etch (30 s) Rinse & air dry Bonding agent scrub (20 s) Air dry Light polymerise (20 s)	Bonding agent scrub (20 s) Air dry Light polymerise (20 s)
Self-etch	Bonding agent scrub (20 s) Air dry Light polymerise (20 s)	Bonding agent scrub (20 s) Air dry Light polymerise (20 s)

2.7.2 Indirect Materials

The intaglio surface treatment stages required to prepare indirect restorative materials for adhesive bonding after final try-in of the restoration are shown (Figs. 2.49, 2.50, 2.51, 2.52, 2.53, 2.54, and 2.55) and are listed in Table 2.10. The use of HF acid and 10-MDP-containing primers where appropriate has been indicated.

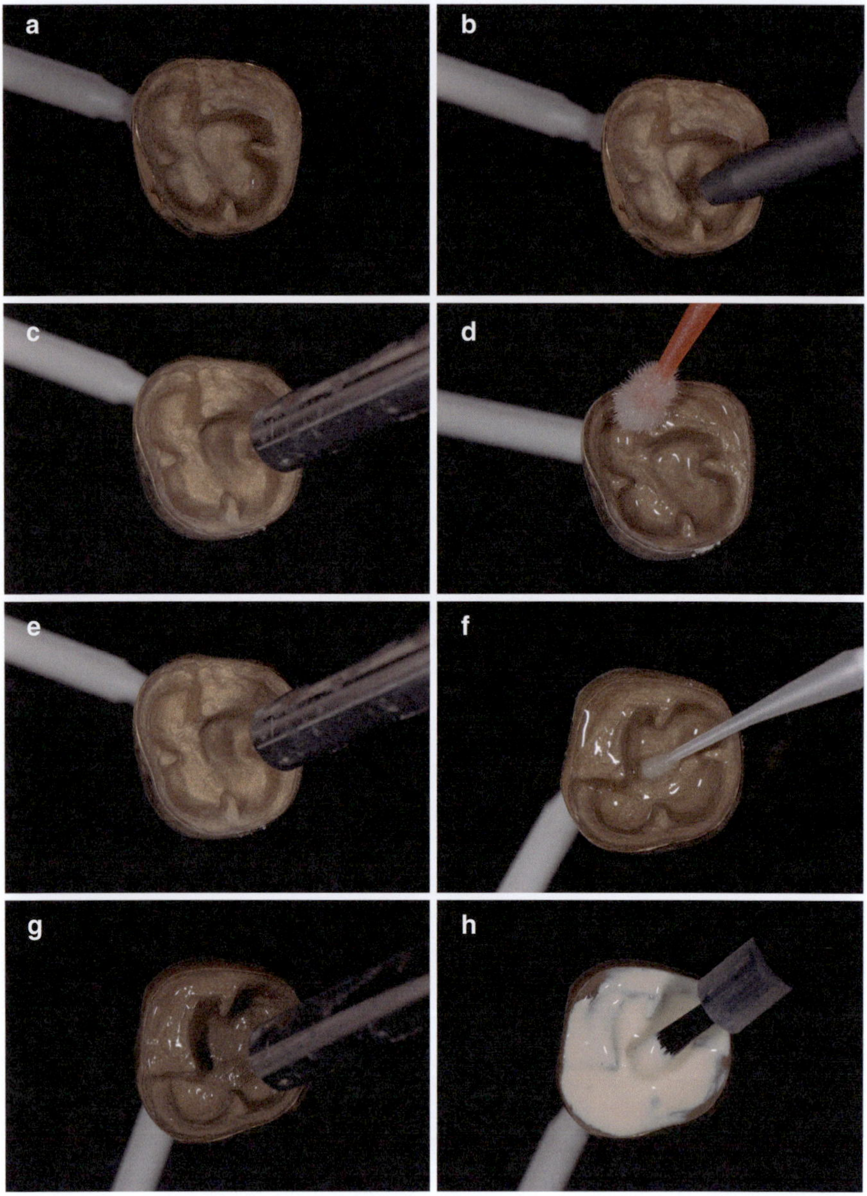

Fig. 2.49 Type III gold alloy onlay restoration surface treatment for adhesive bonding (**a**) Steam cleaned. (**b**) Sand blast. (**c**) Rinse, air dry. (**d**) Alcohol clean. (**e**) Air dry. (**f**) Alloy 10-MDP primer application. (**g**) Air dry. (**h**) Resin cement load

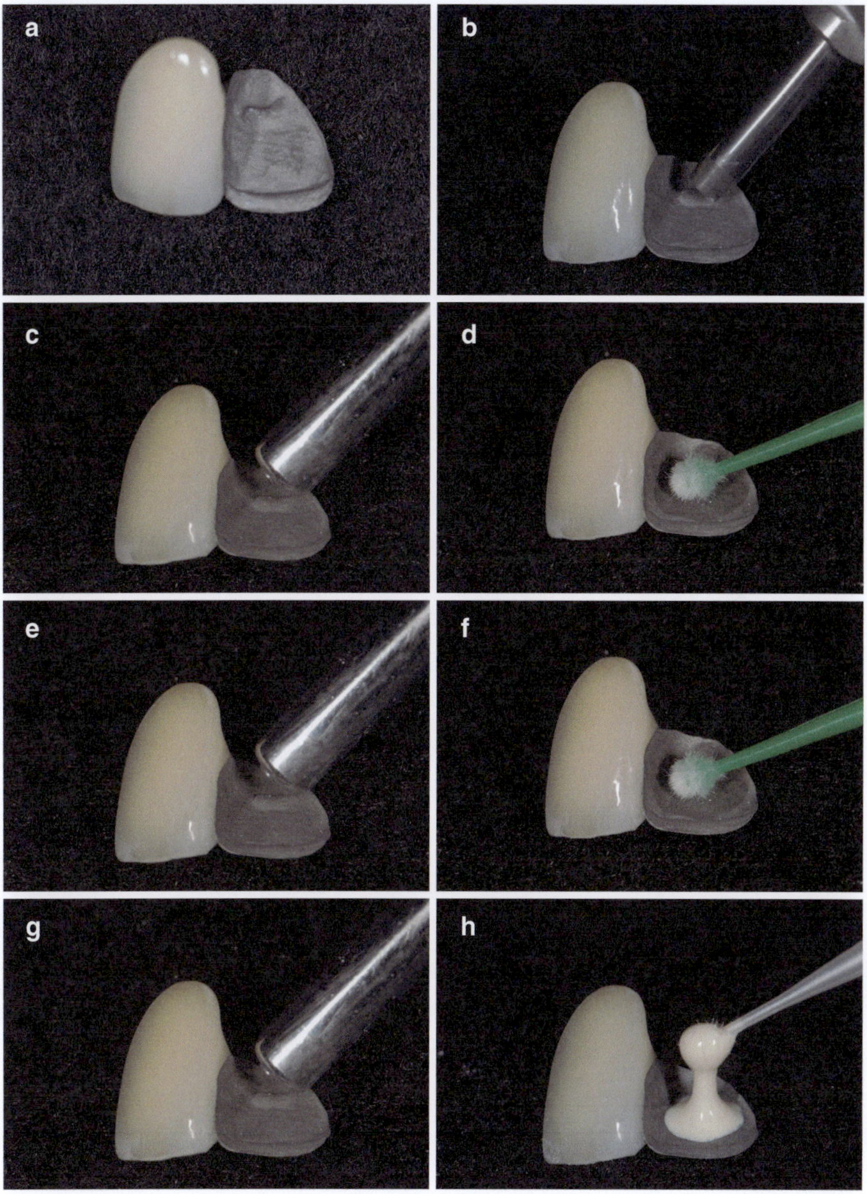

Fig. 2.50 Nickel chrome alloy resin-bonded bridge restoration surface treatment for adhesive bonding. (**a**) Steam cleaned. (**b**) Sandblast. (**c**) Rinse, air dry. (**d**) Alcohol clean. (**e**) Air dry. (**f**) Alloy 10-MDP primer application. (**g**) Air dry. (**h**) Resin cement load

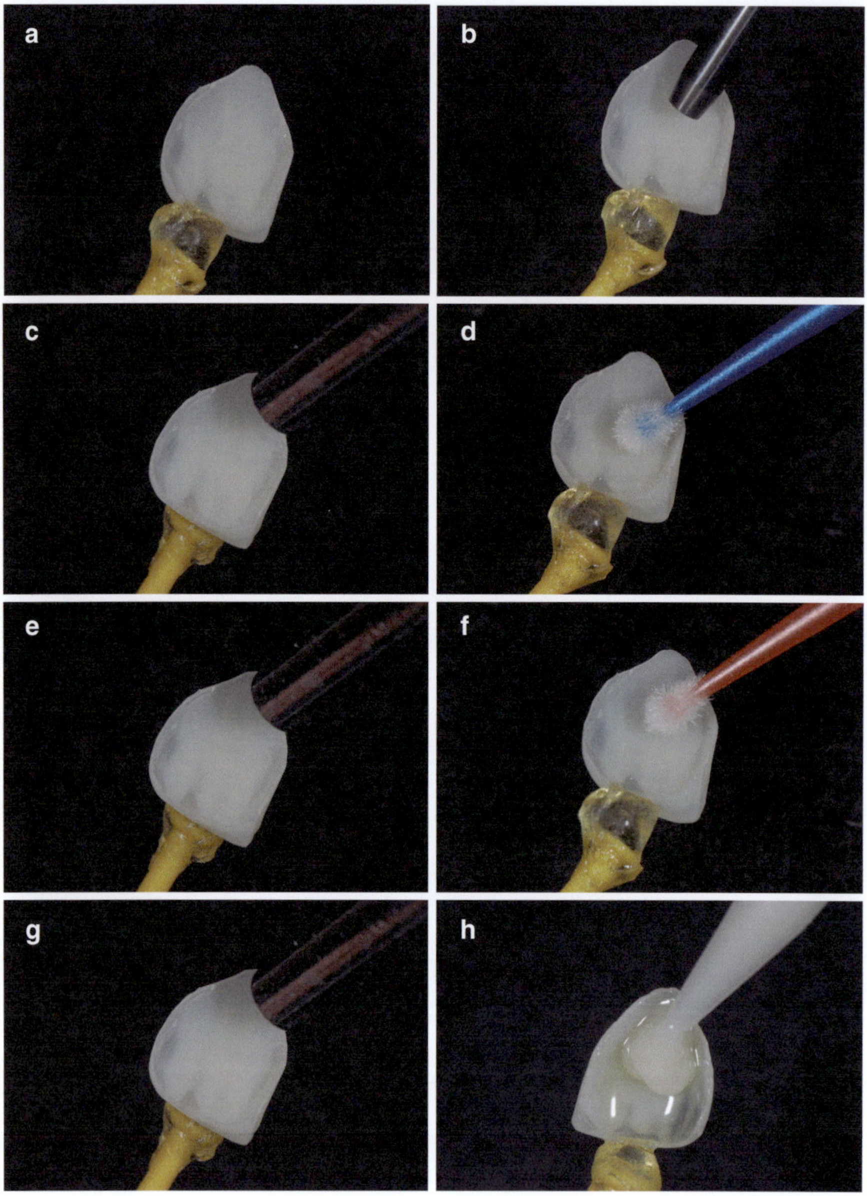

Fig. 2.51 Composite resin veneer restoration surface treatment for adhesive bonding (**a**) Steam cleaned. (**b**) Sandblast. (**c**) Rinse, air dry. (**d**) Alcohol clean. (**e**) Air dry. (**f**) Adhesive application. (**e**) Air dry. (**h**) Resin cement load

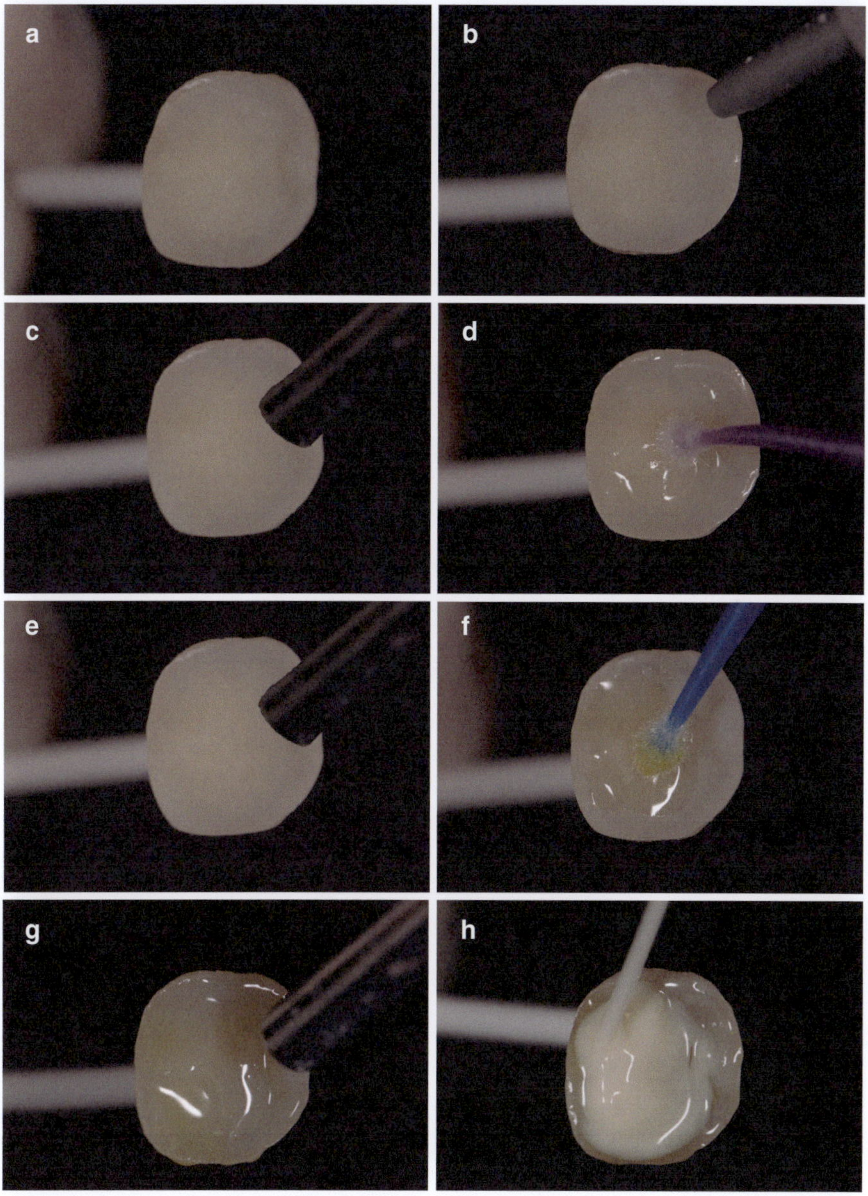

Fig. 2.52 Resin nano-ceramic onlay restoration surface treatment for adhesive bonding. (**a**) Steam cleaned. (**b**) Sandblast (CoJet-Sand). (**c**) Rinse, air dry. (**d**) Alcohol clean. (**e**) Air dry. (**f**) Adhesive application. (**g**) Air dry. (**h**) Resin cement load

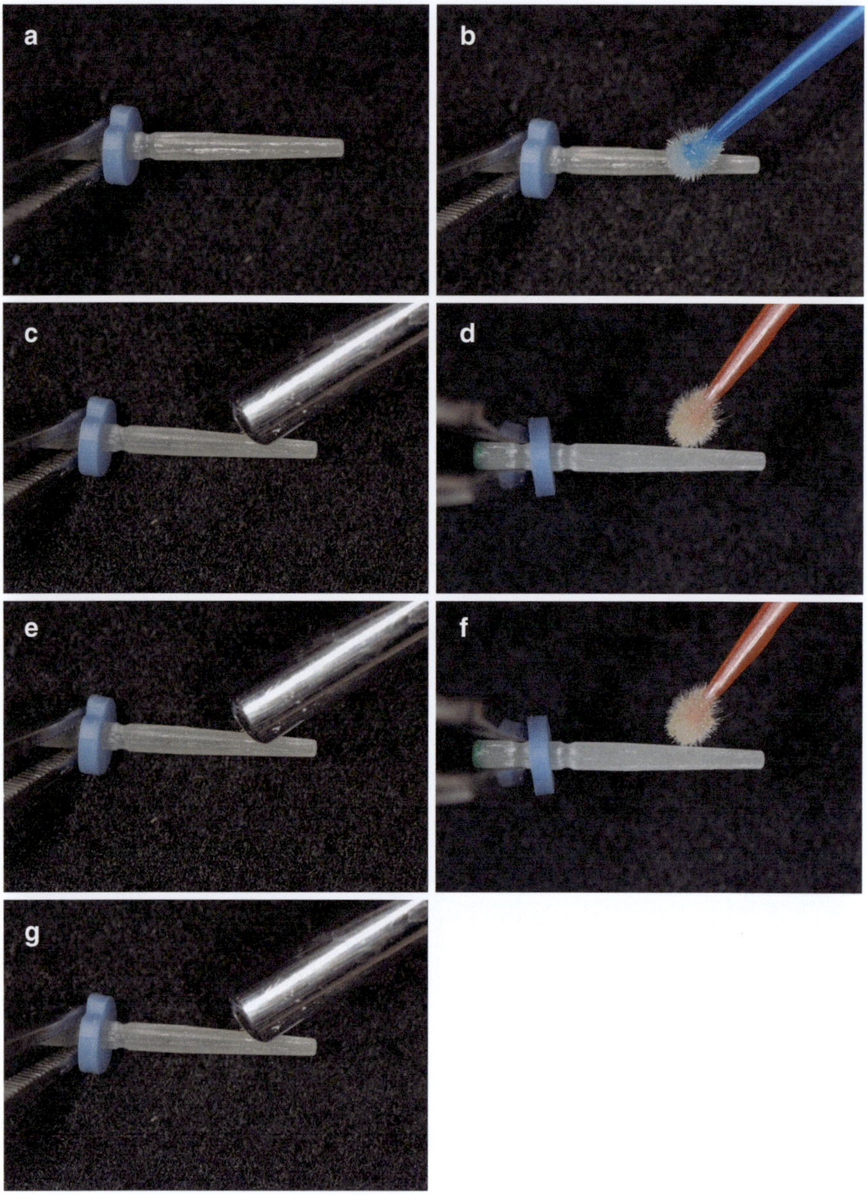

Fig. 2.53 Glass-fibre post-restoration surface treatment for adhesive bonding. (**a**) Steam cleaned. (**b**) Alcohol clean. (**c**) Air dry. (**d**) Silane (60 s if post is not pre-silanated), (**e**) Air dry. (**f**) Adhesive application. (**g**) Air dry

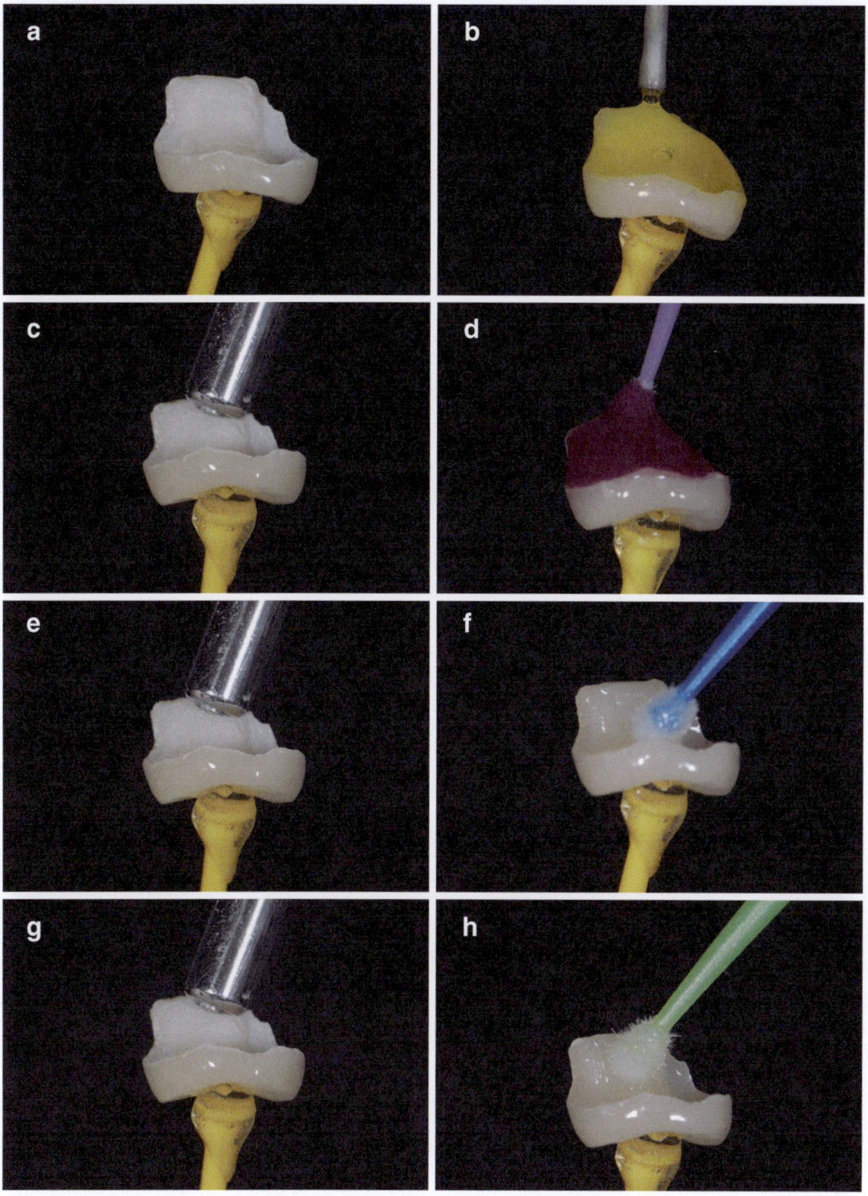

Fig. 2.54 Glass-ceramic lithium disilicate onlay restoration surface treatment for adhesive bonding. (**a**) Steam cleaned. (**b**) 5% or 9.5% HF acid etch (10 or 20 s). (**c**) Rinse, air dry. (**d**) 37% Phosphoric acid etch (15 s). (**e**) Rinse, air dry. (**f**) Alcohol clean. (**g**) Air dry. (**h**) Silane application (60 s). (**i**) Air dry. (**j**) Adhesive application. (**k**) Air dry. (**l**) Resin cement (composite resin restorative paste) load

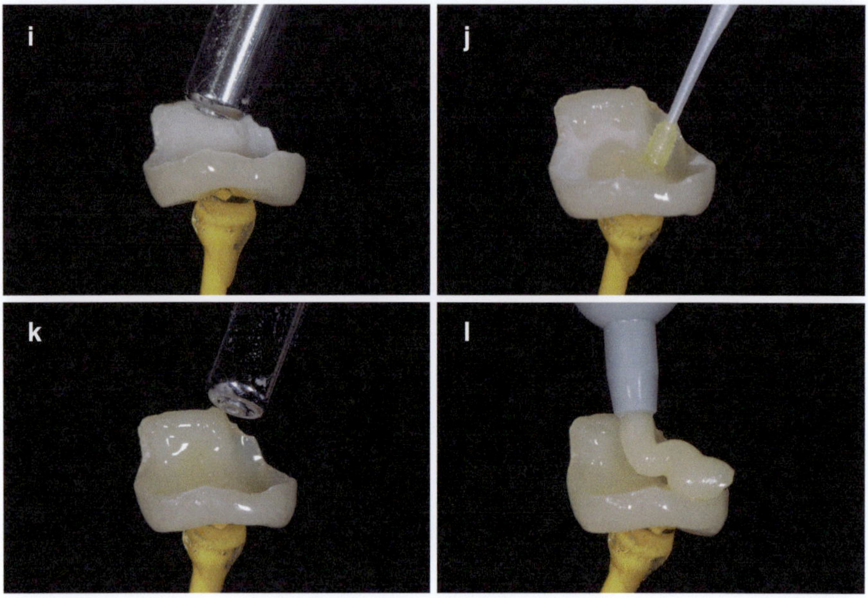

Fig. 2.54 (continued)

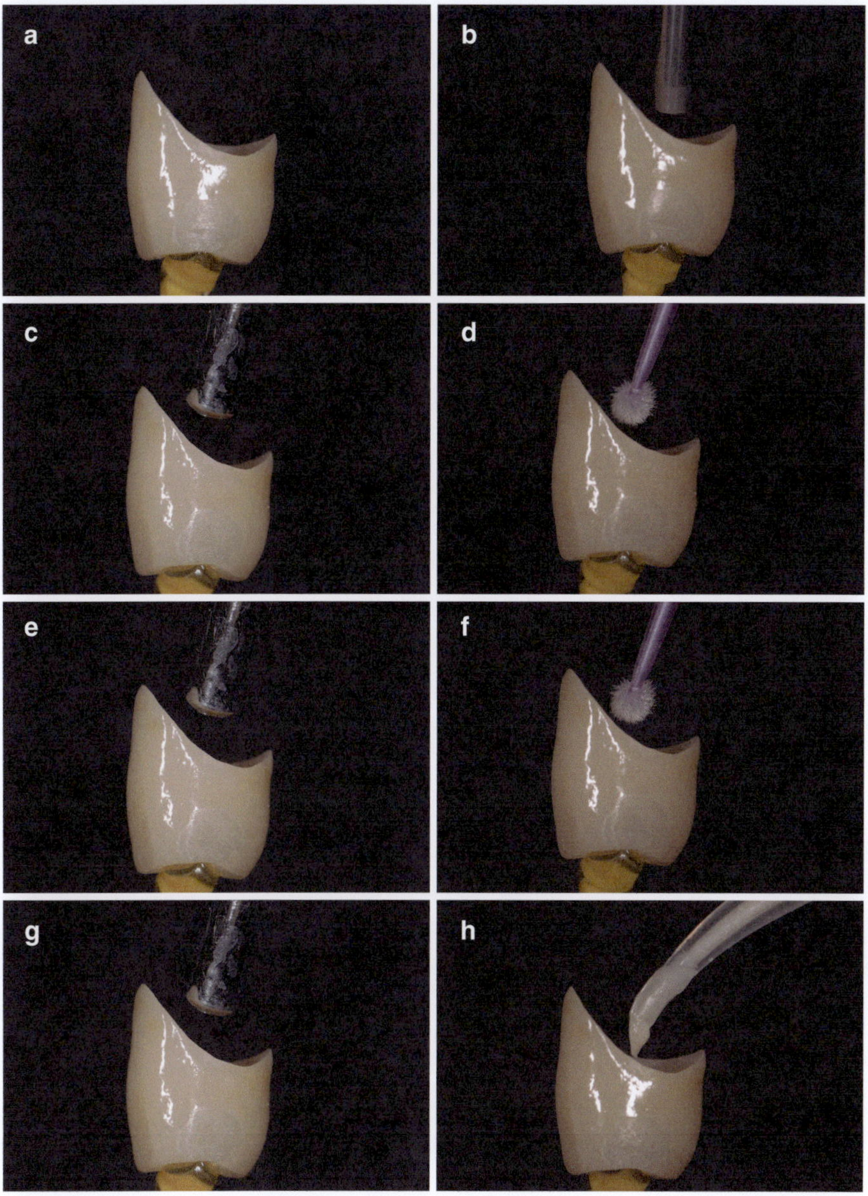

Fig. 2.55 Polycrystalline ceramic zirconia crown restoration surface treatment for adhesive bonding. (**a**) Steam cleaned. (**b**) Sandblast. (**c**) Rinse, air dry. (**d**) Alcohol clean. (**e**) Air dry. (**f**) Ceramic 10-MDP primer application (60 s). (**g**) Air dry. (**h**) Resin cement load

Table 2.10 Adhesive intaglio surface treatments for indirect restorations

Material & restoration type		Restoration surface treatment
Metal alloys	*Gold* *(Type III)* Veneer Crown Onlay Post	1. Steam clean 2. Alumina blast, rinse, air dry 3. (Heat treat—optional) 4. Alcohol clean, air dry 5. Alloy 10-MDP primer application, air dry 6. Resin cement load
	Chrome *(nickel or cobalt)* Resin-bonded bridge Crown Onlay Post	1. Steam clean 2. Alumina blast, rinse, air dry 3. Alcohol clean, air dry 4. Alloy 10-MDP primer application, air dry 5. Resin cement load
Resin-based materials	*Composite resin* Veneer Crown Onlay	1. Steam clean 2. Alumina blast, rinse, air dry 3. Alcohol clean, air dry 4. Adhesive application, air dry 5. Resin cement load
	Resin nano-ceramic Veneer Onlay	1. Steam clean 2. Alumina blast (CoJet-Sand), rinse, air dry 3. Alcohol clean, air dry 4. Adhesive application, air dry 5. Resin cement load
	Glass-fibre Post	1. Steam clean 2. Alcohol clean, air dry 3. Silane (60 s if post- not pre-silanated), air dry 4. Adhesive application, air dry
Ceramics	*Glass* *(Feldspathic or Lithium Disilicate)* Veneer Resin-bonded bridge Crown Onlay	1. Steam clean 2. 5% or 9.5% HF acid etch (10, 20 or 60 s), rinse, air dry 3. 37% phosphoric acid etch (15 s), rinse, air dry 4. Alcohol clean, air dry 5. Silane application (60 s), air dry 6. (Adhesive application, air dry—only required if composite resin restorative paste is used as the cement) 7. Resin cement load
	Polycrystalline *(Zirconia)* Resin-bonded bridge Crown Onlay	1. Steam clean 2. Alumina blast, rinse, air dry 3. Alcohol clean, air dry 4. Ceramic 10-MDP primer application (60 s), air dry 5. Resin cement load

Further Reading

1. Anusavice K, Shen C, Rawls R. Phillips' Science of Dental Materials. 12th ed. St Louis: Elsevier Saunders; 2013.
2. Burke FJT, Lawson A, Green DJB, Mackenzie L. What's new in dentine bonding?: universal adhesives. Dent Update. 2017;44:328–40.
3. Davidson CL, Feilzer AJ. Polymerization shrinkage and polymerization shrinkage stress in polymer- based restoratives. J Dent. 1997;25:435–40.
4. Garcia D, Yaman P, Dennison J, Neiva G. Polymerization shrinkage and depth of cure of bulk fill flowable composite resins. Oper Dent. 2014;39:441–8.
5. Hyun-Hee Park, In-Bog Lee. Effect of glycerin on the surface hardness of composites after curing. J Kor Acad Cons Dent. 2011;36(6):483–9.
6. Patel M. Evolution of indirect restorations for fixed prosthodontics: planning, preparation and cementation. Prim Dent J. 2019;8(3):48–63.
7. Park J, Chang J, Ferracane J, Lee IB. How should composite be layered to reduce shrinkage stress: incremental or bulk filling? Dent Mater. 2008;24:1501–5.
8. Randolph LD, Palin WM, Watts DC, Genet M, Devaux J, Leloup G, et al. The effect of ultra-fast photopolymerisation of experimental composites on shrinkage stress, network formation and pulpal temperature rise. Dent Mater. 2014;30:1280–9.
9. Tjäderhane L. Dentin bonding: can we make it last? Oper Dent. 2015;40:4–18.

Management of Discoloured Teeth

3

Contents

Learning Outcomes

- Explore the causes of internal and external discolouration of teeth.
- Revise bleaching techniques for the management of discoloured vital and non-vital teeth.
- Consider conservative management of early enamel white spot lesions.
- Understand the possible adverse effects of bleaching treatment on planned adhesive restorative procedures.

A. Alani, M. Patel, *Adhesive Techniques in Restorative Dentistry*, BDJ Clinician's Guides, https://doi.org/10.1007/978-3-032-07346-4_3

3.1 Introduction

Teeth have been shown to be important for self-esteem and confidence. This is largely associated with tooth shape, form, colour and their relative positioning. A common aesthetic concern of patients is tooth discolouration. This can present generally or can be isolated to one unit. Patients with discoloured teeth are more likely to face social challenges, have lower dental self-esteem and may also associate the discoloured tooth with a disturbing time in their life, such as non-accidental injury or a traumatic incident. As such, the management of discoloured teeth may be a priority for the patient, especially when considering their social well-being.

The size, shape and colour of teeth are all critical in the perception of aesthetics. The colour or shade of teeth, which is uniform and 'whiter', provides measurable benefit to the patient regardless of the mode or method of the improvement. In this respect, the utilisation of the most conservative method of colour improvement should take precedence over other more aggressive forms of treatment, which result in the removal of sound tooth tissue or otherwise intact teeth with a minimal amount of restorations.

3.2 Aetiology

There are various causes of tooth discolouration, which can either be internal or external in origin. Internal discolouration arises where there are developmental or congenital defects of the enamel and dentine structure, or physiological and pathological processes that have discoloured the pulpal surface of the tooth, manifesting as discolouration. External discolourations arise primarily from diet and social habits.

3.2.1 Internal Discolouration

The process of enamel and dentine formation provides the basis for the colour of teeth. This process may be entirely without defects, but where dentine deposition is great and enamel is thin, teeth may seem more yellow despite the absence of any developmental abnormality. This can be illustrated by the maxillary canine tooth. The canine tooth has a comparatively thick dentine layer when compared to the adjacent enamel layer, resulting in a significant difference in colour between the canine and adjacent teeth units. The formation of tooth tissue in the unborn, neonate, child and adult can be affected by a number of metabolic, genetic, iatrogenic, traumatic, idiopathic, as well as natural ageing processes which can modify the perceived colour of teeth.

Metabolic disorders resulting in physiological changes can manifest in teeth depending on the stage of development and the severity of the disturbance. In conditions where changes in the natural turnover of cells and the release of waste products occur, discolouration may manifest. In alkaptonuria, the lack of enzymes to break down homogentisic acid results in brown discolouration as it becomes incorporated into the dentine on deposition. Similarly, congenital erythropoietic porphyria results in the absence of an enzyme, which in turn results in porphyrin being incorporated into dentine, resulting in red/purple/brown discolouration of teeth. In contrast, patients with hyperbilirubinaemia have increased circulation of bile pigments, resulting in incorporation into dental hard tissues and manifesting as a yellow-green discolouration.

Genetic defects resulting in altered function of odontoblasts or ameloblasts produce defects in dentine and enamel formation, which may manifest on eruption. The first complaint from the patient may be associated with discolouration, but it is also likely to result in further complications of tooth structure (Fig. 3.1).

Amelogenesis imperfecta occurs where enamel is either poorly mineralised or organised. As a result of the differences in aetiology, problems in colour are likely to manifest in different ways. Where enamel is thin, such as in hypoplastic amelogenesis imperfecta, the underlying yellow/brown tinge of the unaffected dentine is likely to be a source of apparent discolouration (Fig. 3.2). Hypoplastic areas can also manifest as pitting or striations in the enamel surface (Fig. 3.3). This in itself is unlikely to be a source of discolouration, but as these areas can harbour bacteria and food products, resulting in external staining, patients report concerns relating to colour. Where mild hypomineralised enamel presents with intense white areas coronally, it is likely to be the significant contrast with the remaining body of the crown that patients are more concerned about than the area of whiteness itself. If hypomineralisation is severe, the discolouration is likely to be significantly darker and more uniform as a result compared to milder forms.

Dentine-related malformations such as dentinogenesis imperfecta and dentine dysplasia may present with the obliteration of the pulp chambers, resulting in a greater intensity of the underlying dentine colour through the enamel. The enamel itself commonly fractures away from the dentine, which can result in expediting the need for treatment. Clinically, the appearance is amber, grey, to purple blue (Fig. 3.4). If the enamel fractures away from the dentine and is exposed to the oral environment, the intensity of discolouration may increase as chromogens are absorbed into the dentine surface more readily.

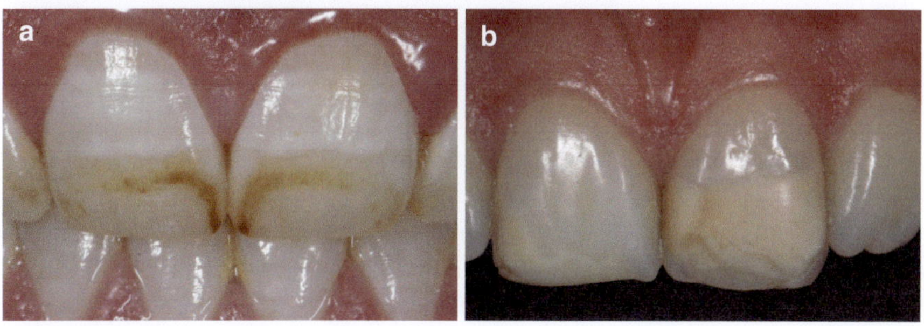

Fig. 3.1 (**a**, **b**) Inherent developmental defects of maxillary incisor teeth showing compromise in colour and form

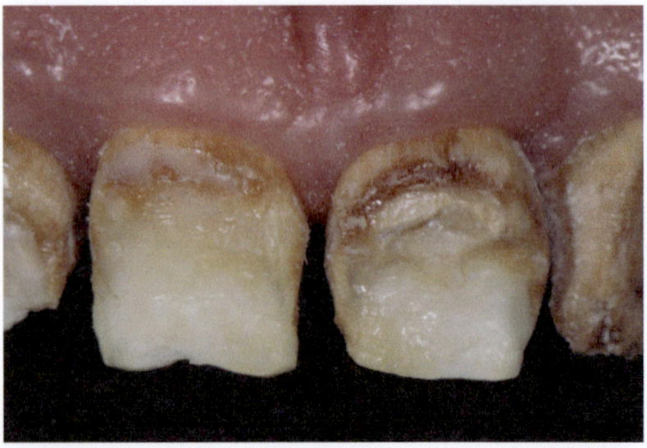

Fig. 3.2 Amelogenesis imperfecta showing thin poorly mineralised enamel exposing the underlying yellow/brown tinge of the unaffected dentine

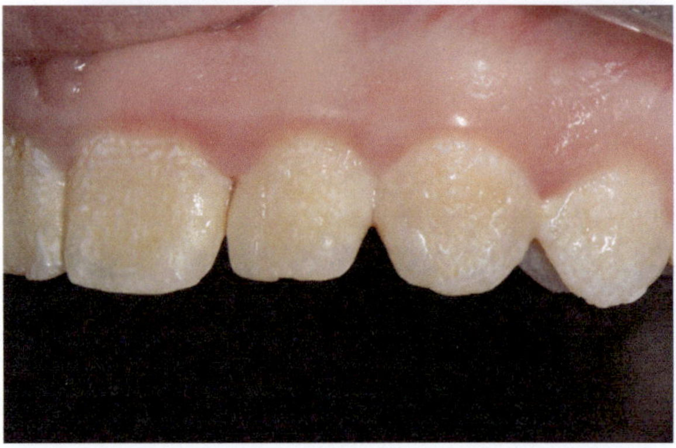

Fig. 3.3 Hypoplastic amelogenesis imperfecta resulting in characteristic pitting exposing thin areas of enamel exposing underlying dentine shade

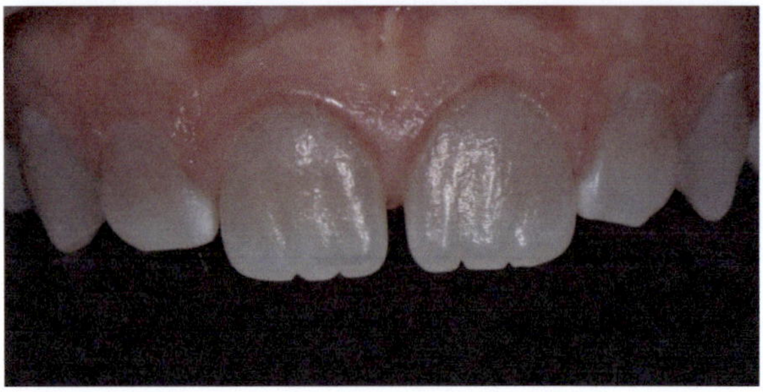

Fig. 3.4 Dentinogenesis imperfecta presenting concurrently with hypodontia

The ingestion of antibiotics during the formative stages of tooth development can result in the incorporation of compounds into the mineralised matrix of the tooth. Most commonly, this occurs with tetracycline. Systemic use of tetracycline results in chelation, which results in the formation of a tetracycline calcium ion complex on the surface of hydroxyapatite crystals, which occurs more often in dentine than in enamel (Fig. 3.5). Due to these issues and other more general medical reasons,

Fig. 3.5 A patient presenting with tetracycline staining with characteristic banding across teeth 43, 42, 41, 31, 32, 33. Note the uniform position of banding across all units

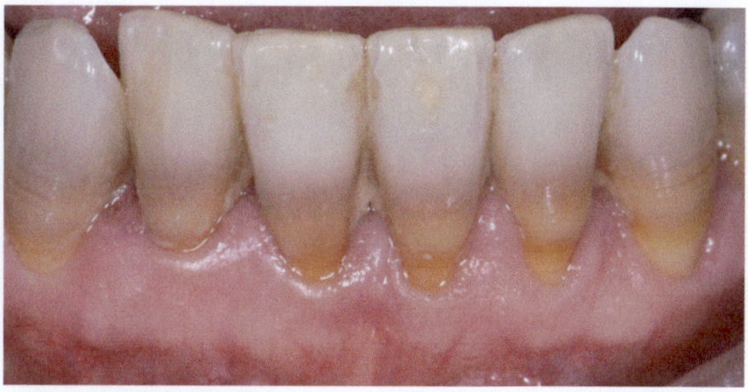

tetracycline is not recommended for expectant mothers, those nursing neonates and children up to the age of 12 years. The intensity, pattern and distribution of the resulting discolouration are dependent on the timing of antibiotic usage, the amounts ingested and the length of time of administration. The teeth appear yellow, brown or grey. The change in colour may coincide with banding across the teeth, reflecting the chronology of antibiotic ingestion. These teeth can be treated with bleaching, although the duration of treatment may be significantly longer when compared to other, more common conditions.

Dental fluorosis occurs when excessive amounts of fluoride are ingested during the formative stages of tooth development. The ideal times to avoid high fluoride exposure are between 1 and 4 years of age, with the critical time between 20 and 30 months. Risk diminishes completely by the age of 8 years. The ingestion of fluoride results in the formation of fluoroapatite, which is beneficial due to its greater ability to withstand acid dissolution. Unfortunately, greater amounts of fluoroapatite result in a greater chance of fluorotic-related tooth discolouration. In its milder forms, fluorosis may be difficult to delineate from normal tooth tissue. Small white spots, flecks or streaks may go unnoticed (Fig. 3.6). Where fluorosis is more severe, resulting from long exposure to high amounts of fluoride, the enamel seems pitted, rough with discolouration and chalky white or brown markings. The discolouration itself may be a manifestation of chromogens being incorporated into the now more porous tooth structure post-eruption.

During early carious lesion development, there will be a balance of mineral loss and gain within the enamel tissue lesion, the balance of which determines disease activity. The enamel surface layer initially demineralises with mineral loss and subsequent porosities, which could break down further to form cavities. If there is further mineral gain in the enamel surface layer (up to 200 microns), the lesion will arrest with the body of the lesion still remaining porous. This leads to the clinical appearance of an opaque white spot due to the scattering of light between the enamel pores and prisms. Clinical presentations of established white spot lesions may prove to be an aesthetic challenge for the managing clinician and often occur in cases of fluorosis, molar incisal hypomineralisation, post-orthodontic treatment after bracket removal and dental trauma (Figs. 3.7 and 3.8). The management of a white spot lesion clinical case is described and depicted in Sect. 3.3.2.

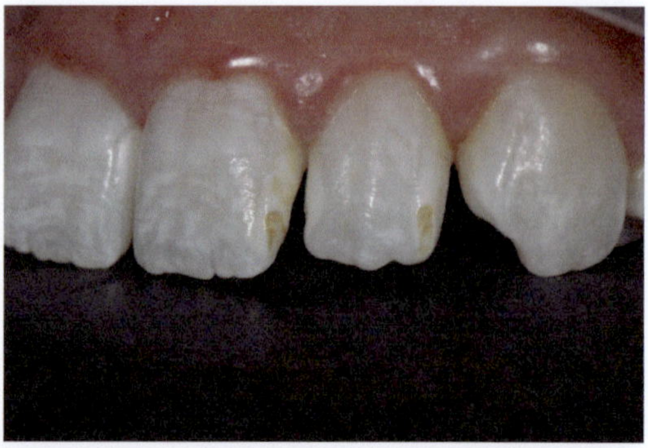

Fig. 3.6 Fluorosis showing white spots, flecks and streaks. Note the more severely affected brown areas disto-incisally on the 21 and 22

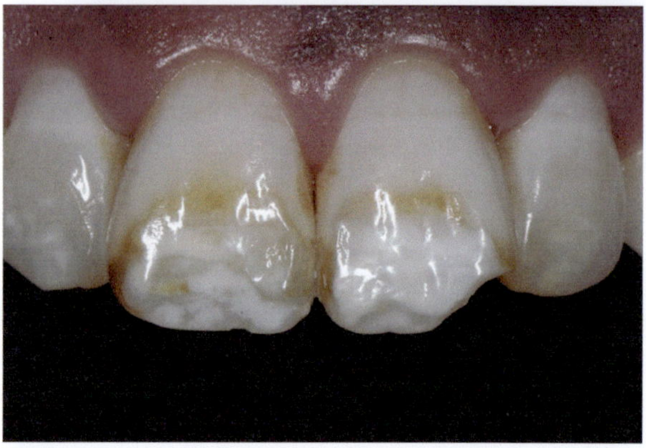

Fig. 3.7 Patient presenting with molar–incisor hypomineralisation and distal incisal fracture of tooth 21 provides asymmetry between the central incisor teeth

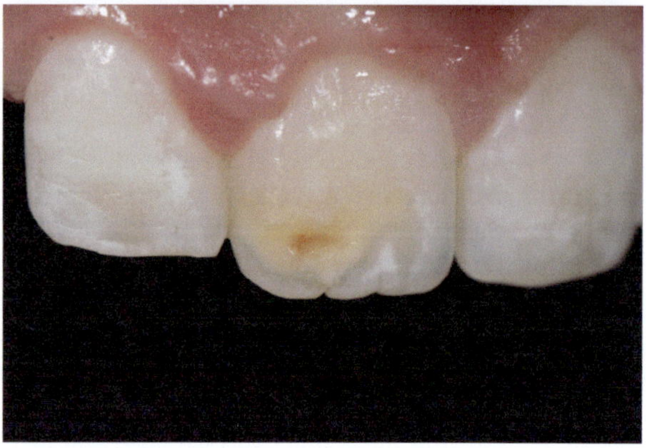

Fig. 3.8 Tooth 11 with a localised area of enamel hypoplasia (white and brown discolourations) in a patient with a history of intrusion of the predecessor deciduous tooth

Dental trauma, which can result in the disruption of the vascular supply to the tooth, is widely recognised as the most common reason for loss of vitality of anterior teeth with concurrent discolouration (Fig. 3.9). Traumatic blows to the face and mouth can cause the rupturing of blood vessels resulting in intra-pulpal haemorrhage causing a significant colour change in the coronal portion of the tooth. The blood vessels can sever at the apical portion or within the coronal portion of the

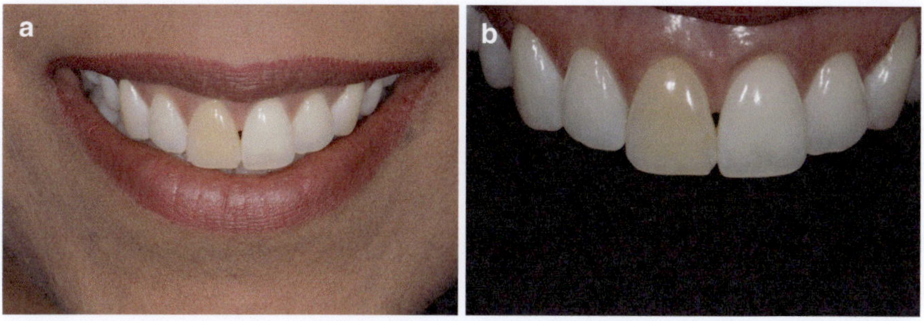

Fig. 3.9 (**a, b**) Internal discolouration of tooth 11 following loss of vitality due to trauma

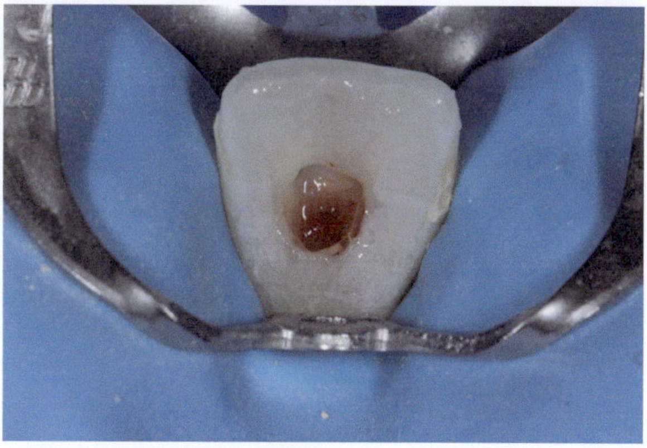

Fig. 3.10 Tooth 11 intra-pulpal haemorrhage causes colour change in the coronal portion of the tooth. Note how the blood products engage the pulp horns and isthmus

tooth (Fig. 3.10). The extravasated blood cells may undergo a breakdown process of haemolysis and release haemoglobin. Iron in haemoglobin combines with hydrogen sulphide produced by bacteria to form iron sulphide. This is a naturally dark compound. Other potential avenues for discolouration include haemorrhage into the patent dentinal tubules by way of the capillary effect, which subsequently progressively degrade, culminating in the deposition of chromogenic by-products. These chromogenic chemicals include hemosiderin, hemin, hematin and hematoidin. Immature teeth with wide-open tubules are more likely to discolour readily.

In contrast to acute pulpal haemorrhage, dental trauma can induce changes in the vital pulp which can result in chronic progression of discolouration and potentially pulpal death. In response to trauma, the odontoblasts can lay down additional layers of reactionary dentine, which can be misinterpreted as physiologic ageing of the pulp (Fig. 3.9).

Existing restorations, microleakage and the formation of secondary caries may contribute to the discolouration of teeth (Figs. 3.11, 3.12 and 3.13). The use of amalgam alloy within an access cavity, as well as metal-based post restorations, can also discolour teeth by way of corrosion or the release of metal ions (Fig. 3.12). Where root canal treatments exist, discolouration may occur through incomplete removal

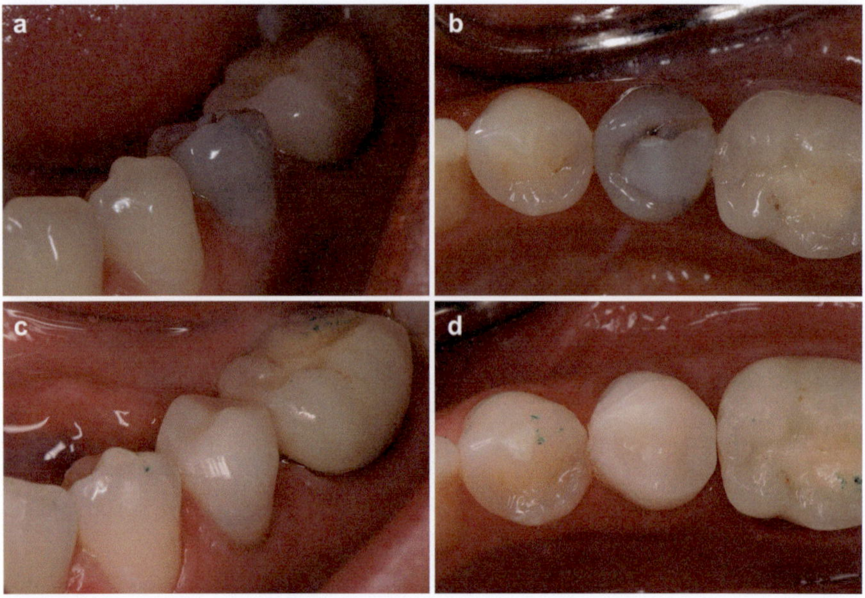

Fig. 3.11 (**a**, **b**) Tooth 35 showing composite resin restoration failure and discolouration due to microleakage and secondary caries. (**c**, **d**) Subsequent management of tooth 35 with restoration and caries removal, internal bleaching and provision of a direct composite onlay restoration

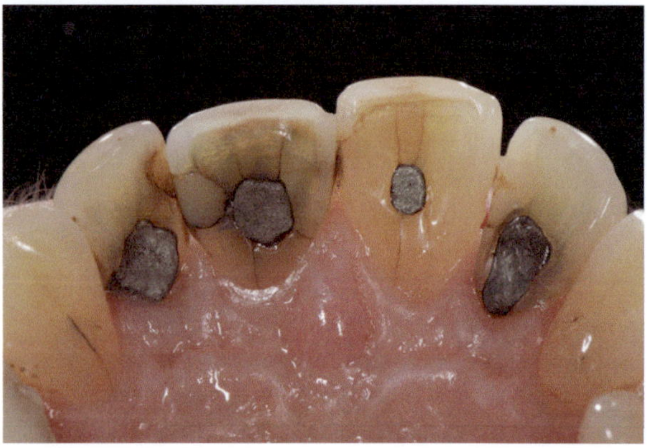

Fig. 3.12 Maxillary incisor teeth showing amalgam and composite resin restoration failure and discolouration due to corrosion, microleakage and secondary caries

of the pulp chamber harbouring pulp remnants that degrade over time (Figs. 3.13 and 3.14). Common areas of tissue stagnation include the pulp horns (Fig. 3.15). Slow degradation of necrotic pulp tissue remnants is complicated by bacterial presence and associated breakdown products and egested toxins. The staining is likely to be much more embedded onto the dentine surface and into the tubules and show through the translucent enamel structure (Figs. 3.13 and 3.14).

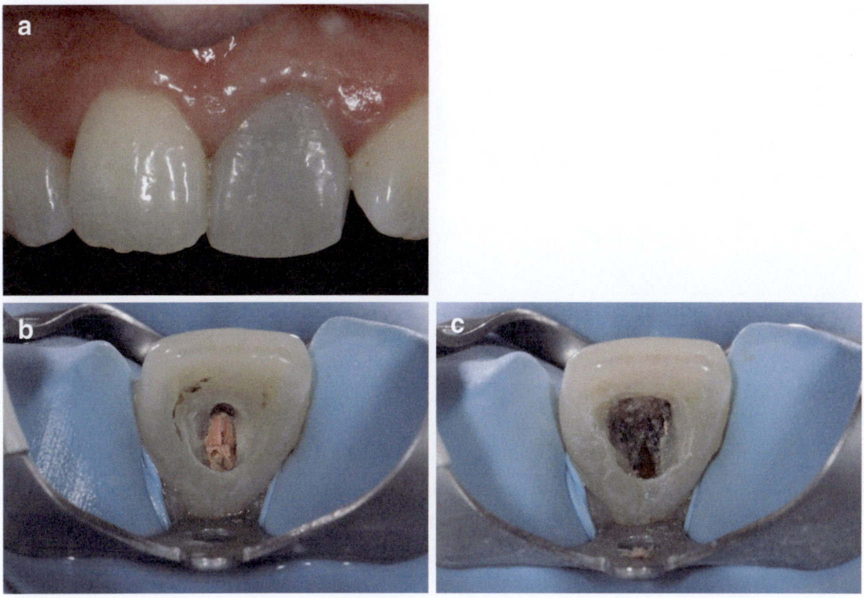

Fig. 3.13 (**a**) Discolouration of previously root-canal-treated tooth 21. (**b**, **c**) Discolouration is evident due to a lack of complete access and debridement of the pulp chamber in conjunction with microleakage of the coronal composite resin restoration

Fig. 3.14 (**a**) Maxillary incisor tooth. (**b**) Palatal access cavity and inadequate removal of pulp chamber roof harbouring pulp remnants that cause discolouration through the dentinal tubules in the coronal aspect

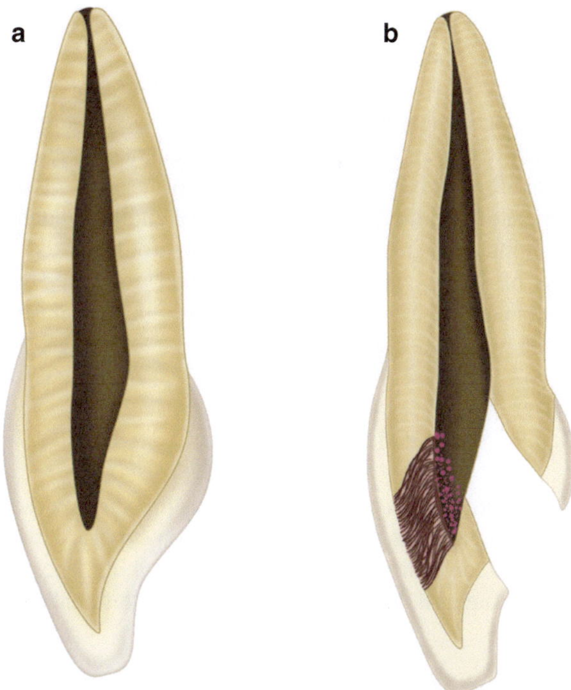

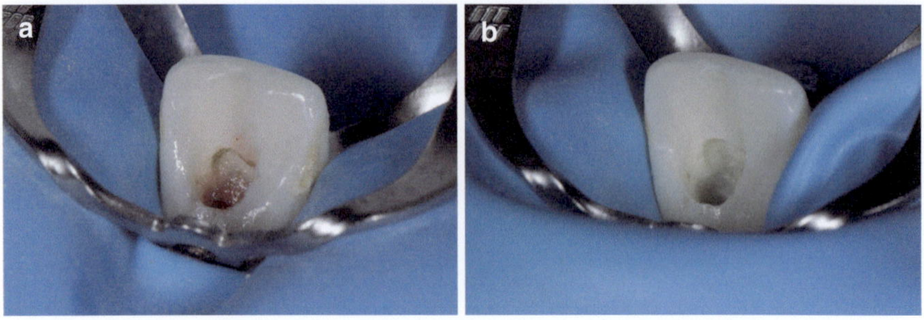

Fig. 3.15 (**a**) Pulp horn harbouring pulpal remnants manifesting as discolouration. (**b**) The pulp horn was instrumented using an ultrasonic scaler and a small rose head bur until these areas were fully exposed and clean

Intracanal medicaments such as those containing tetracycline constituents may also discolour tooth structure. Root canal sealers can cause gradual discolouration of teeth through penetration of the dentinal tubules, resulting in a yellow hue. In contrast to sealants, a starker change in colour is caused by mineral trioxide aggregate (MTA). This discolouration has been attributed to the iron oxidation that chemical setting MTA undergoes (Fig. 3.16). The effect of MTA is especially relevant in teeth that have been dentally traumatised. MTA apexification for non-vital immature incisors is an established method for the management of wide-open apices. As such, the use of MTA should be confined to the apical 3 mm without filling the whole canal length. In such situations, the clinician may consider utilising thermoplastic GP as the more aesthetic alternative despite the potential lack of seal and bioactivity that MTA provides.

Other more natural modes of discolouration include natural ageing of teeth, where secondary and tertiary dentine deposition results in darkening of the tooth, which may be more apparent as the enamel concurrently thins due to functional wear. Reactionary dentine is less porous and more mineralised than naturally deposited dentine. The laying down of additional dentine layers increases the contribution of the naturally more yellow-brown dentine (due to an increased percentage of yellow phosphoprotein) when compared to the static or diminishing thickness of the enamel. This intensifies the chroma of the tooth and reduces translucency (Fig. 3.17).

3.2.2 External Discolouration

Teeth naturally discolour over time as they are exposed to the oral environment. In function, the changes in colour occur on exposure to chromophores from food, liquids and social habits such as cigarette smoking. The prolonged use of chlorhexidine-containing mouth rinses may also be an additional cause.

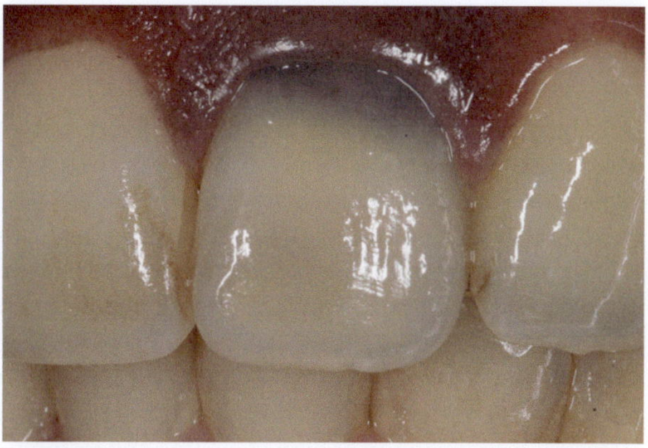

Fig. 3.16 Previously traumatised 21 obturated with MTA exhibiting discolouration in the cervical region

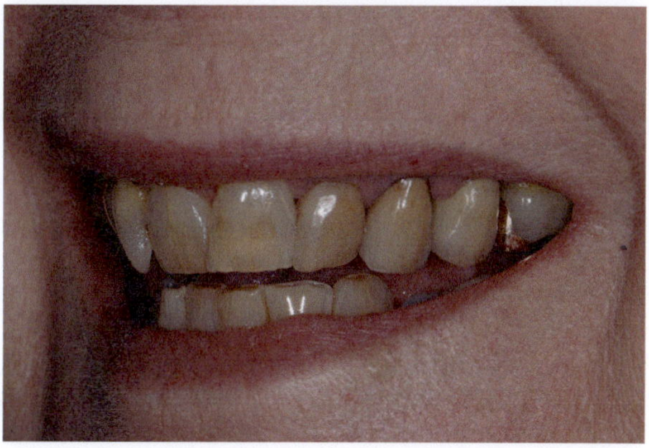

Fig. 3.17 An elderly patient presenting with generalised natural ageing discolouration of her teeth

The process is yet to be fully understood, but it seems as though the constituents of food and drink, such as polyphenols, which provide the colouring to foods or tannins present in tea, coffee and red wine, contribute to the process. Enamel is not impervious, and its porosities can absorb these molecules present within food and drink beverages. There are broadly two sources of discolouration. Those molecules that have coloured constituents which may not attach to or be able to reside within the porosities of enamel. These are known as pigments. In contrast, and of greater significance, 'dyes' have reactive components that allow them to connect to organic material. Common foods and drinks that contain dyes include tomato and cocoa-based products, tea, coffee and red wine.

The presence of a biofilm and the acquired pellicle seems to contribute as bacteria react to the presence of the chromogens, whilst also potentially causing dissolution of enamel, resulting in a greater propensity for deep discolouration. Other less common sources of discolouration include the presence of chromogenic bacteria with green and orange staining in patients with poor oral hygiene and black/brown staining in those with good oral hygiene.

3.3 Tooth Bleaching

The technique of bleaching teeth has long been described as a method of improving anterior aesthetics. Since this time, the delivery of tooth bleaching has undergone some modifications which have been driven by changes in legislation, increased experience, greater scientific knowledge of the process, demand for aesthetic treatments and changes in social attitudes toward dental treatment.

The alternatives to tooth bleaching treatment involve the removal of sound but discoloured tooth tissue to provide either direct or indirect veneer or crown restorations to disguise the appearance of the colour of the tooth (Fig. 3.18). This approach will inevitably weaken the remaining tooth tissue, providing less tooth tissue for future replacement or refurbishment of the restoration as and when this is needed. However, a combination of both bleaching and restoration treatment modalities may be used in certain clinical cases where the colour change treatment may be challenging with bleaching techniques alone.

3.3.1 Colour Mechanisms

A number of different compounds have been utilised to bleach and lighten discoloured teeth. The most commonly utilised bleaching agent gel substances are 10% carbamide peroxide and 6% hydrogen peroxide. The former breaks down into the latter during a process of degradation. A solution of 10% carbamide peroxide results in approximately 3% hydrogen peroxide over a period of 4 h.

Hydrogen peroxide is a colourless liquid that is soluble in water to produce an acidic solution. This solution contains reactive oxygen species that act to oxidise the large complex molecules responsible for discolouration through the formation of free radicals. The net effect of this reaction is the production of smaller molecules. These smaller molecules are able to diffuse through the tooth and are less able to reflect light than the previous large chromophore molecules. Highly coloured large carbon rings are cleaved into large double carbon bond chains, which are lighter in

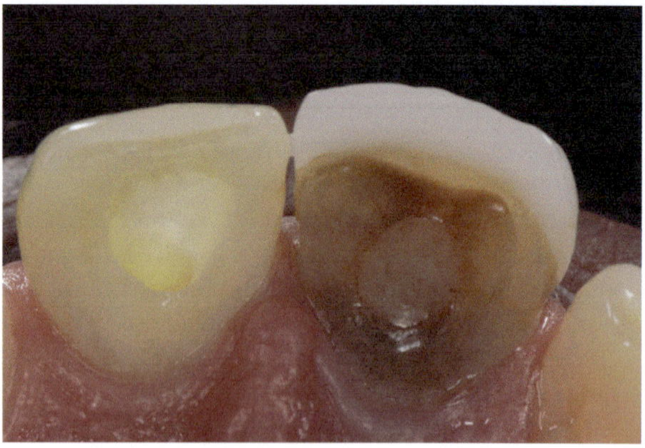

Fig. 3.18 Tooth 21 presenting with loss of vitality and discolouration secondary to trauma where a veneer restoration has been provided to disguise the dark discolouration

colour. These large chains are then broken down into hydroxyl-containing molecules, which are progressively lighter. The process continues until the degradation products of these repeat chemical reactions are colourless, resulting in lightening the shade of the tooth.

The presenting colour of the tooth provides an indication of how successful the prospective bleaching process will be. As would be expected, the lighter the tooth initially, the greater potential for improvement, although this does depend on the patient's presentation. An individual who attends with otherwise light teeth or someone who has been whitening chronically at the time of presentation is unlikely to have a broad scope for further measurable improvement. In contrast, a yellow appearance or stain is likely to be easiest to manage, and black is the most difficult; the latter may be a result of residual products from existing restorations, dental caries, degraded pulpal products or developmental processes.

Indicators of bleaching success also include a consideration for the internal structure of the teeth, and more specifically related to age where physiological and pathological processes play a role. Older teeth, with a greater likelihood of secondary and tertiary dentine deposition, will be inherently more challenging to lighten as penetration of the bleach into the more mineralised tissues is challenging. Older teeth are also likely to have stains and degradation products for longer periods, which may also equate to the severity and intensity of the unsightly colour. These dentinal processes make the tooth more densely coloured in addition to the tubular processes being more erratic resulting in less porosity through which the bleach can penetrate. Conversely, younger teeth, where tubules are more patent and less secondary or tertiary dentine, are likely to lighten more rapidly and predictably. Teeth that are pathologically aged, such as those with attritive or erosive toothwear, may also present with similar issues as dentine is deposited in a similar process.

3.3.2 Patient Assessment

A detailed history should be taken from the patient, and an appreciation of the patient's expectation of treatment needs to be balanced against the current shade of teeth and the desired improvement. Patients who consume strongly coloured foods and drinks should be made aware that the outcome may be compromised as a result, as well as the need for treatment due to a relapse of colour. Discussions on previous treatments may give some indication as to the patient's motivations and expectations.

The clinical examination may reveal marked differences in the shades of each individual tooth, resulting in the need to carefully plot the scheme of bleaching whereby certain teeth would undergo a greater bleaching period than others for purposes of achieving an equal result by the end of treatment (Fig. 3.19). Due to their inherent thickness, canine teeth are likely to require more bleaching than their neighbouring lateral incisor teeth.

Existing plastic or indirect restorations may be retained through the bleaching process and can provide some indication of how successful the process has been (Fig. 3.20). However, teeth exhibiting caries or failing restorations will require

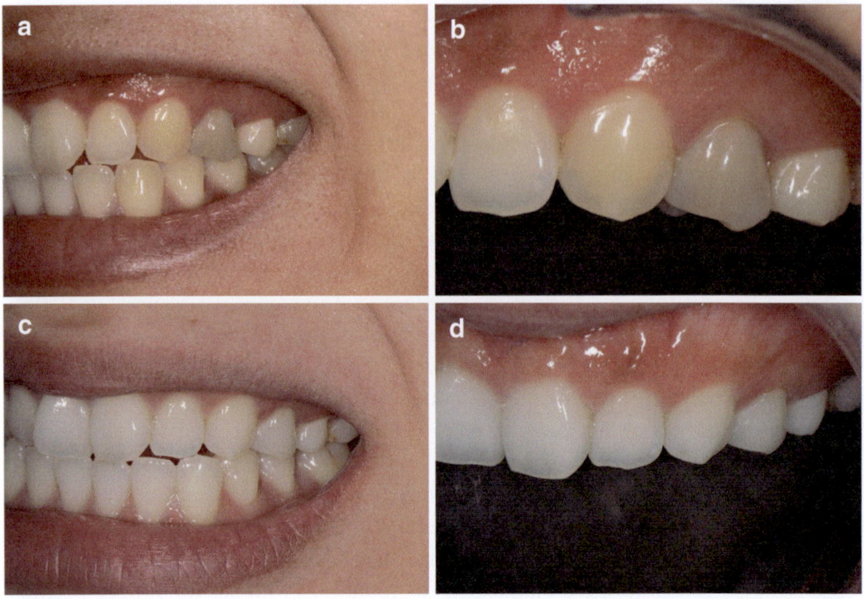

Fig. 3.19 (**a**, **b**) Pre-operative situation with marked differences in the shades of the individual teeth. (**c**, **d**) Post-operative after extended bleaching treatment to tooth 24 prior to bleaching treatment of the adjacent teeth

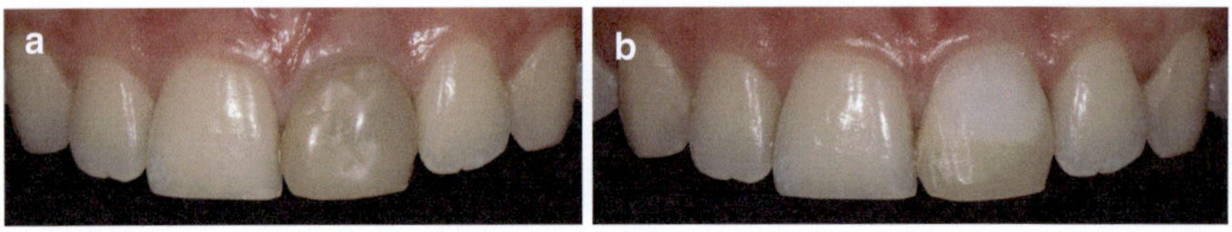

Fig. 3.20 (**a**, **b**) Tooth 21 bleaching treatment where the existing plastic restoration has been retained through the bleaching process to provide baseline reference. The Class IV restoration will be replaced

remedial stabilisation treatment prior to bleaching. Teeth with exposed dentine will be inherently more susceptible to the development of sensitivity and may require restorative intervention prior to beginning bleaching treatment. Patients also need to be made aware that existing plastic and indirect restorations (veneers, crowns and onlays) will not change in colour and that this may result in the need for restoration replacement on completion of the bleaching treatment, which is likely to result in further biological and financial cost.

To provide a contemporaneous record of the presenting complaint, digital photographs of the patient smiling and intra-oral views will aid in assessing the improvements achieved compared to the baseline records (Fig. 3.21). Colour photographs

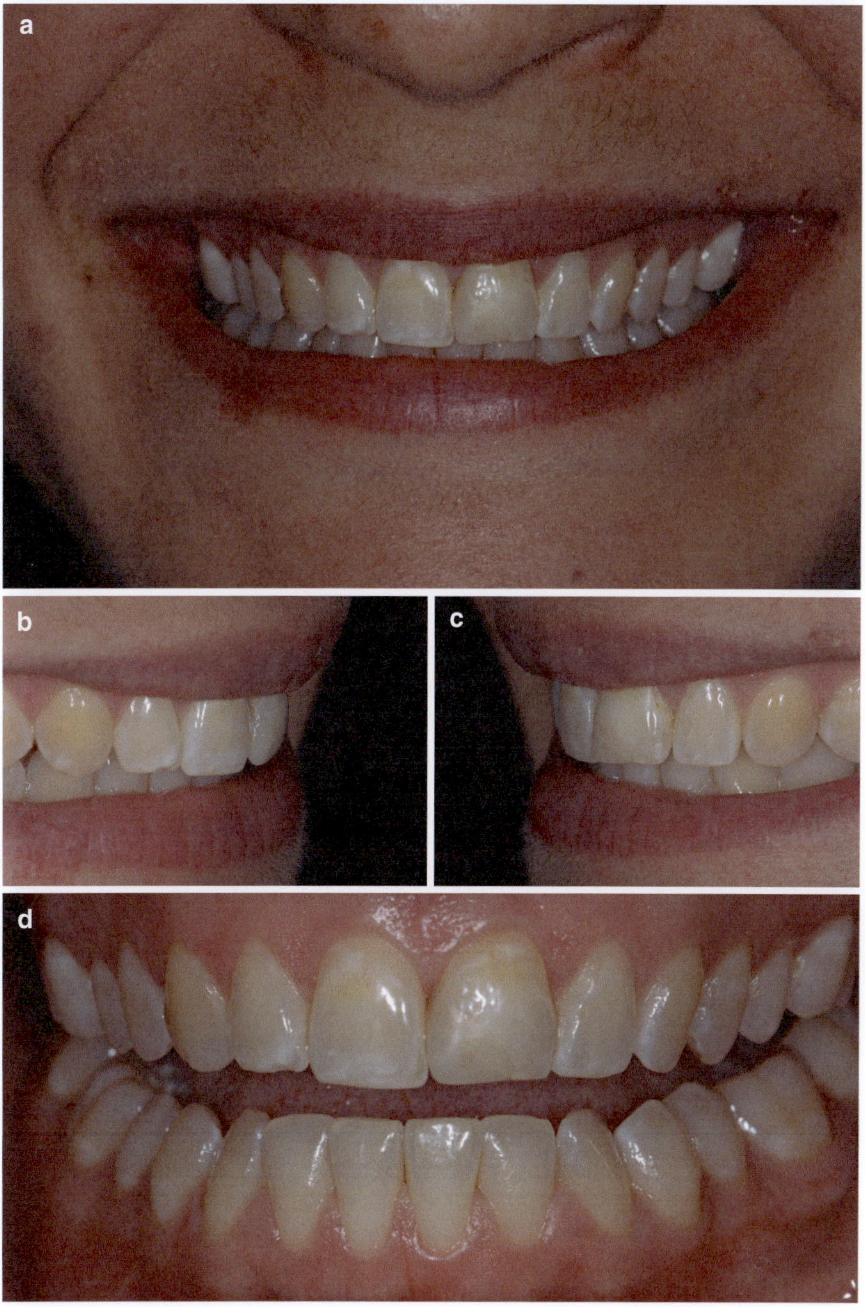

Fig. 3.21 (**a**–**d**) Baseline photographic records

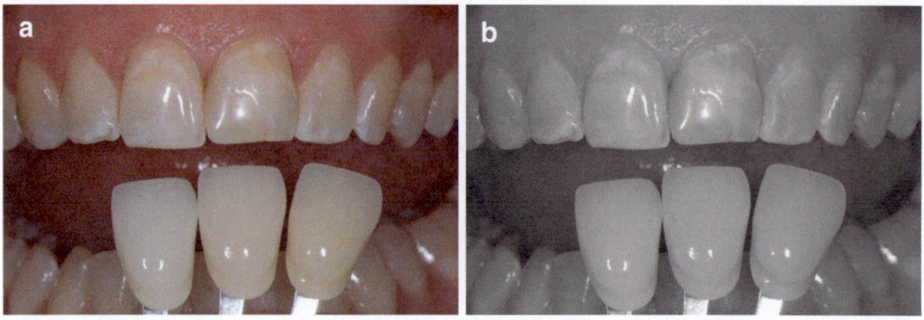

Fig. 3.22 (**a**, **b**) Colour and black and white digital photographs with reference shade tabs to aid shade and value assessment

with reference shade tabs adjacent to the teeth in question will provide an optimal data set; black and white photographs will aid assessment of the shade value (Fig. 3.22).

3.3.3 Vital Tooth Bleaching

Vital tooth bleaching treatment is an effective non-invasive method of improving tooth colour. It may be utilised as a sole course of treatment or prior to restorative treatment with adhesive restorations to improve upon the appearance of teeth that have aesthetic indications to be managed further (Figs. 3.23 and 3.24). It may be carried out in two ways: 'in-office' bleaching allows the clinician to bleach the teeth immediately in a single appointment for the patient. The soft tissues are isolated using a combination of lip retractors, cotton gauze and light polymerised resin. The teeth are cleaned, and the bleaching agent gel is applied directly to the teeth and activated using an activation blue spectrum light. The gel is replenished in 3–4 cycles of 15 min. This procedure has the advantage that the results are immediate for the patient in a short period of time (Fig. 3.25). The 'home bleaching' process allows the patient to carry out the process themselves at their discretion on instruction from the clinician and requires multiple appointments. The bleaching process may be carried out during the day or at night whilst the patient is asleep. This requires the production of a bleaching tray (bleaching agent gel carrier), which is fabricated from intra-oral impressions or digital scans (Fig. 3.26). The laboratory prescription needs to identify key areas, including the teeth planned for bleaching, the design and material of the bleach tray. Generally, bleaching trays are constructed from thermoplastic ethyl-vinyl acetate, and the general minimum thickness should be 1 mm. At the current time, there is no definitive evidence to show that the presence of bleach reservoirs (spacers) is more or less beneficial than in the absence of reservoirs. As the bleaching gels are viscous, the likelihood of material exchange between the gel approximated on the surface of the tooth and the main body of the reservoir is unlikely, as such, it may seem a waste of gel material to prescribe this. Reservoirs

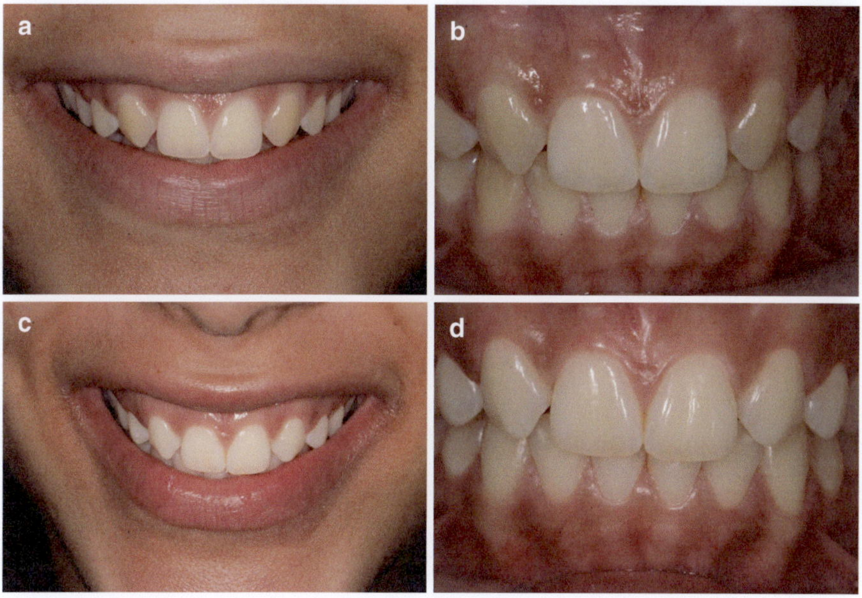

Fig. 3.23 (**a**, **b**) Vital tooth bleaching before and (**c**, **d**) after where improvements have been made to the inherent darkness of the 13 & 23. The patient can consider further restorative treatment for aesthetic improvements

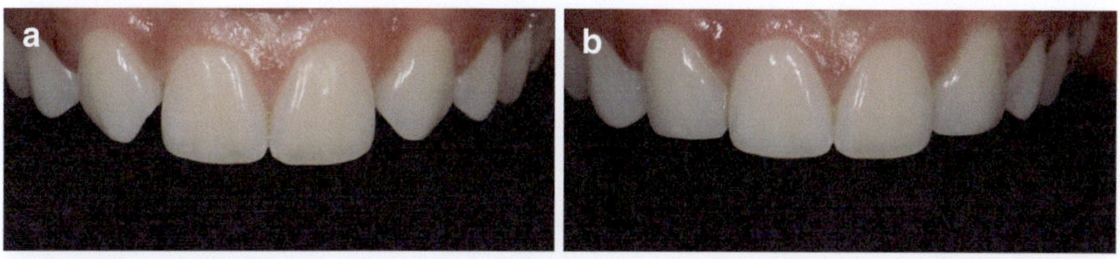

Fig. 3.24 (**a**) Teeth 13 & 23 after bleaching treatment and (**b**) subsequent restorative treatment utilising additive composite resin restorations to camouflage their shape into lateral incisor teeth

may be of greater value where patients have defined areas or islands of discolouration on individual teeth that require preferential bleach exposure to the remaining body of the tooth. Where specific teeth or areas of teeth are being bleached, windows can be cut in the tray to prevent bleach from flowing onto adjacent surfaces, so any shade changes are isolated (Figs. 3.26 and 3.27).

The cervical area of a tooth is notoriously the most difficult area to bleach successfully. If the bleach tray is short in these areas or is not approximated against the tooth, the bleach may not reach or contact the area required. In this respect, the tray should extend just over the visible gingival margin by approximately 1 mm (Figs. 3.26 and 3.27). As long as the tray is not rigid and does not blanch the tissues

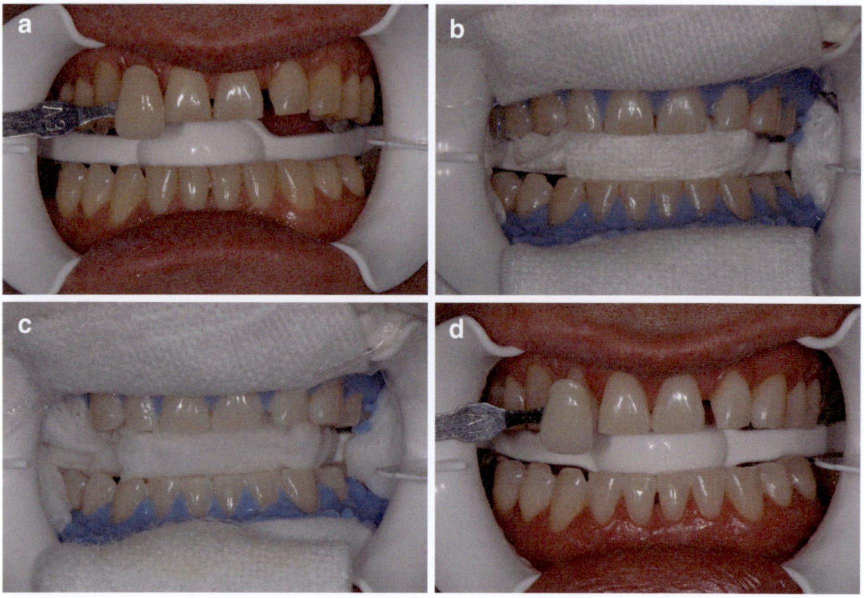

Fig. 3.25 'In-office' bleaching (**a**, **b**) before and (**c**, **d**) after shade tab comparisons, showing isolation using a combination of lip retractors, cotton gauze and light-cured resin

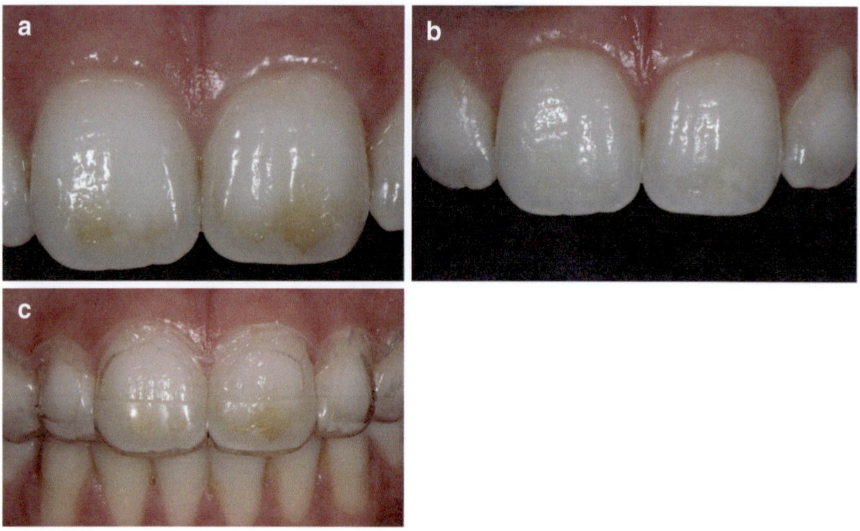

Fig. 3.26 (**a**, **b**) Vital tooth bleaching before and after where improvements have been made to the brown discolouration of teeth 11 & 21. (**c**) The bleach tray has been modified to localise the bleach to the areas of brown discolouration with windows created in the tooth 12 & 22 sites

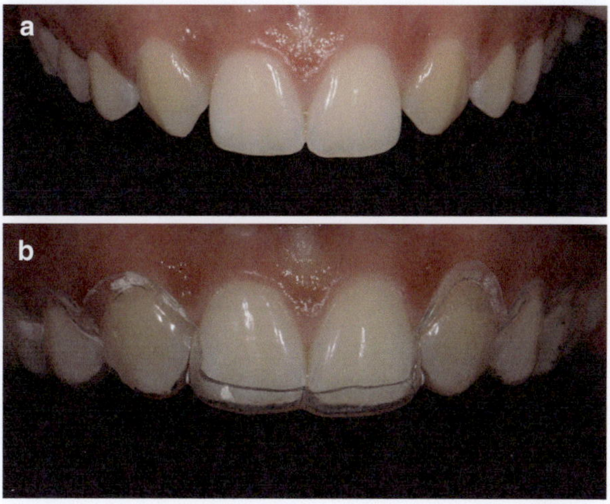

Fig. 3.27 (**a**, **b**) Bleach tray design with scalloped gingival extension and modification to aid external bleaching treatment of specific teeth

on insertion, there should be no risk of causing recession as a result. A cautious approach is required in patients presenting with established gingival recession, associated cervical dentine exposure and existing teeth sensitivity.

3.3.4 Non-vital Tooth Bleaching

Non-vital tooth bleaching treatment encompasses the exact same ethos as the home bleaching method described for vital teeth, the difference being that the internal aspect of the tooth will be treated in conjunction with the external part. It has been described as the 'inside-outside' bleaching technique as it applies a two-fold application of the bleaching agent into the root canal system in addition to the external surface of the tooth via a bleaching tray (Fig. 3.28). The required clinical stages for this treatment are depicted diagrammatically (Fig. 3.29).

Prior to considering 'inside-outside' bleach treatment, optimal root canal treatment should be completed. During endodontic instrumentation and irrigation, the tooth may lighten as a result of antibacterial disinfection treatment with sodium hypochlorite. Chemo-mechanical debridement followed by GP obturation should be concluded with a well approximated coronal restoration in the access cavity under normal circumstances, where teeth are not discoloured. Where bleaching is planned, the clinician may decide to progress to prepare the tooth to receive bleach without a period of monitoring of the endodontic outcome. This may be more of a consideration where the general restorative and endodontic prognosis of the tooth is good in the absence of a periapical lesion.

The non-vital tooth is likely to be the most discoloured unit in comparison to its vital neighbours, and as such, this tooth needs to be treated first, prior to bleaching adjacent teeth. The onus of improvement in shade needs to fall on the patient to conform to the directions, but also tempered with what is realistically achievable, as

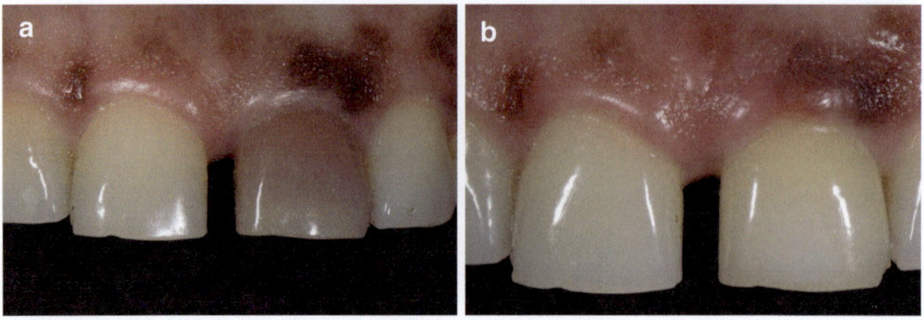

Fig. 3.28 (**a**) Non-vital tooth 21 pre-operative situation and (**b**) after 'inside-outside' bleaching

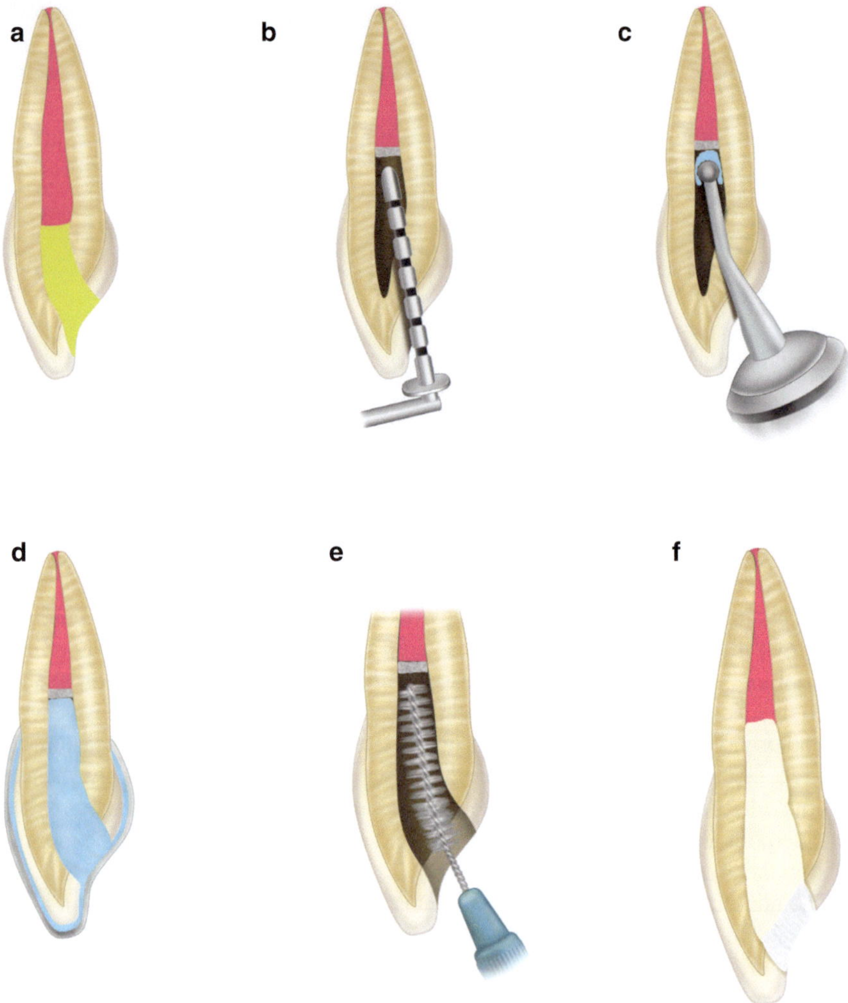

Fig. 3.29 Stages of non-vital tooth bleaching. (**a**) Access cavity. (**b**) GP sub-seal restoration placement. (**c**) Bleach application. (**d**) Fitting of bleaching tray. (**e**) Cleaning of access cavity. (**f**) Access cavity restoration with IRM, GIC and composite resin

expressed by the dentist. Once an acceptable shade has been achieved for the non-vital tooth, attention can turn to the adjacent vital teeth. These can be bleached in isolation from the non-vital tooth until a similar shade is reached. Once attained, a delayed period of no bleach treatment is required after which the shade can be reassessed, and the reapplication of bleach can be considered if necessary (Figs. 3.30 and 3.31).

From an intra-coronal aspect to achieve optimal shade improvement, the access cavity and dentinal tubules should be made free of any restorative or resin material (Fig. 3.32). Bonding resin within the tubules is highly likely to reduce the efficacy

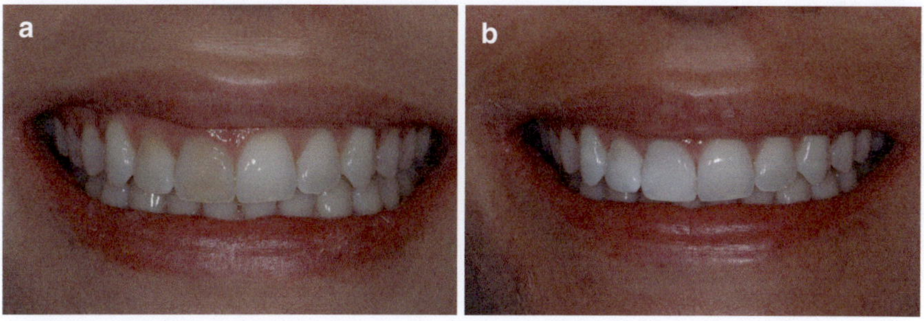

Fig. 3.30 (**a**) Non-vital teeth 12 & 11 before and (**b**) after 'inside-outside' bleaching of in combination with bleaching adjacent vital teeth

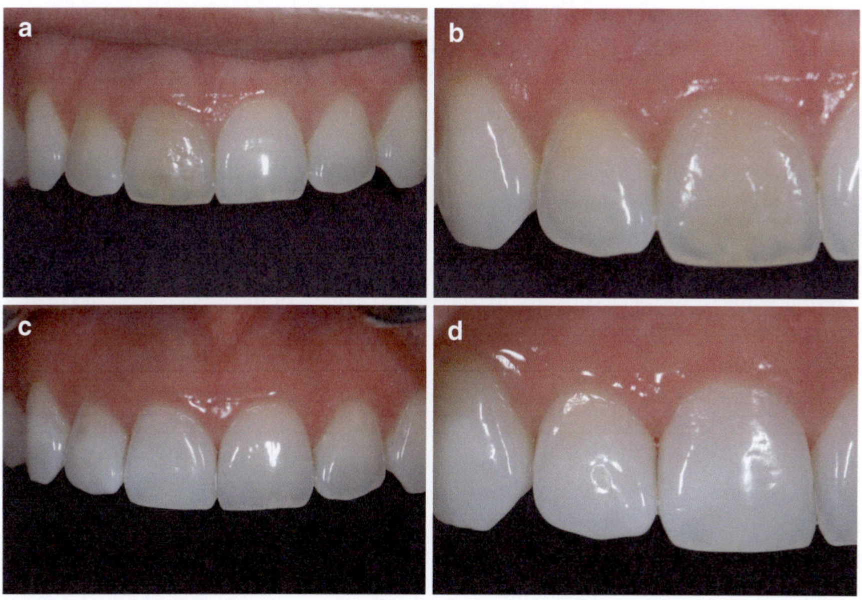

Fig. 3.31 (**a**, **b**) Non-vital teeth 12 & 11 before and (**c**, **d**) after 'inside-outside' bleaching in combination with bleaching adjacent vital teeth

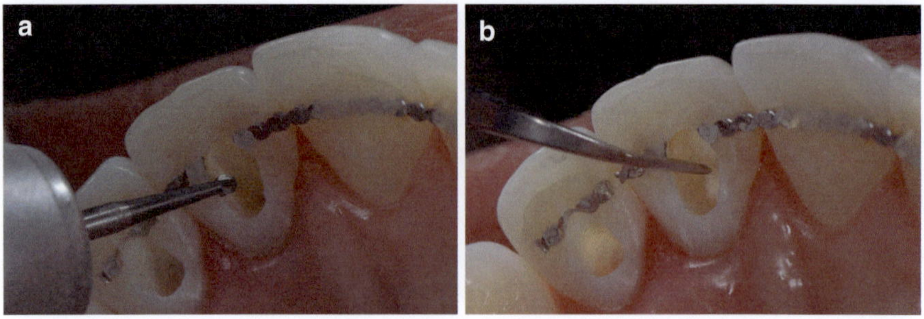

Fig. 3.32 Preparation of access cavities on teeth 12 & 11 through orthodontic retainer with (**a**) tungsten carbide bur and (**b**) ultrasonic scaler to remove existing restorative materials, endodontic debris or pulpal remnants

of bleaching, and the patient should be notified of this prior to the beginning of treatment. The root filling material Gutta Percha (GP) is removed below the visible gingival margin or cemento–enamel junction (CEJ) (Fig. 3.33), and a root canal sub-seal restoration to cover the GP is placed level or just below the visible gingival margin or CEJ. Zinc oxide-based intermediate restorative material (IRM), resin-modified glass-ionomer cement (RMGIC) or glass-ionomer cement (GIC) materials are frequently used (Fig. 3.34).

The patient with instruction and direction self-administers the bleach utilising the bleach syringe to fill the access cavity whilst also filling a bleaching tray that is localised to apply bleach to the tooth's external surface. The syringe tip utilised to apply the bleach can be modified by a scalpel blade to bevel the lumen to aid direction of dispensation of the bleach agent gel (Fig. 3.35) or changed to a malleable metal tip or a curved plastic tip that can be angulated at the patient's discretion for convenience (Figs. 3.36 and 3.37).

Patients are also instructed in the use of single tufted brushes or interproximal brushes to use within the access cavity to prevent food impaction (Figs. 3.37 and 3.38). This provides the patient with the onus to apply and reapply the bleach for the non-vital tooth until they are pleased with the aesthetic outcome. One technique to maximise aesthetic outcome would be to design the bleaching tray to engage the internal walls of the access cavity to maximise contact of the bleach with the discoloured internal walls of the pulp chamber.

One clinical concern with this technique is the presence of the open access cavity, which renders the tooth weaker and allows the possibility of reinfection of the root canal system. The presence of a root canal sub-seal restoration, patient-administered cleaning of the cavity, bleaching agent gel being antibacterial and the relatively short exposure time should collectively mean the chance of reinfection is reduced or nullified. Once bleaching treatment is completed, the provision of the coronal restoration to seal the access cavity should follow. The choice of materials needs to be catered for the roles that are required. IRM is white and opaque, as well as being antibacterial. The opacity will prevent light transmission through the tooth, which may result in a darker crown. Due to its white appearance, it is readily

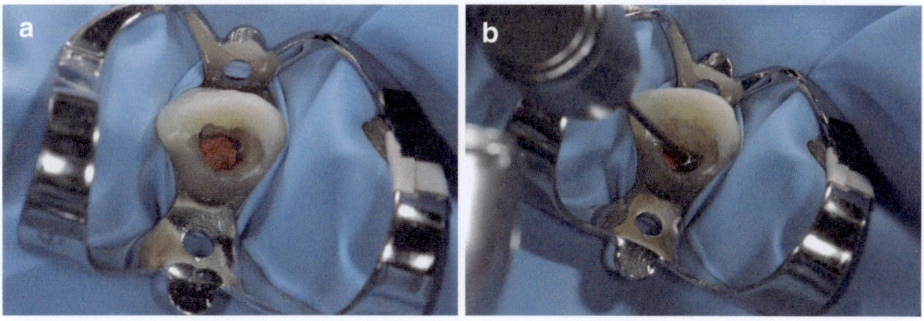

Fig. 3.33 (**a**, **b**) Goose-neck burs of an appropriate size are ideal for removing gutta-percha from the obturated root canal system

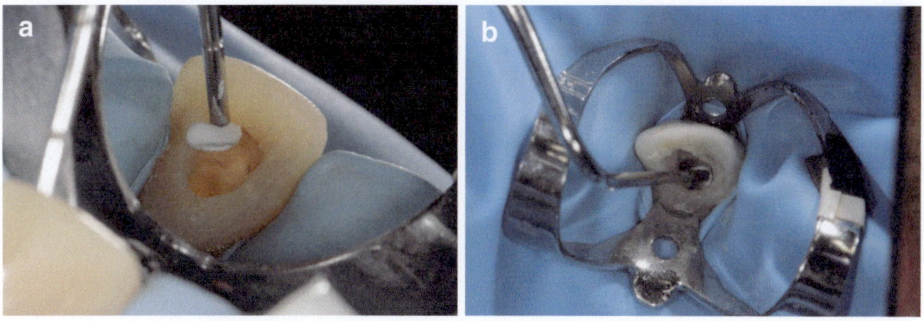

Fig. 3.34 (**a**, **b**) Subsequent placement of IRM sub-seal restoration with an endodontic plugger

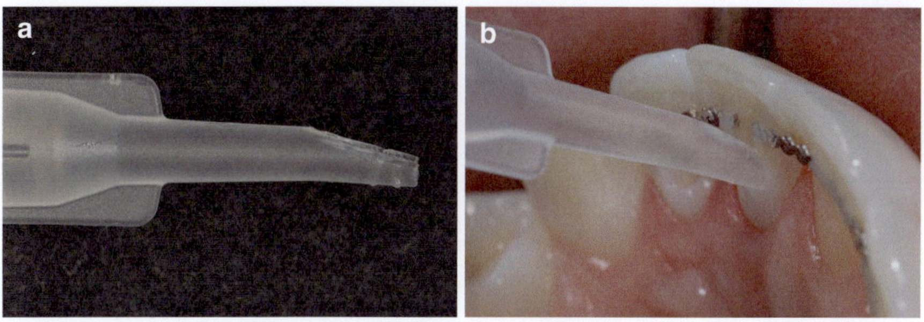

Fig. 3.35 (**a**, **b**) Obliquely trimmed bleach syringe tip utilised to apply the bleach agent gel into the access cavity

identified from the surrounding enamel and dentine, making re-access without iatrogenic damage to the surrounding tooth tissue easier. The root canal and pulp chamber should be filled with this material, leaving approximately 2 mm of space at the entrance of the access cavity. The clinician must be aware that Eugenol may inhibit the polymerisation of resin materials due to its ability to scavenge free radicals. In particular, it may affect self-etch bonding systems and composite resin

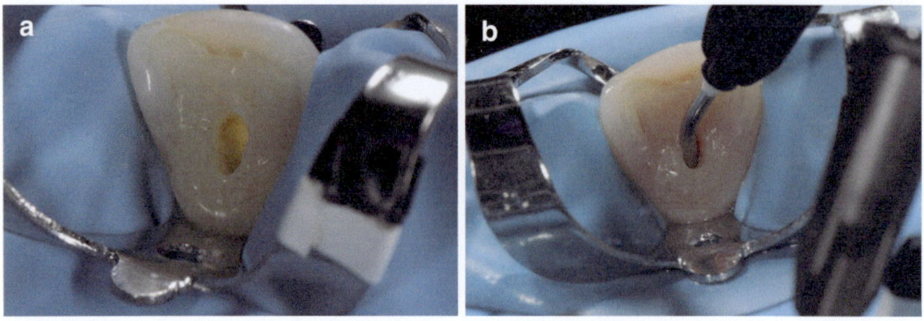

Fig. 3.36 (**a**, **b**) Curved metal bleach syringe tip utilised as an alternative method to aid application of bleach into a small access cavity

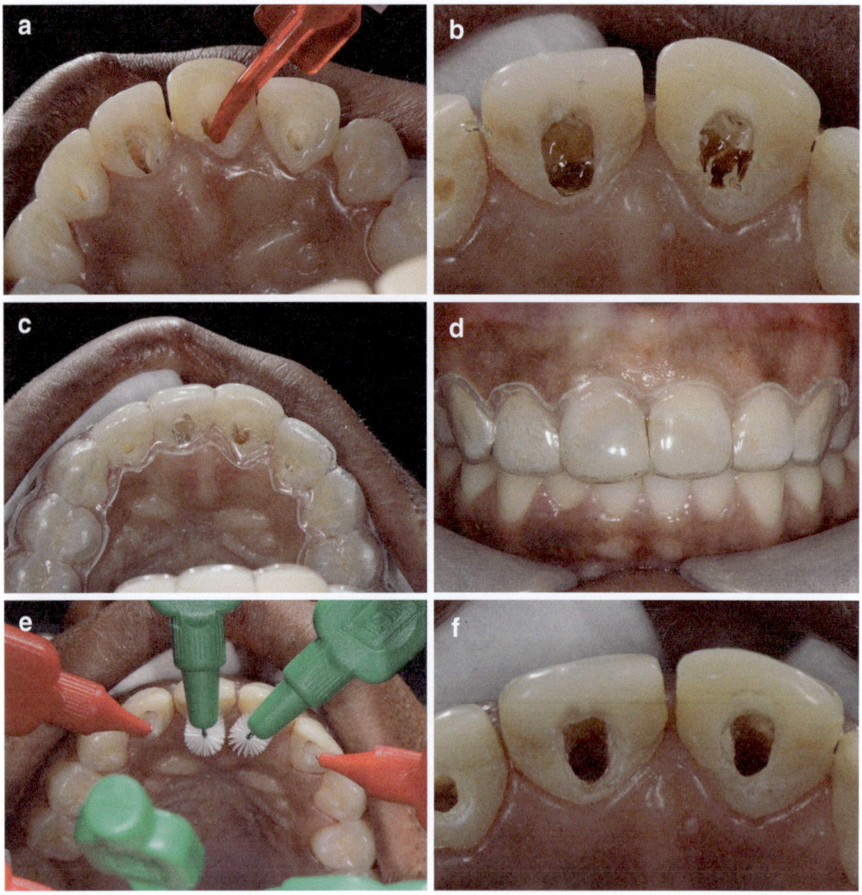

Fig. 3.37 'Inside-outside' bleach treatment of teeth 12, 11, 21 & 22. (**a**, **b**) Curved plastic syringe tip utilised to navigate bleach into the access cavities. (**c**, **d**) Bleaching gel application into the bleaching tray and located over teeth. (**e**, **f**) Interproximal Tepe brush sizes are chosen to aid self-administered cleansing of the access cavities

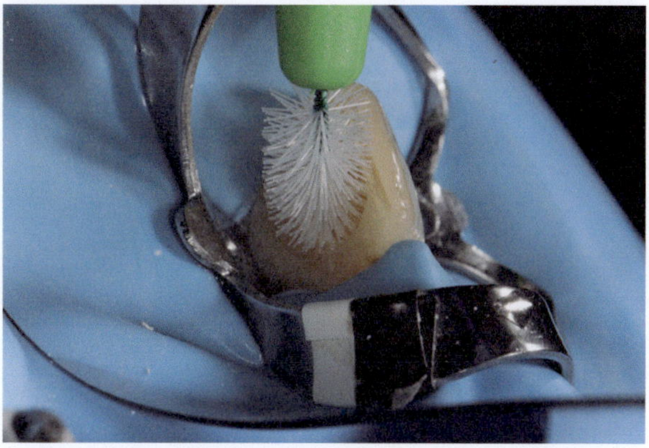

Fig. 3.38 Interproximal brush being assessed for size prior to patient-administered inside-outside bleaching. The aim is to choose a size that fits snugly to the bottom of the cavity and engages the walls to ensure the removal of any debris and residual bleach

materials, therefore, a 1 mm GIC layer must be placed as an intermediate layer to prevent the IRM contacting areas to receive adhesive treatment with resin materials to seal the access cavity. The final 1 mm of space should be restored with composite resin due to its superior aesthetic properties and ability to provide a predictable bond to the enamel (Fig. 3.39).

The coronal restoration in this cohort has a twofold significance. An optimal coronal seal will prevent the regress of bacterial infection into the root canal system to jeopardise apical health. An optimal seal will also prevent leakage of chromogenic materials or bacteria that could cause shade rebound of the initial bleaching outcome. This therefore requires a balance between a restoration that will seal, maintain colour and be easily removed and reapplied depending on the needs of the patient. Unfortunately, composite resin does have some drawbacks and is likely to jeopardise and complicate any further treatment the tooth requires in the future. Etching and bonding procedures will infiltrate the dentinal tubules and seal them. Any future need to revise bleaching will be made almost impossible without the complete removal of these. Polymerised composite resin will be very difficult to delineate from root dentine and will result in a higher chance of removal of tooth tissue if access is attempted in the future. This is likely to be the case even if microscope magnification is utilised. There may be a possibility of perforation, or the tooth may be rendered too weak for successful restoration in the long term. These issues can be mitigated by utilising the trio combination of IRM, GIC and composite resin.

The management of a single isolated discoloured previously crowned tooth is a challenge where a translucent glass-ceramic crown material is to be considered. A provisional crown can be used as an alternative bleach agent gel carrier for the bleaching treatment.

Once the existing crown restoration has been removed and the tooth has been definitively prepared, revealing the discoloured tooth tissue, the clinician should make a provisional crown restoration, ensuring adequate marginal fit and coronal stability. The provisional crown can then be loaded with the bleaching agent gel and utilised to deliver it to the abutment tooth preparation. The patient is instructed in

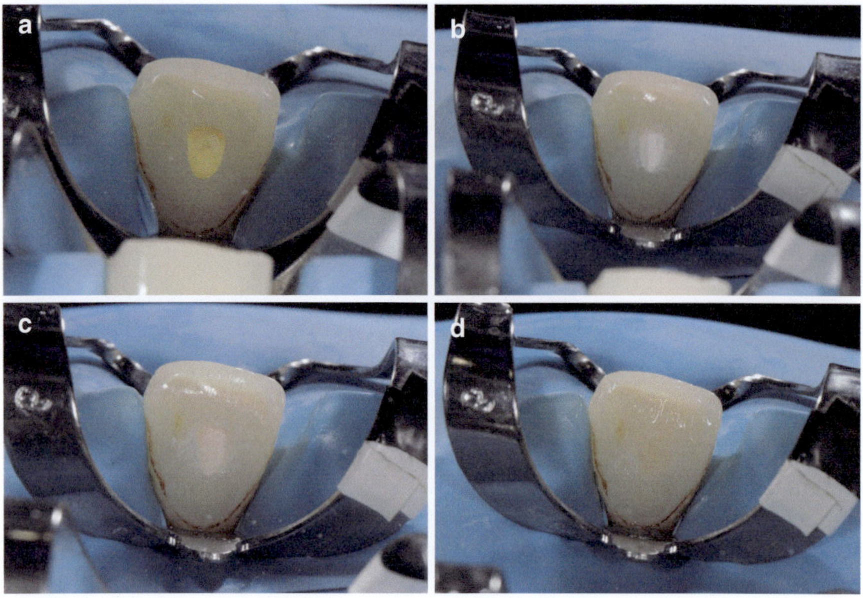

Fig. 3.39 (**a**) Access cavity (**b**) zinc-oxide eugenol IRM base placed over sub-seal restoration, leaving adequate space for (**c**) GIC restoration and (**d**) the superficial capping composite resin restoration

how to load the provisional crown with the gel and locate it over the abutment tooth. Once located, the excess gel expressed can be removed. The patient, much in the same way as they would administer bleach tray-based bleaching, removes the crown, cleans the remnant bleach gel from the provisional crown and tooth and repeats the process. Once a satisfactory base shade of abutment tooth is achieved, the provisional restoration can be cemented in preparation for subsequent review and provision of the definitive coronal restoration (Fig. 3.40).

3.3.5 Treatment Management

The patient should be encouraged to take a lead on how they manage their bleaching treatment. Self-assessment of progression provides the patient with the impetus to either continue or to cease treatment, depending on improvements in colour, but also the development of any tooth sensitivity. Once the bleaching treatment has stopped, the patient should be made aware that there will be some rebound or relapse in colour approximately 2 weeks after. This may be due to residual free radicals remaining, affecting the optical properties of the tooth, and the patient should be reassured that the tooth shade is merely stabilising during this period.

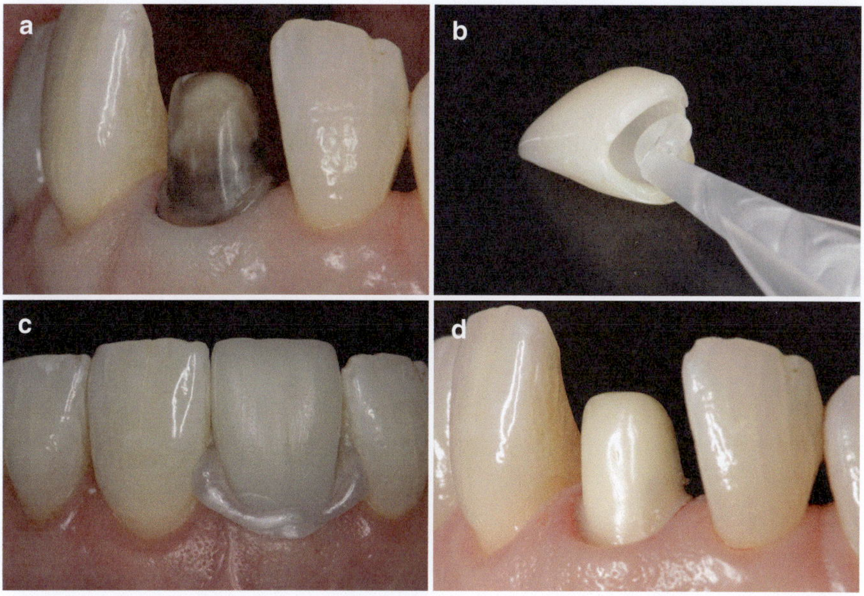

Fig. 3.40 (**a**) Discoloured abutment tooth 11. (**b**) Provisional crown bleaching treatment where the provisional crown is loaded with the bleaching agent gel and (**c**) delivered to the abutment tooth preparation until (**d**) a satisfactory base shade of abutment tooth is achieved

3.3.6 Treatment Complications

Vital tooth bleaching can present with local adverse effects such as tooth sensitivity and gingival/mucosal irritation. Utilising hydrogen peroxide as the bleaching agent over carbamide peroxide results in a faster process but also likely to result in a greater risk of adverse effects to the patient.

A complication issue more specific to non-vital tooth bleaching is the development of external cervical root resorption (ECRR). This condition can be very difficult to treat and in some cases, can render the tooth unrestorable. The presence of hydrogen peroxide within the tooth and diffusing towards the root surface via dentinal tubules has been identified as a possible mechanism causing the inflammatory resorptive process. The more patent the dentinal tubules, the increased amount of diffusion. If the tooth has been previously traumatised, cementum may be absent in the cervical region, especially where a luxation or avulsion injury has occurred, making the tubule patent through and through. An association may exist with patients with immature teeth, and so wider tubules and less than fully developed root walls provide a portal for hydrogen peroxide movement.

There is limited evidence in the dental literature illustrating a significant clinical effect of bleaching on the enamel tissue. Some studies illustrate loss of the aprismatic layer of enamel whilst others have shown decrease in surface hardness, the actual clinical relevance of these changes has not been entirely quantified.

There is some evidence to show that bleaching can reduce the adhesive bond strength of composite resin to previously bleached enamel, and by up to 60% if the bonding procedure is carried out immediately after tooth bleaching treatment. This has been attributed to either the change in enamel structure and organic composition, which weakens the adhesive interface, or possibly to the release of oxygen- and hydroxyl-free radicals that occur by the breakdown of hydrogen peroxide. The interprismatic residual oxygen can result in a reduction of infiltration and polymerisation of the resin. The reduction in bond strength has been shown to be transient and returns to normal after approximately 4 weeks. It is recommended that composite resin restorations (replacement or new) should be delayed for at least 2–4 weeks after the bleaching treatment to allow for optimal adhesive bonding strength (Fig. 3.41).

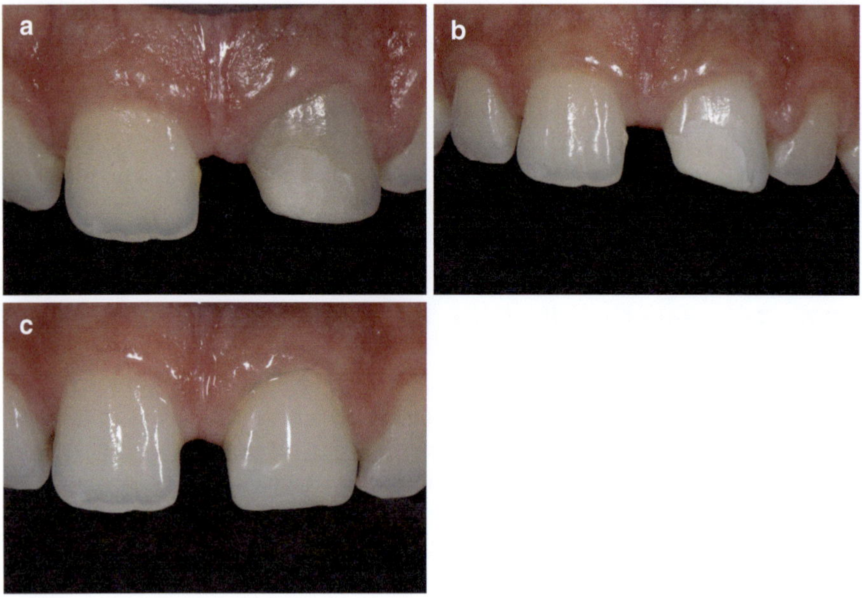

Fig. 3.41 (**a**) Tooth 21 with existing composite resin restoration. (**b**) 'Inside-outside' bleaching treatment completed. (**c**) Provision of definitive Class IV composite resin restoration 4 weeks after completion of the bleaching treatment

3.4 Adhesive Technique

3.4.1 Non-vital Bleaching Sub-seal Restoration

The sub-seal restoration overlying the exposed GP will provide a barrier against reinfection during the bleaching process. Materials that can be used for this are IRM, RMGIC or GIC.

A case highlighting the clinical stages required is shown (Figs. 3.42, 3.43, 3.44, 3.45, 3.46 and 3.47) and the clinical stages and tips are listed in Table 3.1.

3.4.2 Icon® Treatment

The treatment of white spot lesions can be successfully managed by employing conservative methods without the requirement for gross macro removal of the enamel structure. Acid etching of the white spot lesion followed by resin infiltration will stop lesion progression, also reducing light scattering by changing the refractive index and therefore camouflaging the white spot appearing on the enamel surface. This may be carried out in conjunction with the aforementioned bleaching techniques where appropriate. A case highlighting the clinical stages is shown (Figs. 3.48, 3.49, 3.50, 3.51 and 3.52), and the clinical stages are listed in Table 3.2.

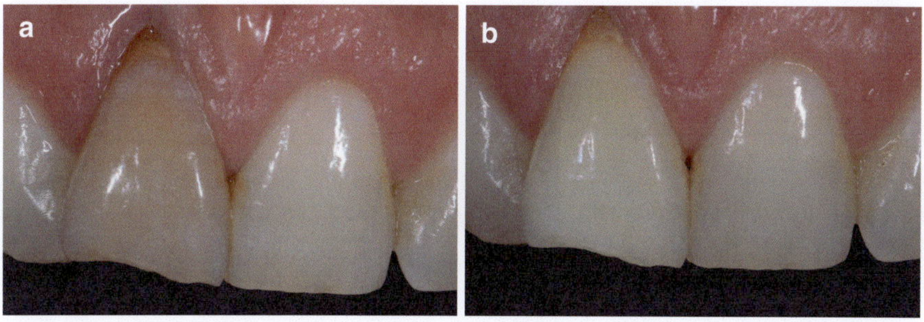

Fig. 3.42 Tooth 11 (**a**) before and (**b**) after "inside-outside' bleaching technique. The patient can now consider restoration of the incisal edge with direct composite resin, orthodontic treatment to improve the tooth positional and gingival grafting to correct the recession soft tissue defect

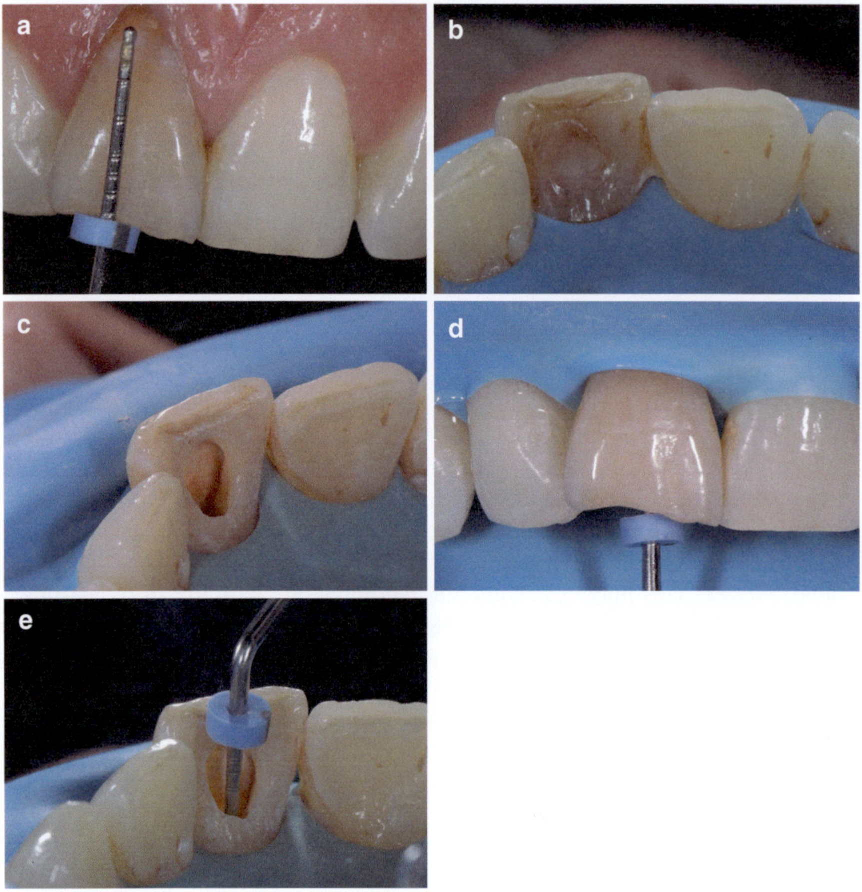

Fig. 3.43 (**a**) Tooth 11 measuring facial crown height from incisal edge reference point to the CEJ. (**b**, **c**) Isolation, access cavity depth and (**d**, **e**) gutta–percha removal comparison to base line CEJ measurement

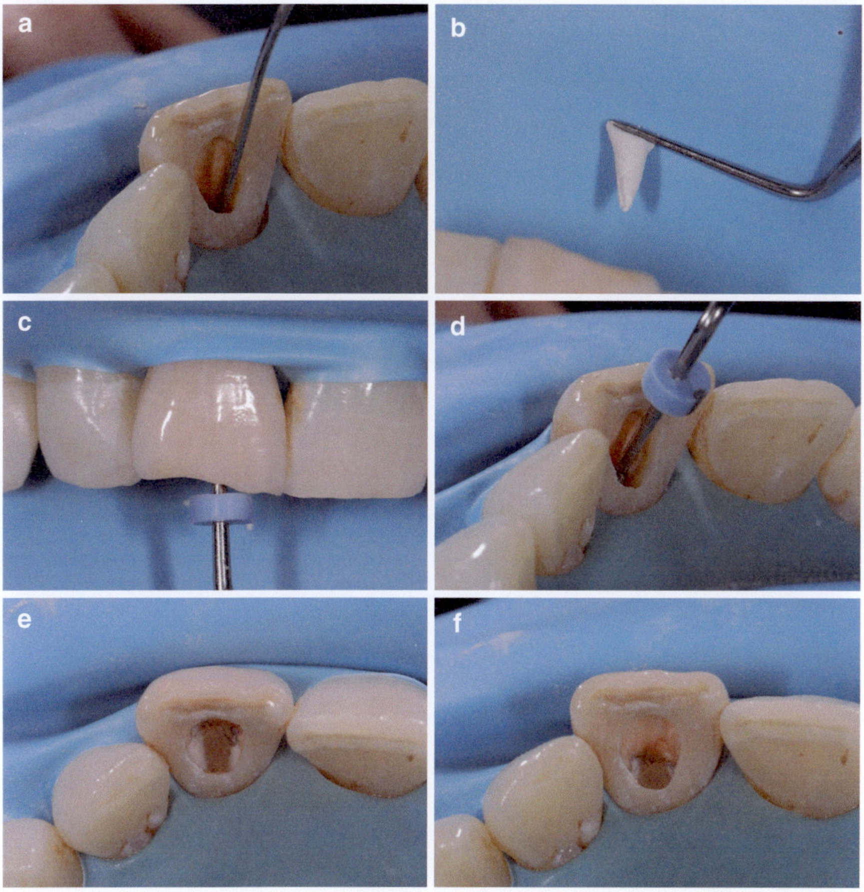

Fig. 3.44 (**a**) Cavity disinfection with sodium hypochlorite and (**b**, **c**, **d**, **e**) placement and packing of IRM sub-seal restoration over exposed gutta–percha, (**f**) ensuring clean cavity walls

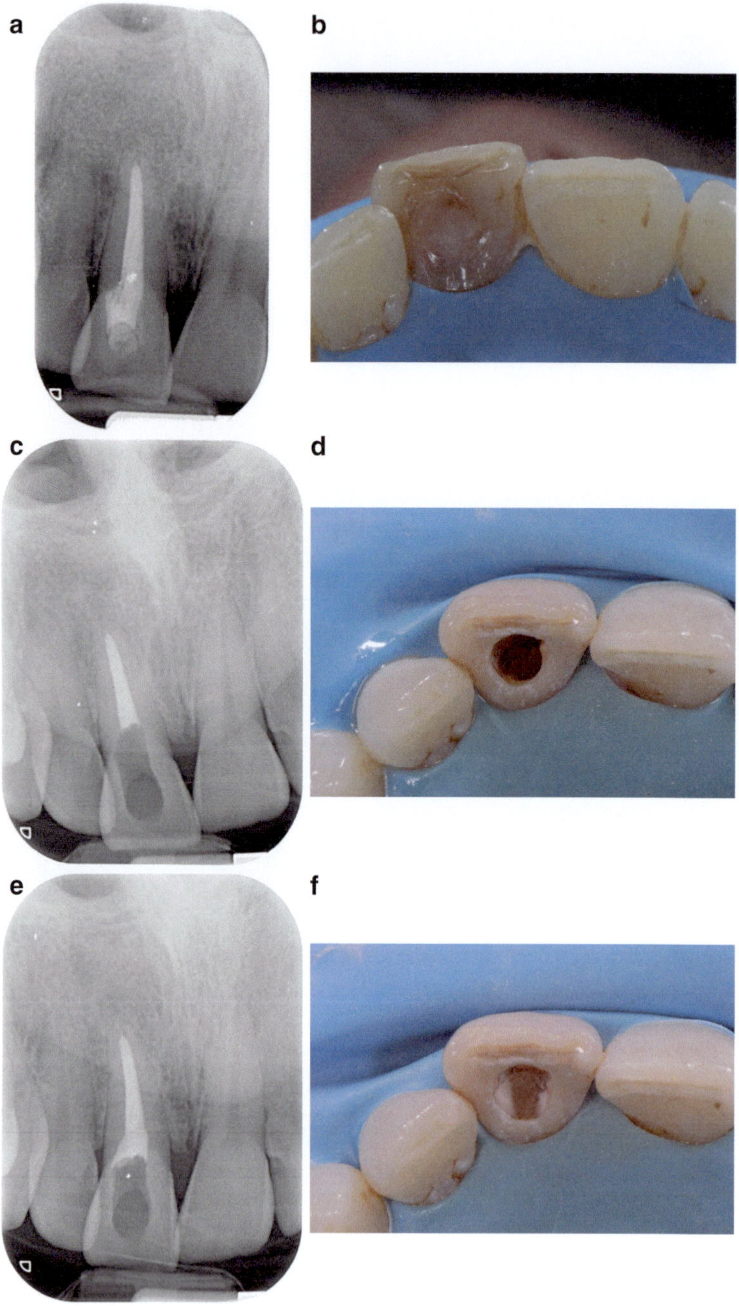

Fig. 3.45 Check radiographs of (**a**, **b**) pre-operative restoration, (**c, d**) gutta–percha removal and (**e**, **f**) IRM sub-seal restoration placement

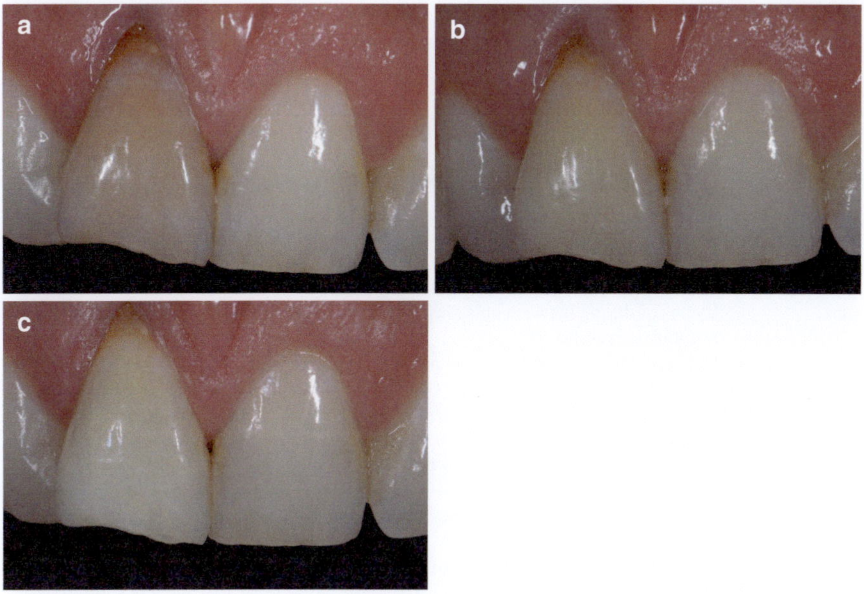

Fig. 3.46 (**a, b, c**) Tooth 11 showing the bleaching effect of gradual lightening of the tooth shade

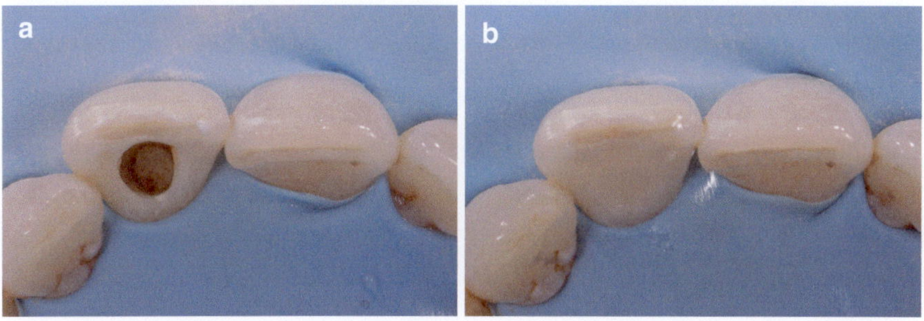

Fig. 3.47 (**a**) Access cavity. (**b**) Restoration with GIC and composite resin once desired tooth shade has been reached

Table 3.1 The clinical stages and tips for sub-seal restorations for non-vital bleaching

Sub-seal restoration for non-vital bleaching	
Stages	Tips
1. Measure crown height	A periodontal probe with a rubber reference stop is placed on the buccal surface
	The crown height is measured from an incisal edge reference point to the visible gingival margin or CEJ
2. Rubber dam isolation	Isolating adjacent teeth can aid angulation of the bur to the tooth's long axis
3. Access cavity and GP removal	Existing restorative material should be carefully removed with diamond or tungsten carbide burs. Ultrasonic scaler tips and sandblasting in deep areas can reduce the amount of extra dental tissue loss and decrease the risk of perforation
	Cycles of drying between episodes of instrumentation will aid identification of restorative material
	Ensure complete exposure of the pulp horns to ensure efficiency of the bleaching
	Safe GP removal utilising Gates–Glidden or Goose neck burs, or with heated tip instruments approximately 1+ mm below the visible gingival margin or CEJ
	Magnification should be utilised to examine the access cavity walls. GP remnants or sealer should be removed to ensure the best contact possible with the bleach and the residual dentine
4. Measure access cavity depth	A periodontal probe with a rubber reference stop is placed into the palatal access cavity
	The extent of GP removal is measured from the incisal edge reference point into the base of the access cavity and compared to the baseline measurement (+1 mm)
5. Radiograph	Checks to ensure maintenance of an axial position in access cavity preparation, restoration removal and depth of GP material removal
6. Cavity disinfection	Disinfection of the exposed GP material and cavity with sodium hypochlorite
	Dry cavity before application of sub-seal restoration
7. Sub-seal restoration	Application of 1 mm thickness of IRM, RMGIC or GIC to the level or just below the visible gingival margin. A thick mix of the material and pre-measuring a plugging instrument (to same length as coronal length of tooth) simplifies this stage
	If RMGIC or GIC is used, the cavity area to be filled should be conditioned first with polyacrylic acid and rinsed
	Magnification utilised to examine the access cavity walls. IRM, RMGIC or GIC remnants should be removed to ensure the best contact possible with the bleach and the residual dentine
8. Radiograph	Checks to ensure adaptation of sub-seal restoration and confirm sealing of GP material

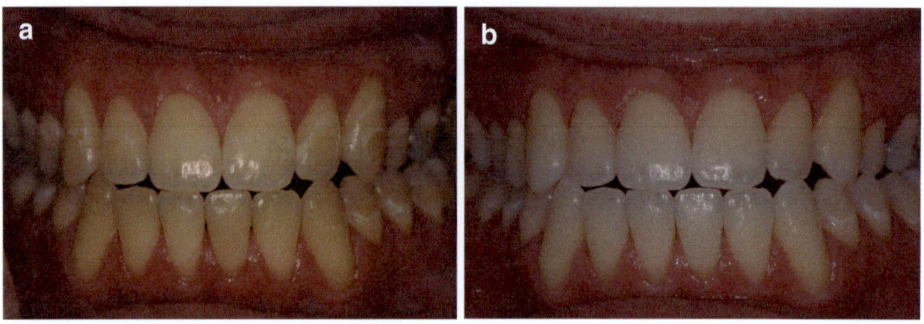

Fig. 3.48 (**a**) Pre-operative situation. (**b**) After vital tooth bleaching, Icon® treatment and provision of direct composite resin restorations

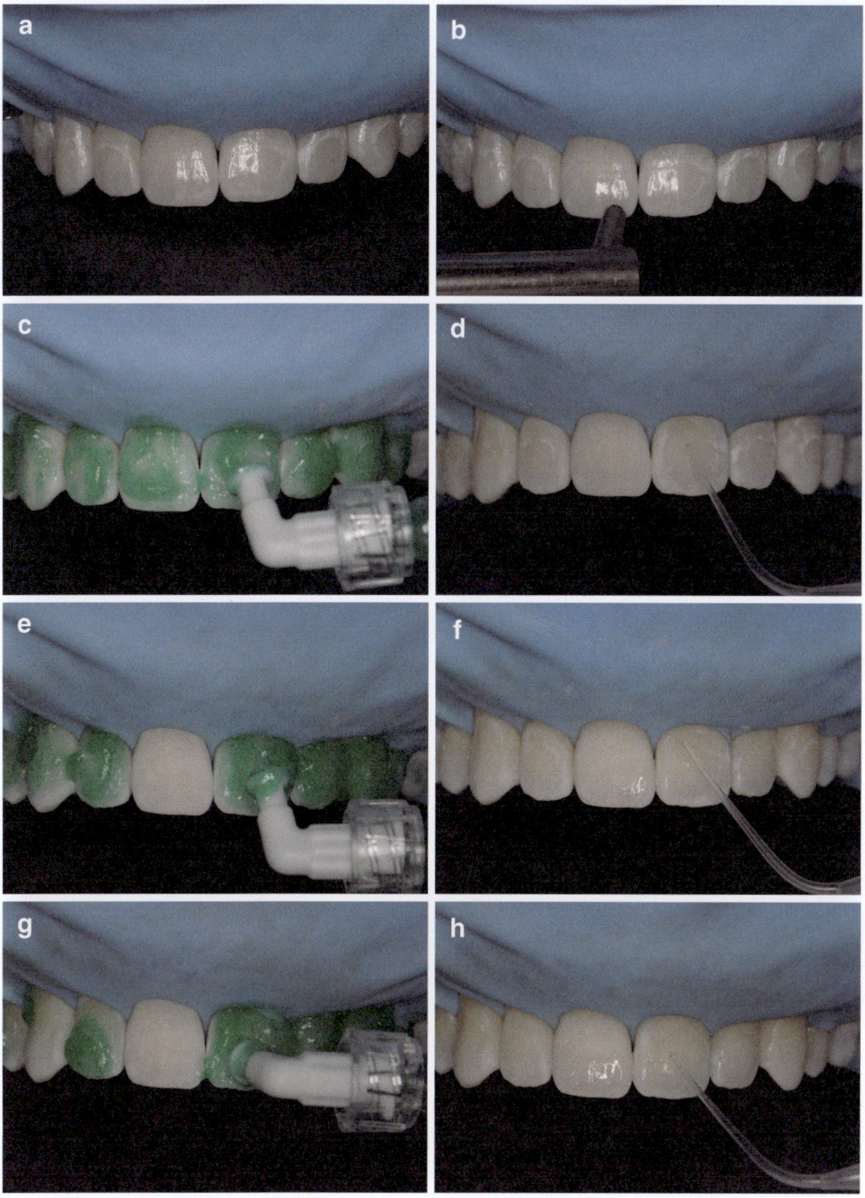

Fig. 3.49 Icon® treatment stages. (**a**) Teeth isolation. (**b**) Surface preparation with sandblasting. (**c–h**) 3 cycles of Hydrochloric acid abrasion with reduced amounts of acid application for each cycle, and drying teeth with Ethanol to preview results achieved

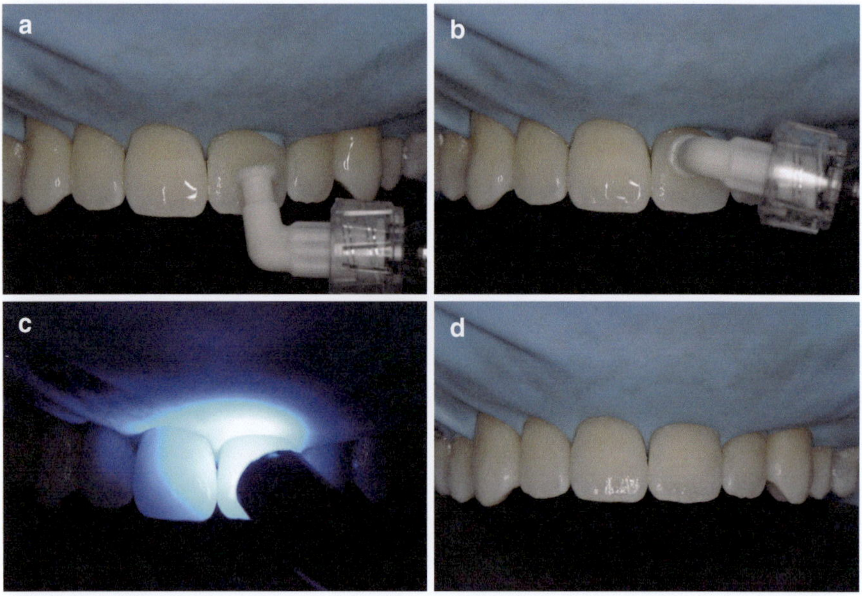

Fig. 3.50 Icon® treatment stages. (**a**, **b**) two cycles of resin infiltration. (**c**) Light polymerisation. (**d**) Completion of treatment

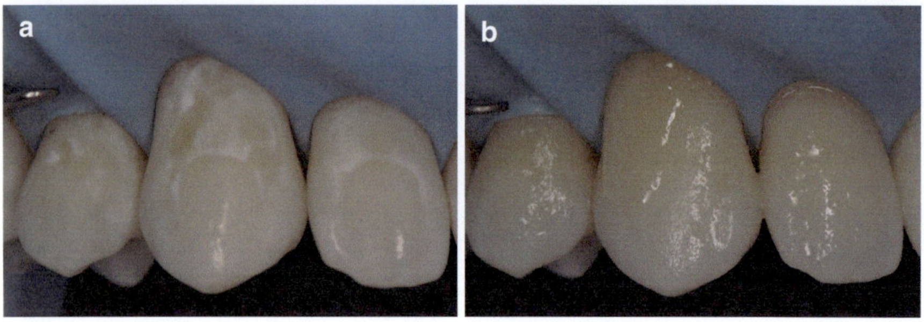

Fig. 3.51 (**a**) Tooth 13 before and (**b**) after Icon® treatment with provision of direct composite resin restoration to the facial surface

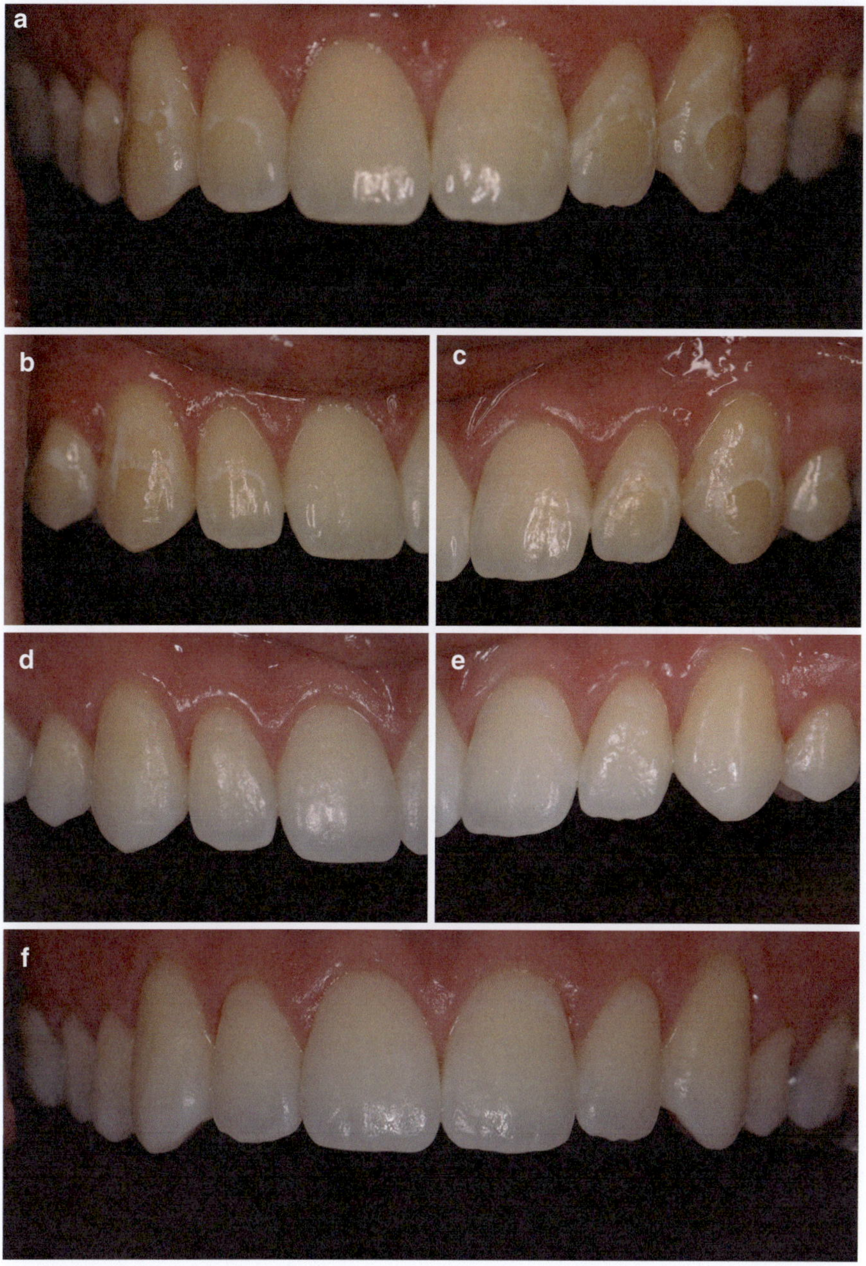

Fig. 3.52 (**a**, **b**, **c**) Pre-operative situation. (**d**, **e**, **f**) After vital tooth bleaching, Icon® treatment and provision of direct composite resin restorations for teeth 13 & 2

Table 3.2 The clinical stages required for Icon® treatment

Icon® treatment
1. Isolation
2. Prophylaxis/Sandblasting/Abrasive disc
3. Hydrochloric acid (icon-etch) scrub for 2 min
4. Rinse with water for 30 s & dry
5. Ethanol (icon-dry) application for 30 s & preview colour change
6. Repeat icon-etch and icon-dry cycles as required
7. Resin infiltration (icon-infiltrant) application for 3 min
8. Remove excess resin and light polymerise for 40 s
9. Repeat resin infiltration (with new applicator tip) for 1 min
10. Remove excess resin and light polymerise for 40 s
11. Polish

Further Reading

1. Dahl JE, Pallesen U. Tooth bleaching - a critical review of the biological aspects. Crit Rev Oral Biol Med. 2003;14(4):292–304.
2. Kunt GE, Yilmaz N, Sen S, Dede DO. Effect of antioxidant treatment on the shear bond strength of composite resin to bleached enamel. Acta Odontol Scand. 2011;69:287–91.
3. Lai SC, Tay FR, Cheung GS, Mak YF, Carvalho RM, Wei SH, Toledano M, Osorio R, Pashley DH. Reversal of compromised bonding in bleached enamel. J Dent Res. 2002;81:477–81.
4. Lee JH, Kim DG, Park CJ, Cho LR. Minimally invasive treatment enhancement of white spot lesions in adjacent tooth. J Adv Prosthodont. 2013;5(3):359–63.
5. Plotino G, Buono L, Grande NM, Pameijer CH, Somma F. Nonvital tooth bleaching: a review of the literature and clinical procedure. J Endodont. 2008;34(4):394–407.
6. Settembrini L, Gultz J, Kaim J, Scherer W. A technique for bleaching non vital teeth: inside/outside bleaching. J Am Dent Assoc. 1997;128:1283–4.

Modifying Tooth Form

4

Contents

Learning Outcomes

- To appreciate aesthetic symmetry, tooth proportion ratio, and the absence of spacing in the aesthetic zone.
- To recognise how clinical presenting factors such as tooth size, shape, angulation and position affect the ability to successfully modify tooth form.
- To realise that a large aspect of tooth modification is to manipulate light reflection.
- Explore the methods used for restoration, aesthetic and functional try-in.

4.1 Introduction

Facial aesthetics, gingival architecture, tooth form and occlusion all combine to provide orofacial harmony. Teeth have functional and aesthetic features that should also be replicated in the restorations that we provide. The contours of any tooth

A. Alani, M. Patel, *Adhesive Techniques in Restorative Dentistry*, BDJ Clinician's Guides, https://doi.org/10.1007/978-3-032-07346-4_4

presenting to the clinician may be restored with individuality, with no strict generic recipe to be followed. This is what makes a smile individual. However, symmetry of tooth and restoration form may override the importance of colour and will enhance the overall presentation in the area of aesthetic interest (Figs. 4.1, 4.2, and 4.3).

In the aesthetic zone, teeth may be healthy but their size, distribution and positioning within the arch may create aesthetic asymmetry. Spacing or multiple diastemas between otherwise intact healthy incisor teeth are commonly considered by patients as being unsightly or unattractive, as the presence of space results in aesthetic disruption in a row of maxillary incisors (Fig. 4.4). The aetiology of the spacing is multifactorial, largely stemming from discrepancies between tooth size and shape in combination with dental arch width (Fig. 4.5). In contrast, patients may find a midline diastema desirable where there is consistent symmetry between both left- and right-hand sides. A solitary diastema remote from the midline may be less desirable as the arch will become inherently asymmetric.

Routinely spacing may not present in isolation; there may be occlusal issues and other considerations that need to be managed within the treatment plan to remedy the problem. Soft tissue factors such as thick and low frenal attachments may also require assessment and consideration. Absent teeth (genetic or acquired),

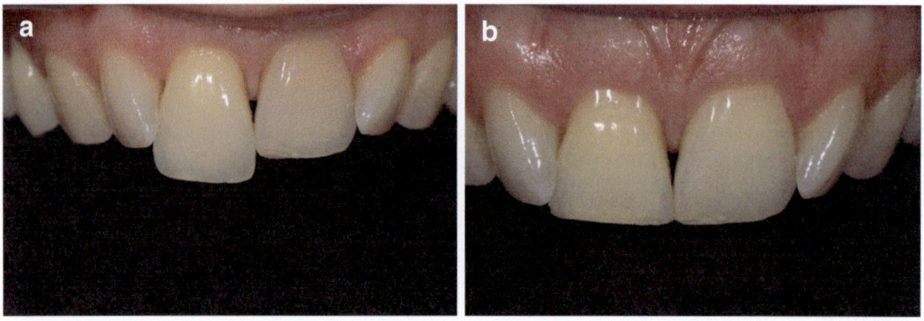

Fig. 4.1 (**a**) Tooth 11 with increased crown length showing asymmetry in the aesthetic zone. (**b**) Incisal length subtractive adjustment allows improved aesthetic harmony with adjacent teeth. Further disto-incisal embrasure adjustment can be made for aesthetic improvement

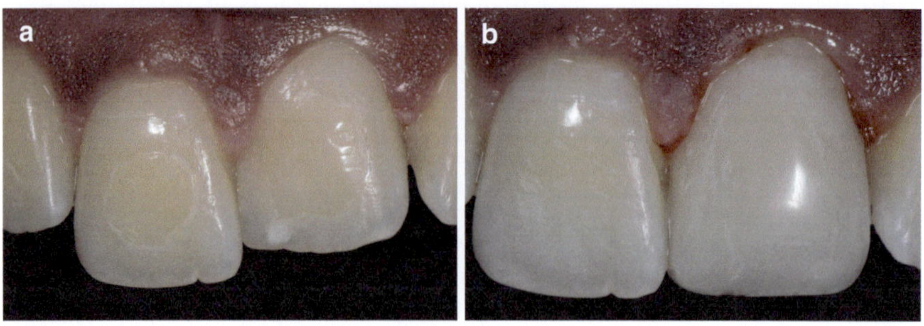

Fig. 4.2 (**a**) Tooth 21 is severely intruded and ankylosed due to trauma. (**b**) Provision of a direct additive composite resin veneer improving the incisal edge profile and aesthetic harmony with adjacent teeth

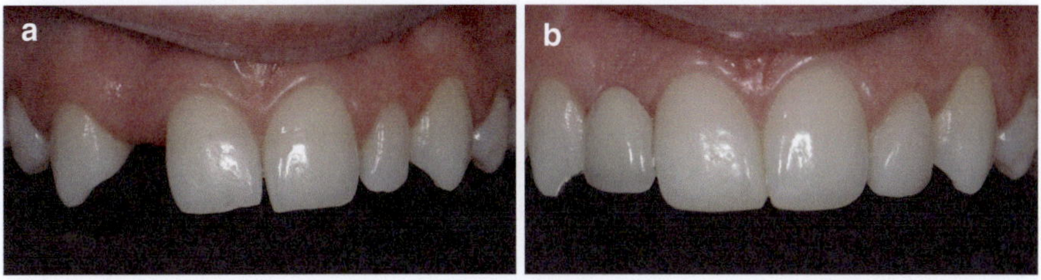

Fig. 4.3 (**a**) A less than optimal orthodontic treatment outcome with position of tooth 11. (**b**) Provision of direct composite resin restorations for teeth 11, 21 & 22 to improve tooth form and incisal edge profile. A resin-bonded bridge was provided to restore the missing tooth 12

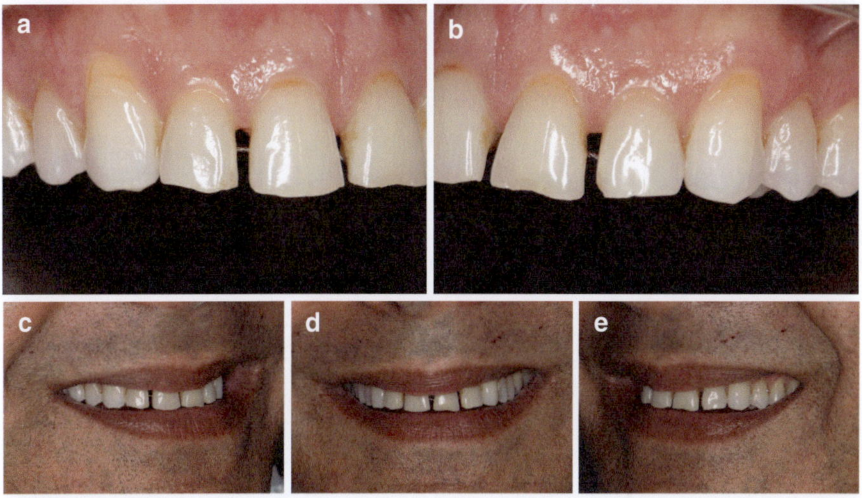

Fig. 4.4 (**a–e**) Multiple diastemas between maxillary anterior teeth post-orthodontic treatment and uneven incisal edges from generalised tooth surface loss (attrition)

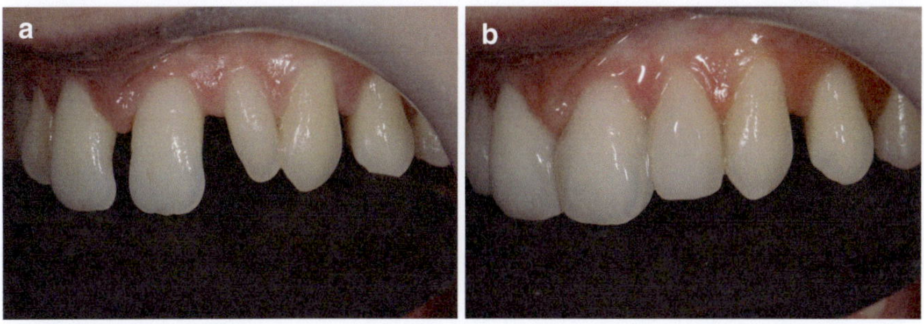

Fig. 4.5 (**a**) Multiple diastemas stemming from generalised microdontia (**b**) Provision of direct composite resin restorations to close diastemas and improve upon tooth size and shape

genetically malformed teeth (Figs. 4.5 and 4.6) and periodontal disease are common aetiologies.

Aesthetic discrepancies mainly arise where teeth are either undersized or oversized for the space or the position within the arch. Two different examples of this within the same position in the maxillary arch are the lateral incisor position. In patients with developmental or congenital anomalies, the canine tooth may develop into the lateral incisor position (Fig. 4.7). In contrast, the lateral incisor may be undersized for the space, otherwise known as the peg-shaped lateral incisor (Figs. 4.7 and 4.8).

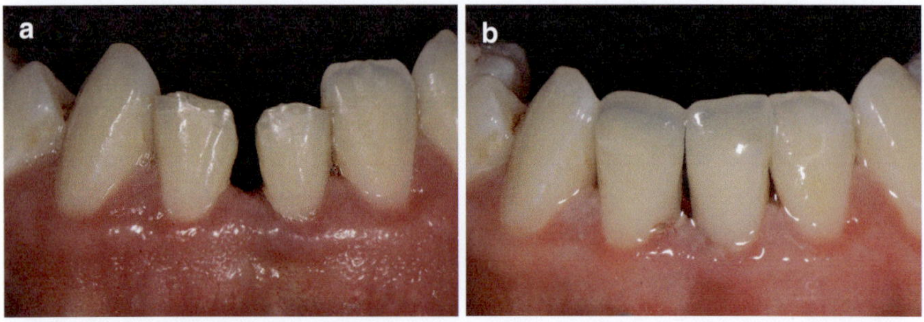

Fig. 4.6 (**a**) Localised spacing between teeth 31 & 42 due to missing tooth 41. (**b**) Direct additive composite resin restorations to close the space and restore the incisal edge profile

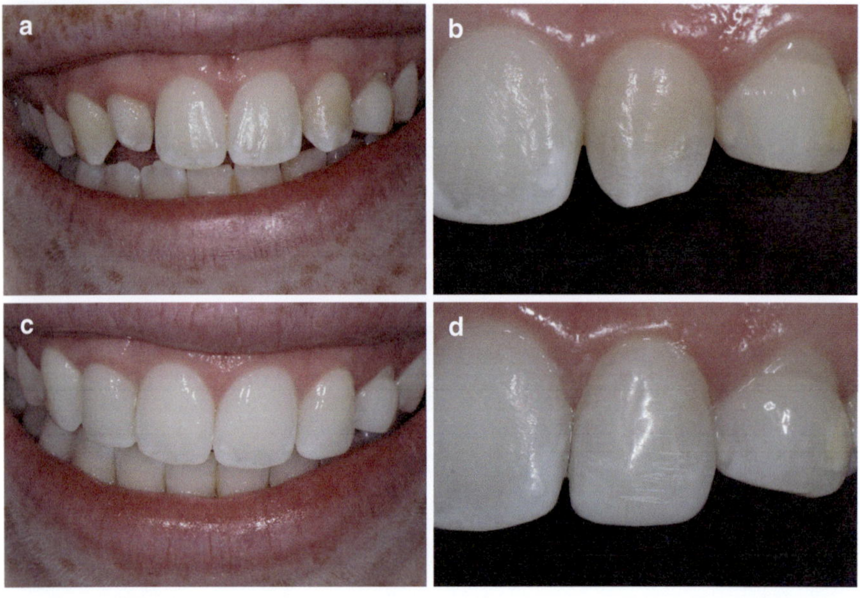

Fig. 4.7 (**a**, **b**) Multiple diastemas presenting with a peg-shaped lateral incisor tooth 12 and a congenitally missing tooth 22 with canine tooth 23 in its position. (**c**, **d**) Both teeth 12 & 23 were augmented through vital tooth bleaching and restoration with direct composite resin to improve symmetry and enhance aesthetics

The gingival margin to incisal edge length of the tooth is also likely to be an issue that patients may be aware of when assessing their smile. Inherently smaller teeth or toothwear processes can give the perception of unevenness and a visual discrepancy between adjacent tooth units (Figs. 4.9 and 4.10). With uneven incisal edge profiles, the common patient complaint of 'my teeth are not straight', can impact significantly on the patient's perception of the problem and they may not be aware of the exact aetiology (Figs. 4.4 and 4.10). Patients exhibiting gingival recession revealed by a high smile line may also complain of tooth size discrepancies. Tooth malpositioning in either buccal or palatal positions will also make teeth appear shorter.

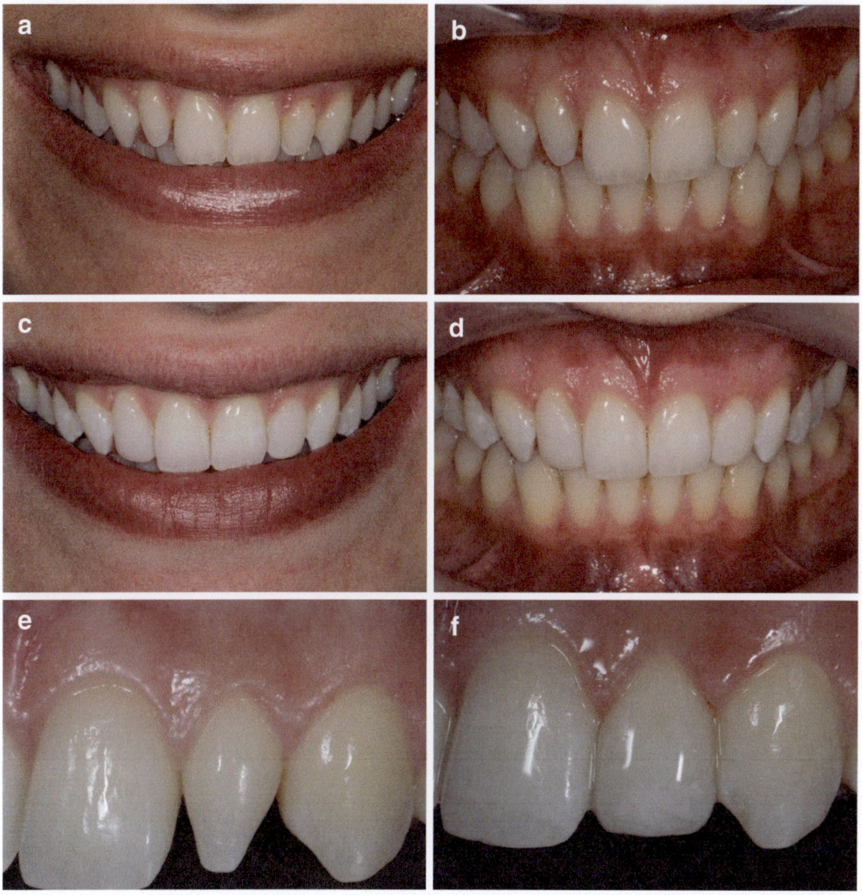

Fig. 4.8 (**a**, **b**) Peg-shaped lateral incisor teeth 12 & 22. (**c**, **d**) Provision of direct additive composite resin restorations improving the incisal edge profile and aesthetic harmony with adjacent teeth. (**e**) Peg lateral incisor tooth (**f**) augmented to improve anatomical contour and aesthetic shape

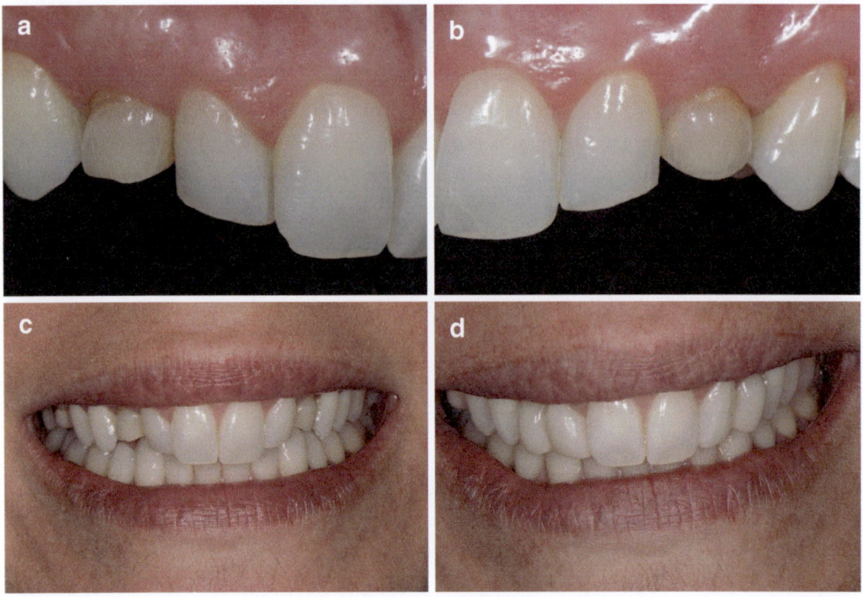

Fig. 4.9 (**a–c**) Retained deciduous canine teeth, diminutive in size resulting in a short appearance and incorrect gingival profile compared to adjacent teeth. (**d**) Provision of direct additive composite resin restorations to deciduous canine teeth and teeth 12 & 22, resulting in improved aesthetic balance in the patient's smile

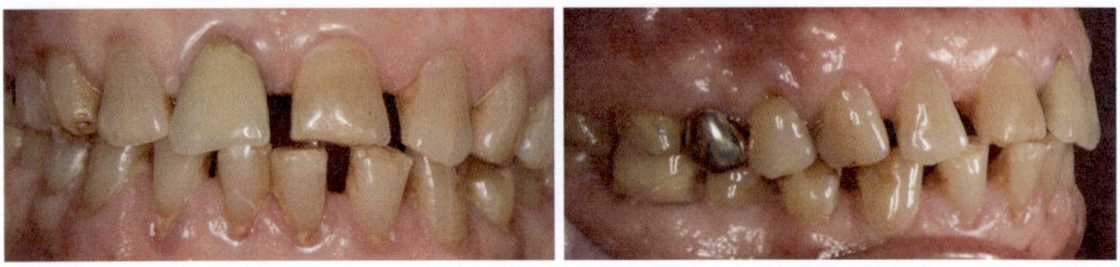

Fig. 4.10 Generalised tooth surface loss (attrition) with shortening of teeth, uneven incisal edges and multiple diastemas

If teeth are missing or worn resulting in drifting of adjacent teeth, the spacing may be uneven and difficult to manage outside of orthodontic bodily tooth movements (Fig. 4.10). Equally, teeth that have drifted may not be perfectly upright in the long axis and may be tilted in mesial or distal directions, compounding the aesthetic and functional issues further.

The manner by which teeth reflect ambient light also plays a role. Remote from spacing along the line of the arch, teeth may present with differences in bucco-palatal positioning. This manifests with buccally positioned teeth reflecting light more readily than their neighbours, which appear darker in comparison. The reflective properties of teeth are not confined to their bodily position. The buccal profile of teeth can be reshaped to more readily reflect light or resorb it. Outside of shape and position, the shade of teeth can also be modified through tooth bleaching treatments, as discussed in Chap. 3.

This chapter will look at techniques in augmenting teeth utilising adhesive dentistry to modify tooth form for aesthetic and functional purposes.

4.2 Treatment Planning

The shape and size of the spacing play a key role in the management of closure or slenderisation. Where a space is too large, restoration with an additive technique can possibly make teeth unnaturally oversized, especially if they are modified in isolation from adjacent units. An example of this is the closure of a large midline diastema, resulting in the proportion ratio (width:length ratio) of the central incisors becoming disproportionate (Fig. 4.11). In contrast, smaller areas of spacing may be considered negligible, and restoration may be considered less beneficial due to the ongoing restoration maintenance burden. In the former, orthodontics could be considered to reduce spacing to make closure with a restoration more amenable; in the latter, the space may be completed with orthodontics alone (Fig. 4.12). The management of spacing through adhesive bonding requires an appreciation of multiple factors. It cannot be crudely measured purely through the distance between the teeth. The size of the teeth, their shape in addition to their gingival profile can make managing spacing challenging to achieve successfully.

Clinical- and laboratory-based diagnostic investigations can be performed to obtain more information on improvements to be made for the tooth proportion, shape and distribution of the spacing.

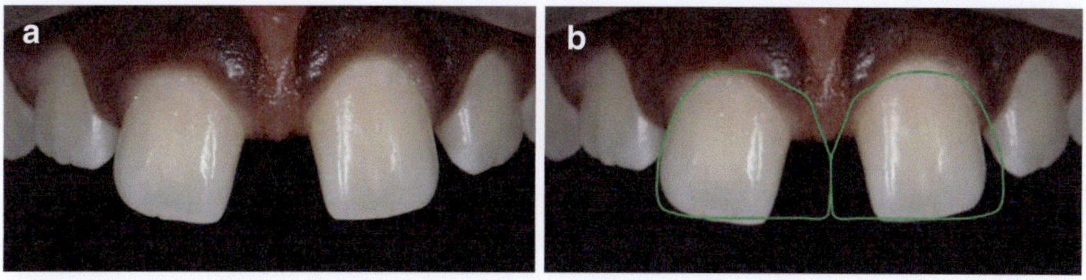

Fig. 4.11 (**a**) Large midline diastema. (**b**) Proposed closure demonstrated via digital silhouette design resulting in teeth 11 & 21 becoming grossly disproportionate with a change in the gingival emergence profile. Orthodontic treatment in conjunction with possible restorative treatment should be considered here to fully close or reduce the size of the diastema

4.2.1 Clinical Assessment

In a variety of ways, chairside clinical investigations may be more valuable than those obtained through the support of technical colleagues. A chairside exercise when assessing spaces and tooth symmetry is the measurement of the spaces and tooth dimensions (Figs. 4.12 and 4.13). This can be utilised to decide upon how to proceed with the treatment, i.e. orthodontically manage the space, augment the teeth or a combination of both treatment modalities. Information may also be used to prescribe a diagnostic wax-up.

A direct intra-oral try-in of the proposed treatment utilising composite resin material provides the patient and clinician with an insight into how definitive restoration provision is likely to progress, and it can also aid the laboratory prescription for a diagnostic wax-up (Fig. 4.14). Both intra-oral and extra-oral assessment of aesthetic and functional parameters of the redesigned teeth and smile must be borne in mind. Considerations are paid to the facial and dental midline; central incisor tooth size and proportion ratio; incisal edge positions in relation to the curvature of the lower lip; long-axis of the displayed teeth; gingival zenith height; interdental papilla shape, interdental contact point location and shape of the interdental embrasures. Assessment of phonetics and occlusal function must also take place. The tooth show and lip line at rest, and the smile line with dynamic tooth show during speech and laughter, provide the patient, the clinician and the technician with further useful diagnostic information. This can be communicated to the technician through digital photographs and complemented by an impression or intra-oral digital scan of the prototype shapes to help guide the diagnostic wax-up. The clinician may consider the diagnostic wax-up an unnecessary stage in the provision and

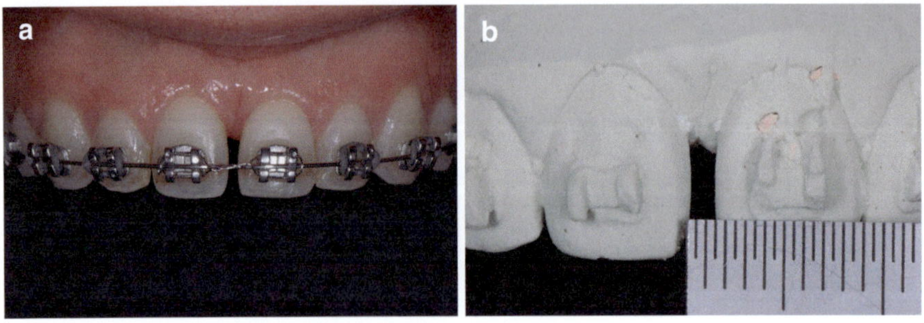

Fig. 4.12 (**a**, **b**) Small midline diastema to be closed with orthodontic treatment

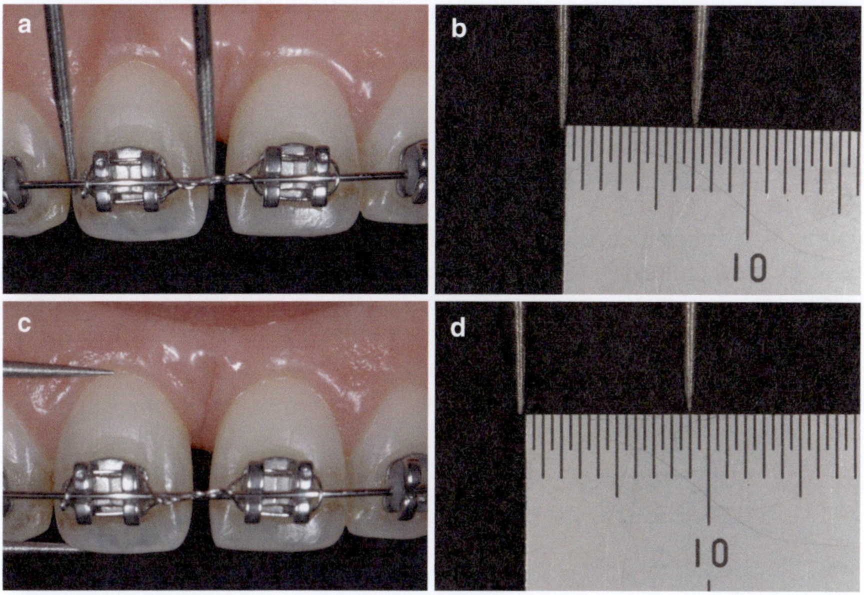

Fig. 4.13 (**a–d**) Measurement of tooth 11 to calculate proportion ratio (width:length ratio), 7 mm:9 mm = 0.77 (77%)

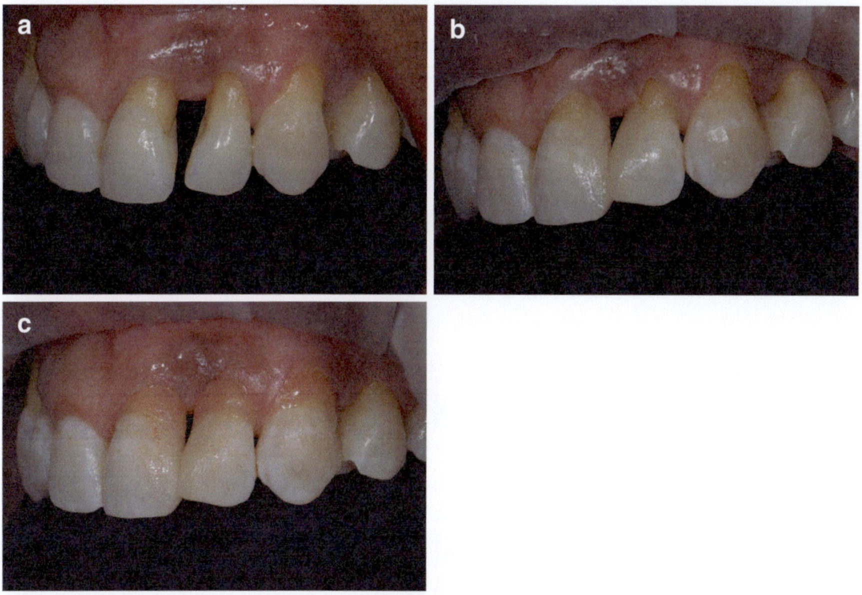

Fig. 4.14 (**a**) Teeth 21, 22 & 23 direct aesthetic try-in with (**b**) tooth coloured and (**c**) gingival coloured composite resin material to demonstrate diastema closure and improvements in tooth form and gingival profile

perform the restorative changes directly based on the findings from the direct try-in stage.

If the wax-up is completed, a prototype provisional try-in is made by the clinician, taking a silicone impression of the diagnostic wax-up to transfer the information to the patient's mouth with a temporary acrylic (Bis-acryl) material, which is trimmed and shaped to allow the patient a preview of the proposed definitive treatment (Figs. 4.15 and 4.16). Alternatively, the laboratory can provide an indirect CAD–CAM milled prototype provisional try-in pattern for this. Adjustments may be made to the prototype provisional try-in at the discretion of the patient and clinician and recorded by way of impression or digital scan for 3D reference of the new tooth shapes (Figs. 4.17 and 4.18). The prototype provisional try-in may be removed or it is proposed that the patient keep it in situ for a short period of time for further self-assessment, at which point they can again reconsider the difference and improvements. This technique is discussed further in Sect. 4.5.1.

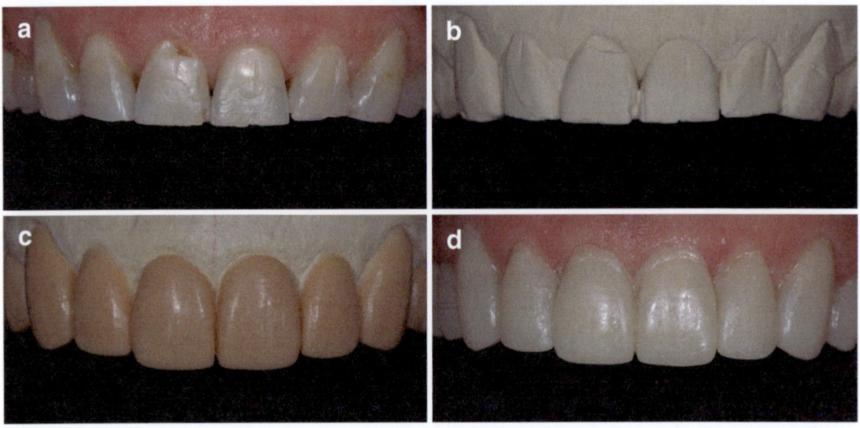

Fig. 4.15 (**a**, **b**) Tooth surface loss (attrition) resulting in shortened teeth. (**c**, **d**) Diagnostic wax-up and prototype provisional try-in information transfer to the patient's teeth 15–25 with a temporary Bis-acryl material to allow preview of the proposed definitive treatment

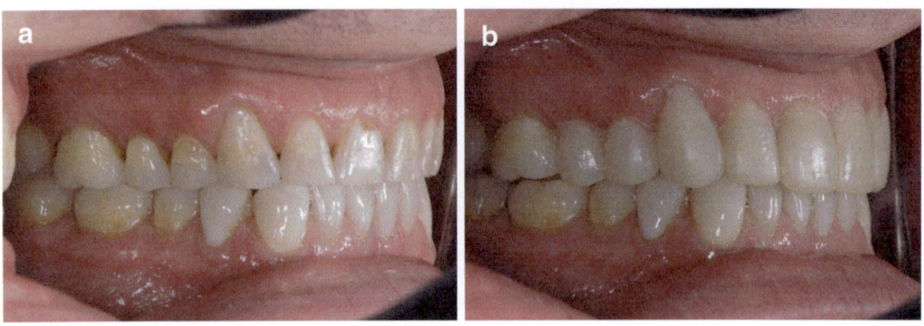

Fig. 4.16 (**a**) Teeth 15–25 with (**b**) prototype provisional try-in to allow preview of the proposed definitive treatment

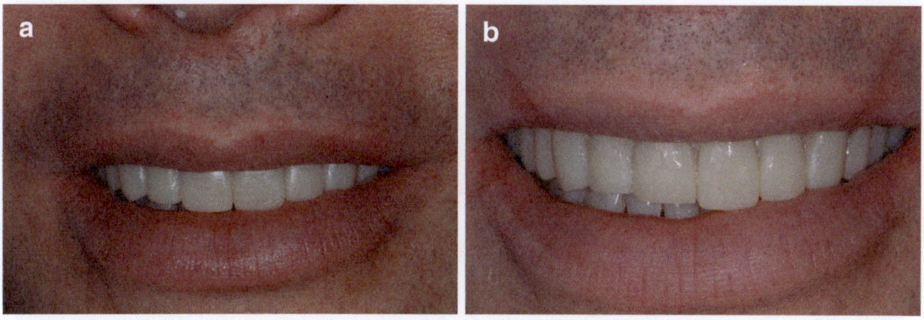

Fig. 4.17 (**a**) Teeth 15–25 prototype provisional try-in. (**b**) Bis-acryl material adjustment on teeth 15–11 to show tooth length differences to the initial proposal on teeth 21–24

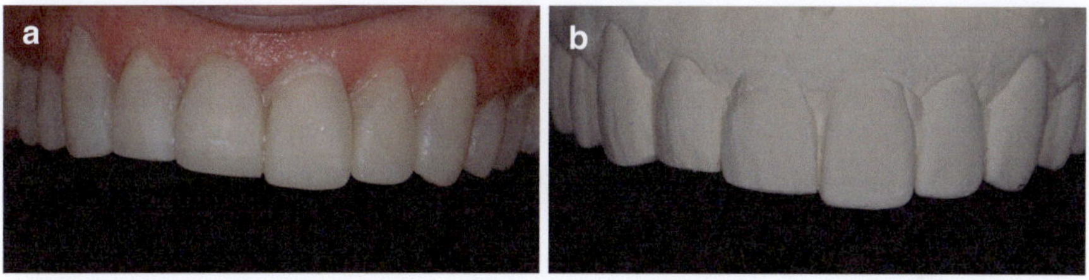

Fig. 4.18 (**a**) Prototype provisional try-in adjustment on teeth 15–11 to show tooth length differences to the initial proposal on teeth 21–24. (**b**) Recording of the new tooth shapes by way of impression and pouring of the reference study cast

An important aspect of either direct composite resin try-in or prototype provisional acrylic try-in as an investigation is the appraisal and assessment of the patient's reaction and feedback. This is valuable in realising the expectations of the patient and whether these can be met through the process of additive direct composite resin bonding or indirect adhesive restoration provision. At this stage, patients whose expectations may be greater than what may be clinically possible, or biologically beneficial to the teeth, are likely to require further explanation of the salient clinical issues to express the risks and benefits of proposed alternative treatment strategies. Despite this, patients with high aesthetic expectations may reflect on the try-in or prototype and feel this may be acceptable. Others may spend longer deciding, and at this point may ask questions as to the changes and what they entail. It may be prudent to suggest to the patient that digital photographs can aid their deliberations prior to a decision on treatment progression. This process can potentially contribute to the consent process.

4.2.2 Laboratory Assessment

Study casts are poured in gypsum from accurate impressions made of alginate or rubber-based materials, or are 3D printed from intra-oral digital scans. Occlusal records, including a facebow record and jaw registration allow mounting the casts to an articulator to individualised anatomic relationships recorded from the patient (Fig. 4.19). This is likely to improve the patient's treatment outcome, especially where extensive procedures and restorations are planned (Figs. 4.20 and 4.21).

In conjunction with photographs, a digital silhouette design may be used to provide further diagnostic information to determine the ideal central incisal proportion ratio and guide diagnostic tooth shapes. Diagnostic waxing may be carried out utilising both digital, analogue or a combination of both processes (Figs. 4.22, 4.23, and 4.24).

What may be counterintuitive for the technician is the nature of the treatment and the modes through which it can be delivered. Technical colleagues may be accustomed to providing wax preview with the perception that future treatment will involve a subtractive technique resulting in wholesale crowns or veneers. As such, the laboratory prescription of the diagnostic wax-up requires more information on the exact pattern of wax addition and how this relates to the teeth with or without any significant subtractive preparation. The use of a contrasting-coloured wax to model material is useful for this assessment (Figs. 4.15, 4.20, and 4.24), the use of 3D printers may be of limited value to this effect due to their mono colour cast print ability.

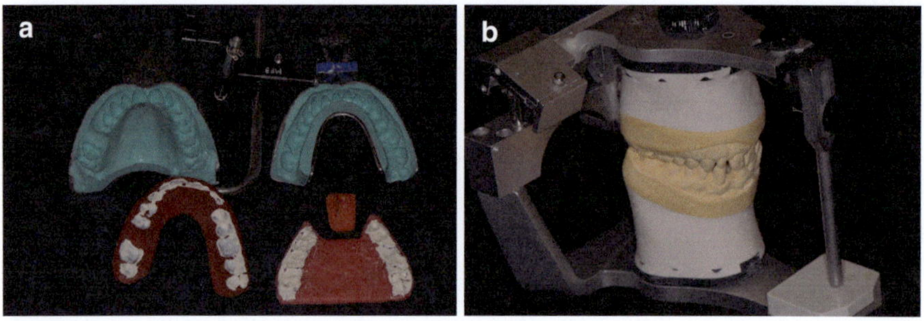

Fig. 4.19 Diagnostic records. (**a**) Alginate impressions, facebow record and centric jaw registration. (**b**) Mounted study casts to a semi-adjustable articulator

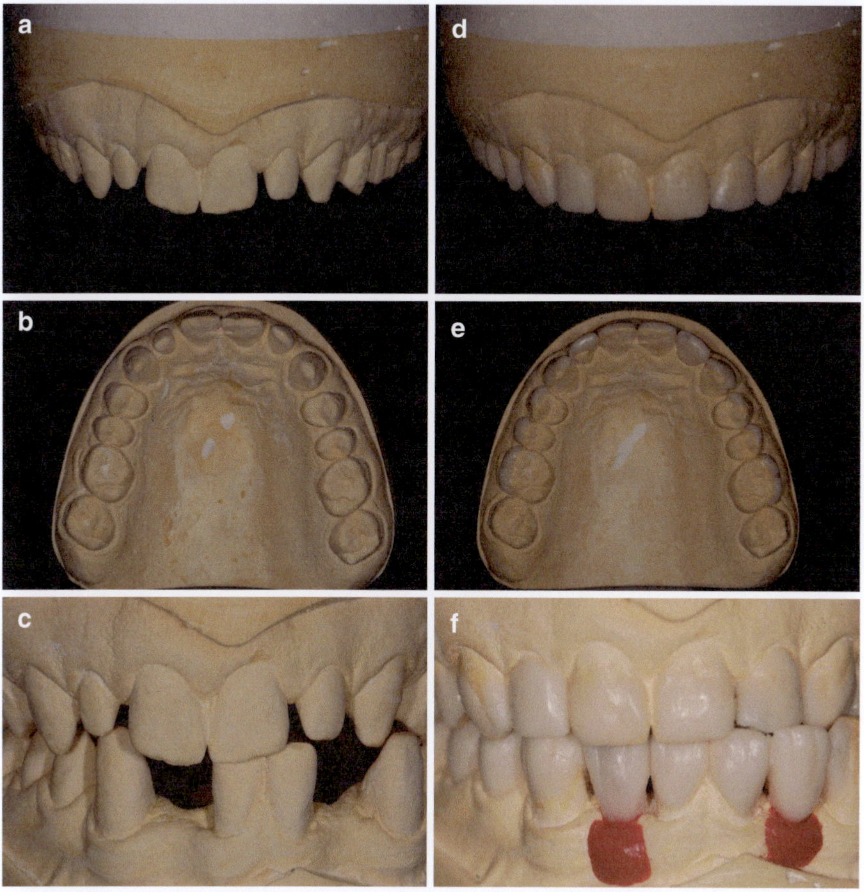

Fig. 4.20 (**a**–**c**) Patient with hypodontia post-orthodontic treatment showing missing teeth, soft tissue defects, peg-shaped lateral incisor teeth 12 & 22 and multiple diastemas. (**d**–**f**) Diagnostic wax-up for planning of extensive composite resin restorations, surgical gingival grafting and implant fixture placement

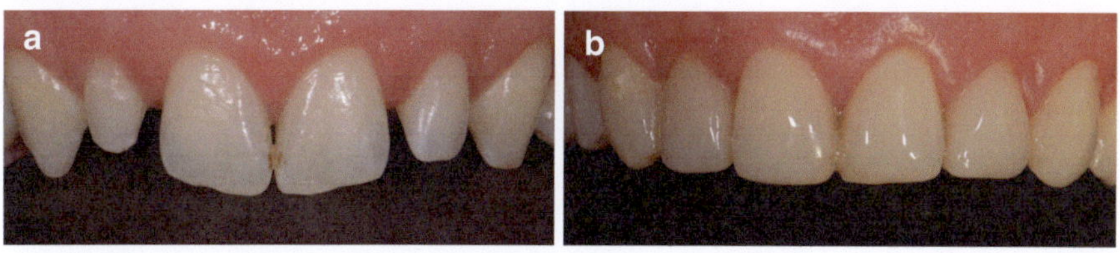

Fig. 4.21 (**a**) Pre-operative situation and (**b**) provision of extensive direct composite resin restorations

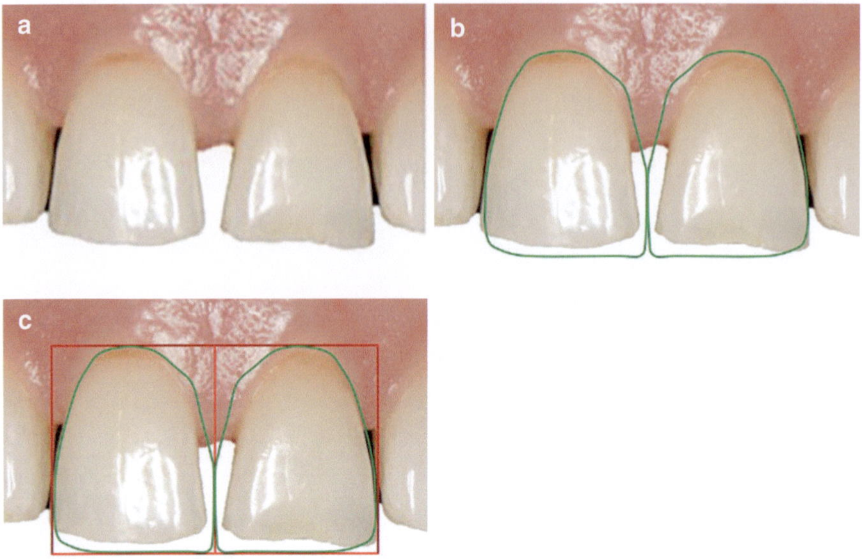

Fig. 4.22 (**a**, **b**, **c**) Digital silhouette design of teeth 11 & 21 to change the length and width proportion ratio for midline diastema closure

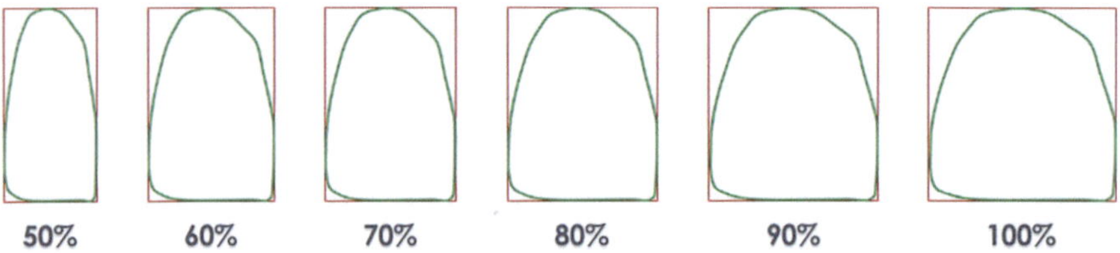

Fig. 4.23 Digital design of tooth 11 to highlight the proportion ratio change influence on tooth shape

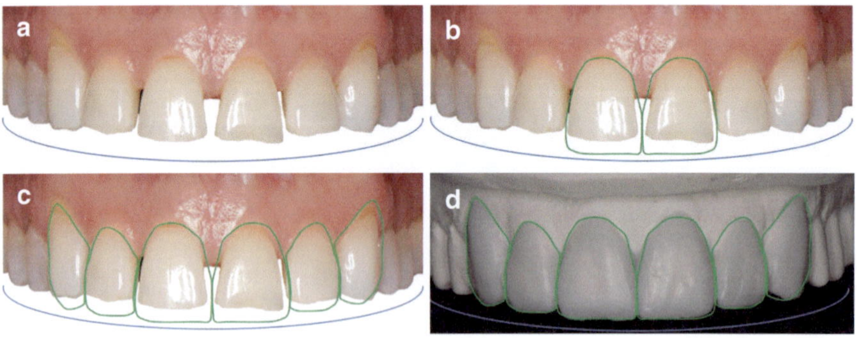

Fig. 4.24 (**a–d**) Digital silhouette design of teeth 11 & 21 to change length and width proportion ratio in relation to lower lip curve to guide analogue diagnostic wax-up of teeth 13–24

4.3 Key Clinical Factors

There should be consideration made of the key clinical presenting factors that affect the ability to successfully modify tooth form.

4.3.1 Gingival Profile

The gingival profile plays an important role in the management of improving the form of teeth. Gingival profile is the superior determinant of shape of the tooth where the body and incisal areas provide the inferior determinants. The lip line, gingival arch and zenith profile frame the cervical portion of the tooth and so dictates the shape of the tooth out with of bonding or adhesion. It has a very specific role when dictating the form of adhesive resin bonding to close spacing between teeth.

A flat gingival profile reduces scope to make a tooth wider. This restricts the margin to widen as the tooth will become larger without an appropriate emergence profile and proportionally out of ratio with the tooth length. As a result of the flat profile, the tooth is square in appearance. Modification of the gingival profile is beneficial to space closure. Recreation of a gingival zenith through planned tissue removal creates an arc for natural widening of the tooth, which gradually progresses to the contact point (Fig. 4.25). The design of the arc depends on the envisaged change in width of the tooth, the size of the space and the length of the tooth. The gradient of the created arc also influences the nature of the widening and thus can make the tooth more triangular if the gradient is steep.

In patients where the smile line is low and the visible gingival margin is not shown, modification to the gingival profile may not be required to achieve a desirable aesthetic result (Fig. 4.26).

4.3.2 Tooth Size and Shape

At the very basic level, the incisor tooth should be longer than it is wide. Taking the central incisor as an example, a desirable proportion ratio is approximately 80% (Fig. 4.23). Proportionally, this ratio is likely to vary depending on a number of factors, including the patient's facial profile, the lips and smile and how these frame the teeth, the general appearance of the teeth and the gingival profiles. This ratio needs to be considered and tailored when teeth size and shape may be modified through augmentation with composite resin bonding or indirect adhesive restoration. If horizontal augmentation is significant resulting in closure of the interdental space, the negative effect on the tooth proportion ratio will be apparent, where the tooth will look too wide and square (Fig. 4.11). Hence, in situations where teeth are widened to close a diastema, length additions can be considered to maintain appropriate proportion ratios of the treated teeth (Figs. 4.22, 4.24, and 4.26). Length additions may be considered at the incisal edge (hard tissue addition) or at the gingival margin (soft tissue removal).

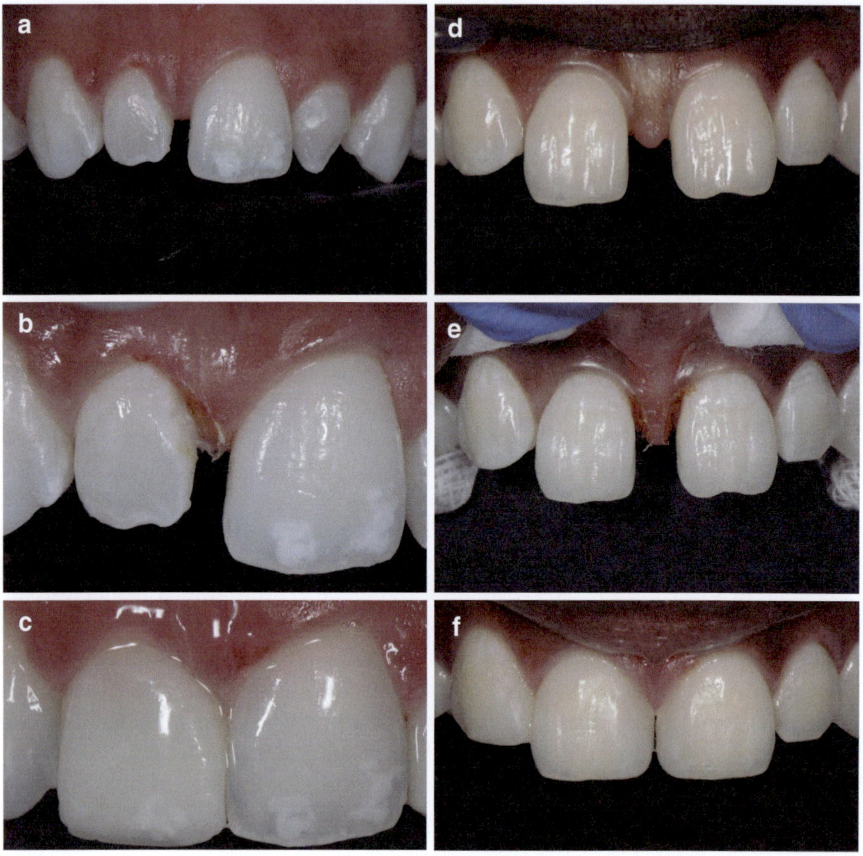

Fig. 4.25 (**a–c**) Tooth 11 sculpting of buccal soft tissue with electrosurgery to increase surface area for the provision of composite resin restoration. (**d–f**) Teeth 11 & 21 modification of the interdental gingival profile with electrosurgery to benefit diastema closure with composite resin restorations

The facial profile of anterior teeth play an important role in the aesthetic perception of one's smile. Light reflectivity can be influenced by modifying the labial surface to manipulate the way light is reflected. The absence of any incisal embrasure and interdental transitions will give the appearance of width and bulkiness. Thus, creating appropriately sized and angulated embrasure spaces can slenderise the tooth and reduce the possibility of a wide tooth from capturing the eye. A large flat profile, where the marginal ridges and transitional line angles are positioned towards the extreme mesial and the distal surfaces, will also give the perception of the width of the tooth. In contrast, repositioning these medially towards the centre of the tooth, or greater curvature in cross or long sections, will give the perceived appearance of narrowness or slenderness

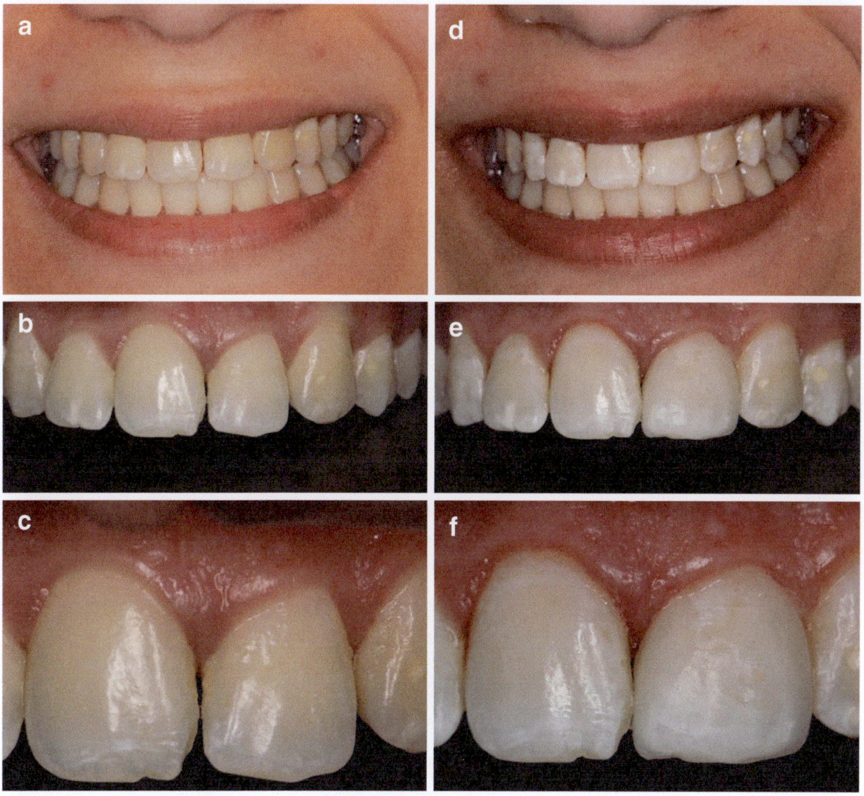

Fig. 4.26 Patient with a low smile line where the gingival profile does not show. (**a–c**) Tooth 21 pre-operative situation. (**d–f**) Provision of direct composite resin restoration to improve upon the width, length and incisal profile. The gingival asymmetry has been accepted without change

and alterations in length. Cervical line angle positions can also modify the passage of light reflection in the same way, where close proximity of the line angle to the gingiva will lighten the tooth and influence its length appearance (Figs. 4.27 and 4.28).

Texture and surface detail can also play a role. Increased surface texture (perikymata) can increase the reflectiveness of teeth and thereby allow them to appear brighter and will give the perception of a greater width and reduced height. In contrast, increasing vertical grooves with give the perception of narrowness or increased height.

Tooth shape augmentation influenced by surface characteristics, the marginal ridge profiles in tandem with the gingival profile will allow greater scope for shape modification. The best example being example with modification of a peg-shaped lateral incisor tooth, which is tapered towards the incisal edge resulting in a diastema on either side. In essence, this provides a large scope to modify the tooth form with play of the transitional and cervical line angles to create a more natural appearance (Figs. 4.29 and 4.30).

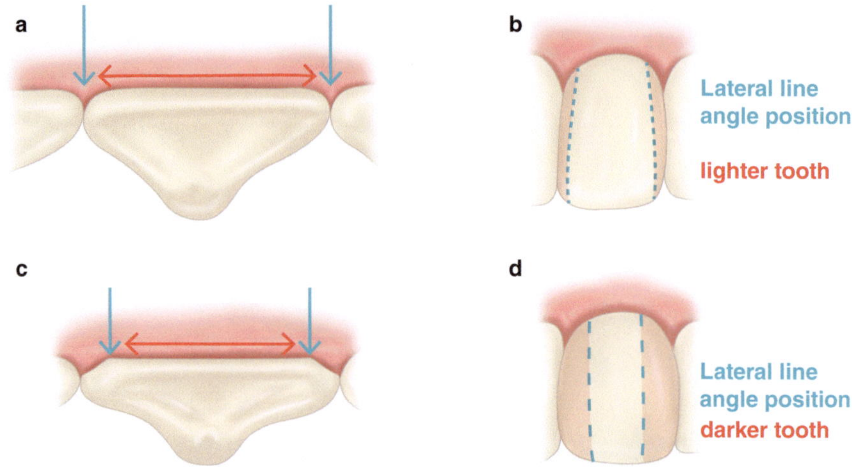

Fig. 4.27 (**a–d**) Buccal profile of anterior teeth modified by enhancing the labial surface to manipulate the way light is reflected to alter perception of the wideness of the tooth

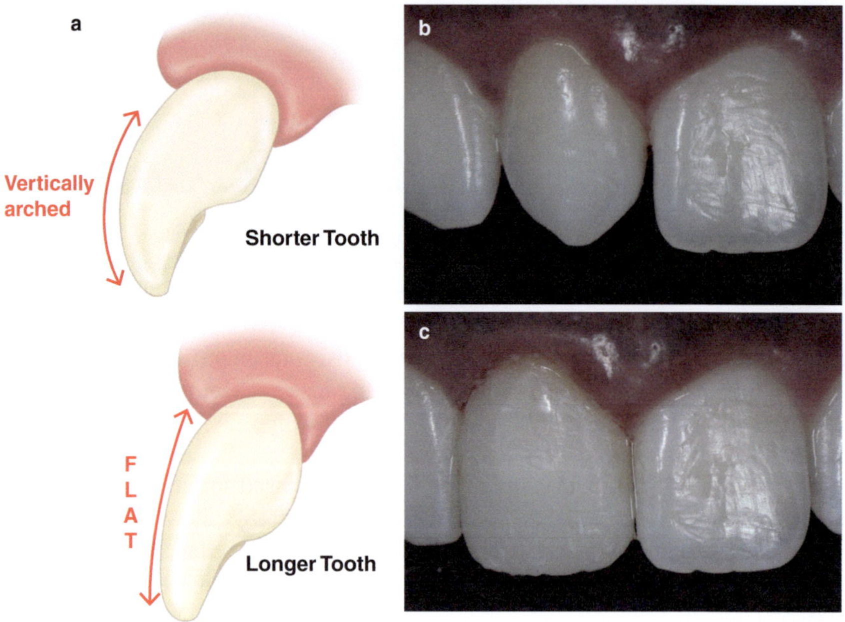

Fig. 4.28 (**a**) Greater curvature in long sections will alter the appearance of length. (**b**) Canine tooth 13 in the position of tooth 11 is naturally bulbous (**c**) and has been made to look longer by flattening the buccal contour in conjunction with composite resin augmentation

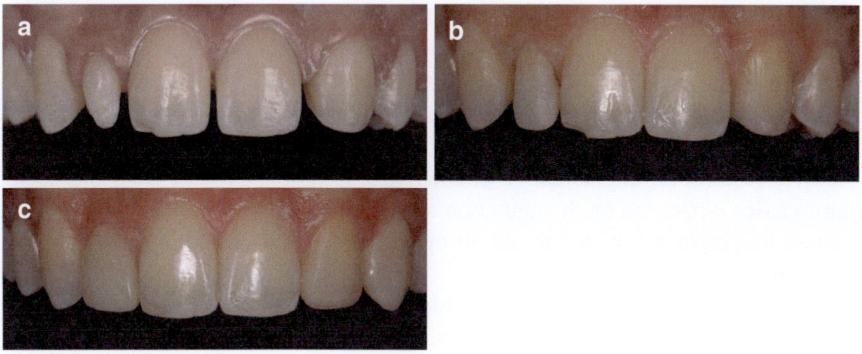

Fig. 4.29 (**a**) Multiple diastemas presenting with peg-shaped lateral incisor tooth 12 and congenitally missing tooth 22 with canine tooth 23 in its position (Image courtesy of Dr. Kaval Patel). (**b**) Patient post-orthodontic treatment with closure midline diastema. (**c**) Provision of composite resin restorations to teeth 12 (anatomical build-up), 11 (distal–incisal edge), 23 (direct veneer) & 24 (direct veneer)

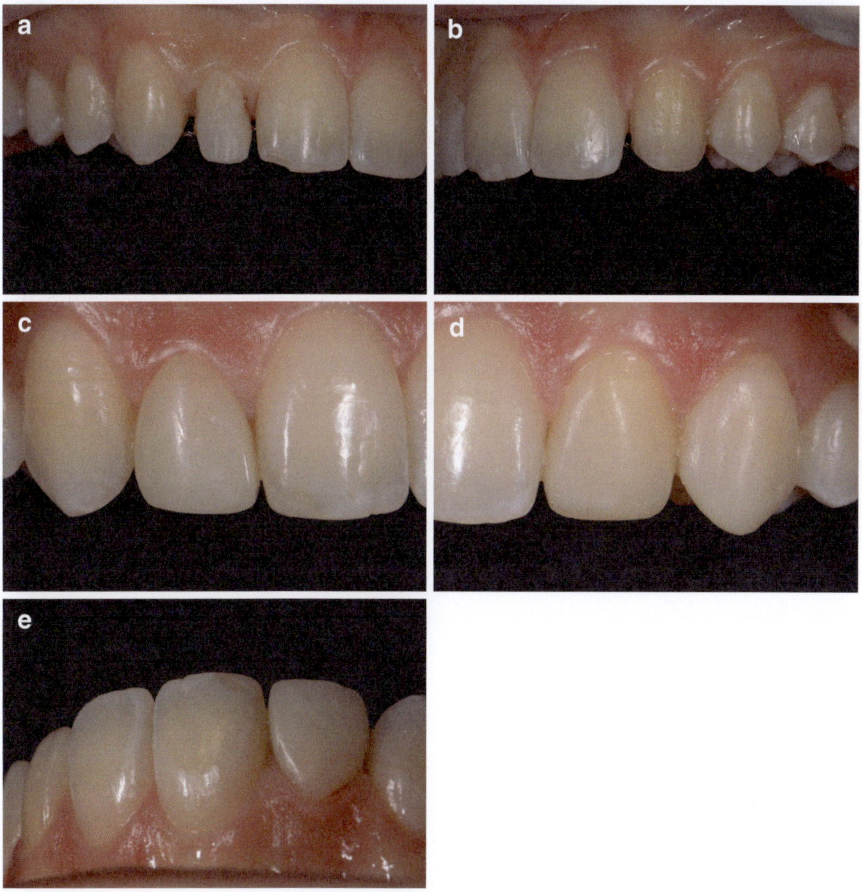

Fig. 4.30 (**a**, **b**) Patient presenting from Fig. 4.29 post-orthodontic treatment with closure of midline diastema. (**c**, **d**) Provision of composite resin restorations to teeth 12 (anatomical build-up), 11 (distal-incisal edge), 23 (direct veneer) & 24 (direct veneer). (**e**) Post-operative situation

4.3.3 Tooth Angulation and Position

In the aesthetic zone, maxillary teeth are generally inclined in a mesial direction where their long axes converge toward the midline. Variations in overjet and overbite complicated by tooth rotations may make restorative tooth modification via adhesive restoration augmentation challenging. It should be said from the outset that in cases where the teeth angulation and position correction is extensive, orthodontic treatment is advised to aid an optimal treatment aesthetic and functional outcome.

In situations where the patient would like a space closed, proclined maxillary anterior teeth exhibiting interdental spacing (Fig. 4.10) are more difficult to manage than those that are otherwise positionally correct or retroclined. Interproximal additions of composite resin material will make the teeth wider, closing the space, but simultaneously making the teeth more prominent. Making the teeth wider will result in more light reflection on the buccal surface, increasing their already prominent appearance. In contrast, retroclined teeth are inherently less likely to present with spacing due to a higher likelihood of crowding. The crowded dentition can provide an appearance that is considered unsightly by patients. Differences in bucco-palatal positioning results in significant differences in the manner with which neighbouring teeth reflect light. The further palatal or lingual a tooth resides, the greater the shadow cast on the buccal surface by the adjacent teeth and soft tissues such as the lips. These appearances may be compounded by inconsistent incisal edge profiles if teeth are angled towards the palatal or lingual.

The appearance of retroclined teeth can be modified by adhesive bonding of direct or indirect composite resin veneers to the facial surfaces, creating the appearance of teeth that are in line or more harmonious, making an aesthetic improvement (Figs. 4.31, 4.32, 4.33, 4.34, and 4.35). However, the restoration gingival emergence profile and contact point areas are likely to be changed and less ideal than the norm. The clinician needs to ensure the cleansability of the contact areas and ensure an adequate embrasure space is created for long-term restoration maintenance.

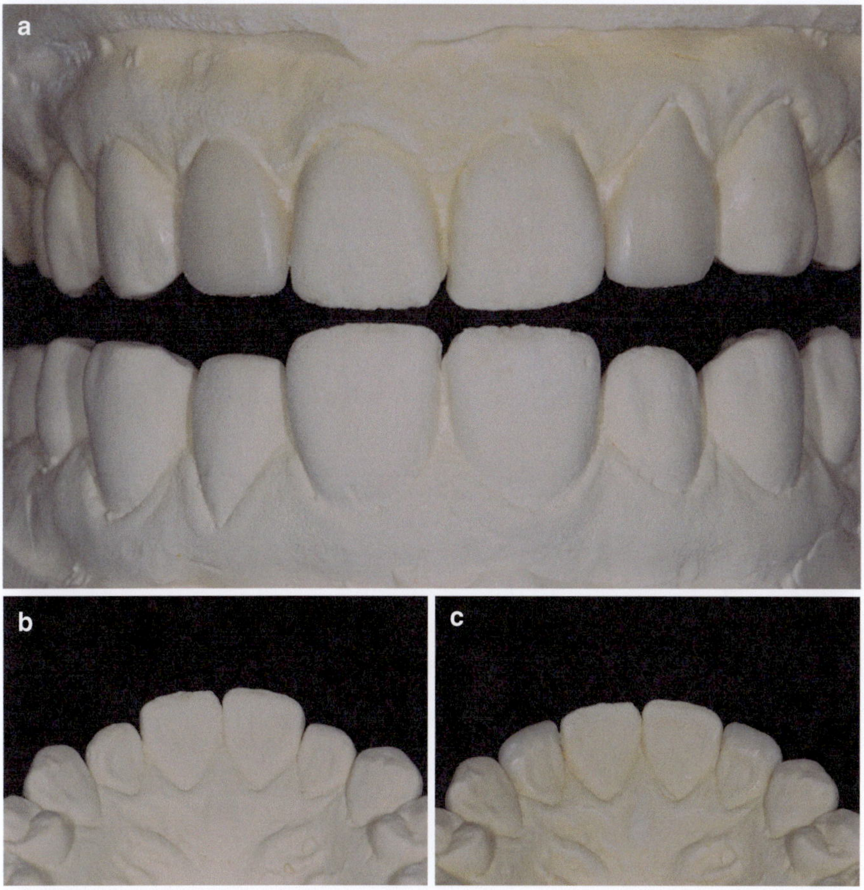

Fig. 4.31 (**a**, **b**) Diminutive retroclined teeth 12 & 22. (**a**, **c**) Diagnostic wax-up to improve appearance of facial profile and incisal length

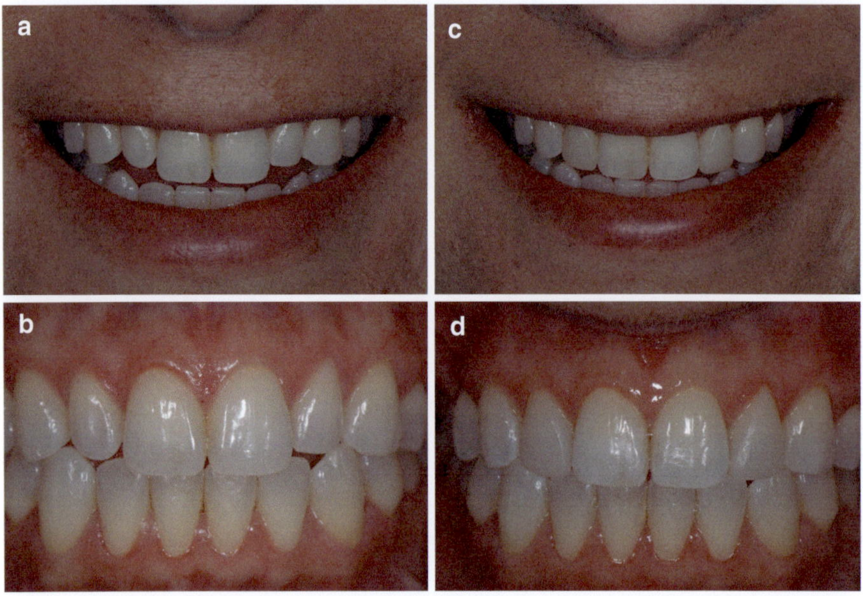

Fig. 4.32 (**a**, **b**) Diminutive retroclined teeth 12 & 22. (**c**, **d**) Direct additive no preparation composite resin veneer restorations to improve appearance of facial profile and incisal length

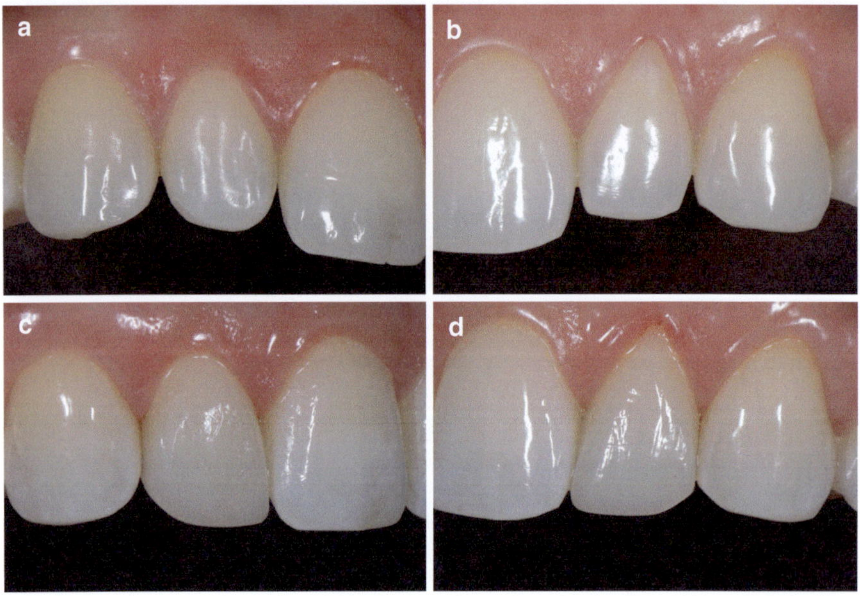

Fig. 4.33 (**a**, **b**) Diminutive retroclined teeth 12 & 22. (**c**, **d**) Direct additive no preparation composite resin veneer restorations to improve appearance of facial profile and incisal length

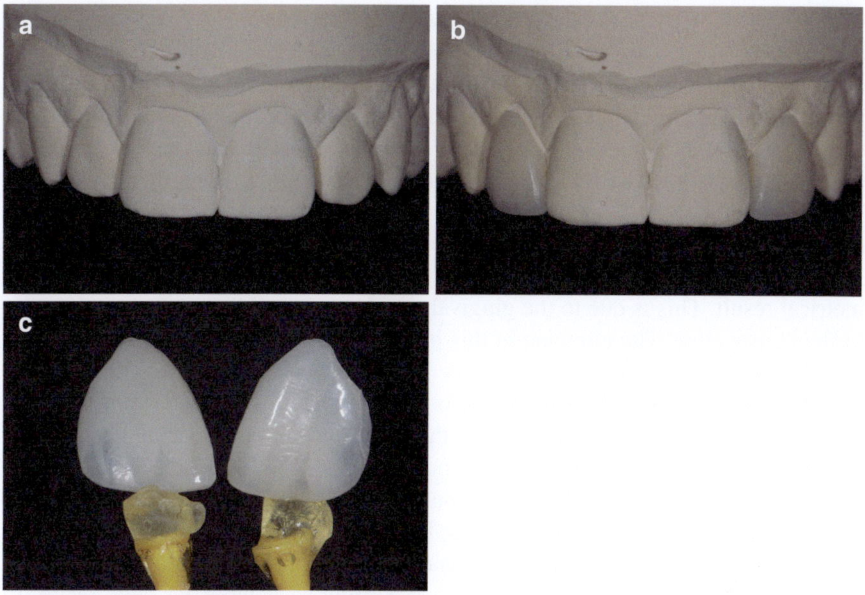

Fig. 4.34 (**a**) Retroclined teeth 12 & 22. (**b**, **c**) Indirect additive no preparation composite resin veneer restorations to improve appearance of facial profile and incisal length

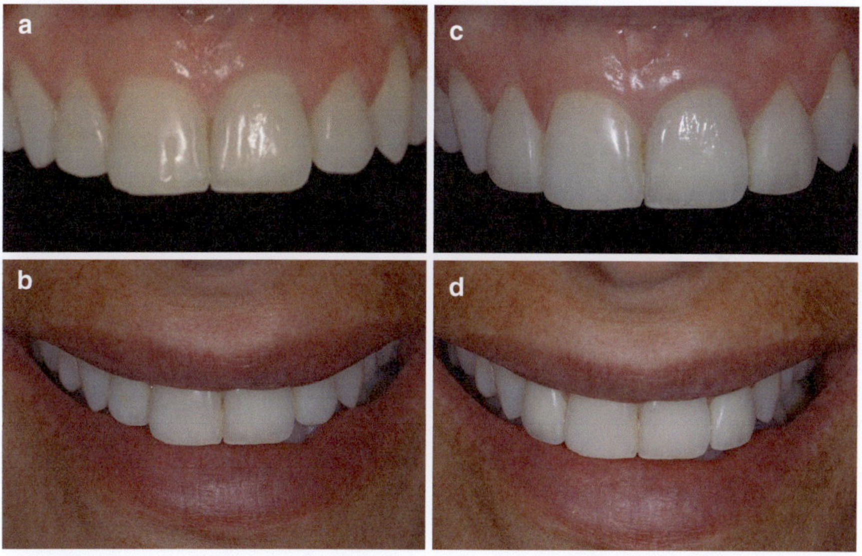

Fig. 4.35 (**a**, **b**) Pre-operative retroclined teeth 12 & 22. (**c**, **d**) Indirect additive no preparation composite resin veneer restorations to improve appearance of facial profile and incisal length

4.4 Managing Spacing and Black Triangles

In isolation, spacing that is evenly distributed may be easier to manage than spacing that is wholly confined to a single interdental space. For example, an anterior tooth that has a distal interdental contact with a 2 mm mesial space may be more difficult to manage than one where there are two spaces of 1 mm on each interdental side. This division of space allows the clinician to maintain some aspect of symmetry of the tooth unit with augmentation on either side. Where the space is wholly on one aspect, the augmentation to one side may result in difficulty in achieving a symmetrical result. This is due to the gingival zenith not coinciding with the mid-point of the incisal edge. The clinician in this instance may consider the option for orthodontic treatment or augment the space and not close it completely to avoid an unsightly appearance. Where the space is large in these instances, the clinician can decide to augment the adjacent tooth to the space and split the spacing between the two adjacent tooth units to avoid the asymmetry (Fig. 4.36). This, however, increases the restoration maintenance burden of the patient for the two teeth.

Where multiple spaces reside, the challenge to close spaces whilst maintaining symmetry is more challenging. If the generalised space distribution is asymmetric, merely closing spaces may not result in an entirely acceptable aesthetic result. In these instances, the need for clinical and laboratory investigative records is greater

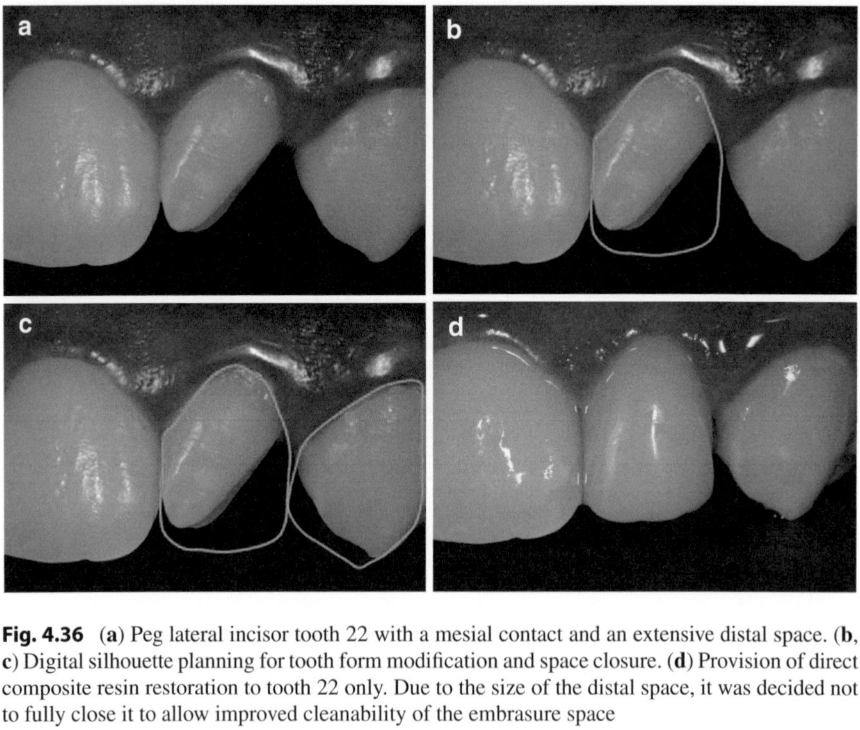

Fig. 4.36 (**a**) Peg lateral incisor tooth 22 with a mesial contact and an extensive distal space. (**b**, **c**) Digital silhouette planning for tooth form modification and space closure. (**d**) Provision of direct composite resin restoration to tooth 22 only. Due to the size of the distal space, it was decided not to fully close it to allow improved cleanability of the embrasure space

for case planning. Spacing issues may be compounded if missing teeth (congenital or acquired) result in either ½ unit or 1 ½ units of space. Other aesthetic and functional challenges include the drifting and progressive migration of teeth into space. Teeth that lie off-axis with mesial or distal inclination will cause changes in the inclination of the incisal edge and gingival zenith position. Again, for an optimal treatment aesthetic and functional outcome, orthodontic treatment must be considered if positional correction is extensive.

Post-periodontal treatment soft tissue changes invariably result in papillary regression and gingival profile change. This culminates in numerous aesthetic issues where black triangles between the teeth reveal the clear discrepancy between coronal enamel and root dentine. The latter is worsened by the change in diameter of the tooth when migrating from the cemento-enamel junction further apically and the difference in colour between the two surfaces (Figs. 4.14 and 4.37). The length of the clinical crown is increased without a proportional increase in width, and the tooth is now longer and proportionately 'narrower'. There are various methods to attempt to remedy these issues. A removable prosthetic gingival veneer engages the embrasure spaces and gives the impression of a healthy gingival profile. The other technique to manage these changes is the provision of composite resin restorations with tooth and gingival coloured

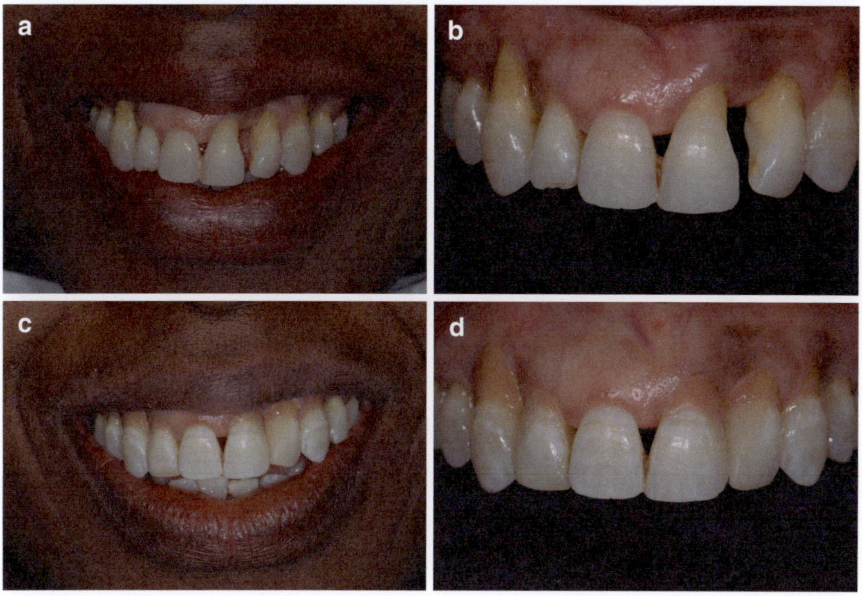

Fig. 4.37 (**a**, **b**) The patient presenting from Fig. 4.14, High smile line exhibiting tooth size discrepancies due to advanced periodontal disease with associated gingival profile change due to recession and presence of a diastema and black triangles. The cemento-enamel junction is seen as well as the difference in colour between tooth and root surfaces. (**c**, **d**) Provision of composite resin restorations to teeth 13, 12, 21, 22 & 23 with tooth and gingival coloured materials to give the appearance of a naturally appearing teeth without root exposure

materials to recontour the tooth to close the spaces and give the appearance of a natural appearing tooth without root exposure (Figs. 4.37 and 4.38). An important aspect to be aware of is the smile line, as by virtue of the teeth being now naturally longer, composite resin material additions may make the teeth more prominent without the use of the gingival coloured material. These restorations can be delivered directly or indirectly with additive 'no preparation' composite resin veneers (Figs. 4.39 and 4.40).

Restoration, cleansability and maintenance are important considerations. Patients are likely to have had extensive periodontal treatment due to well-established periodontitis, resulting in these severe soft tissue changes. Composite resin augmentation to close embrasure spaces automatically creates a greater challenge for the patient to clean and maintain. Where large interproximal brushes were passive in their passage, interdental augmented sites are now more plaque retentive and require greater dexterity to successfully clean. These biological issues need to be balanced against the aesthetic improvement in appearance. The patient and clinician should consider the extent to which the embrasure is closed, retaining an accessible embrasure, be it smaller than previously, may be the most sensible approach.

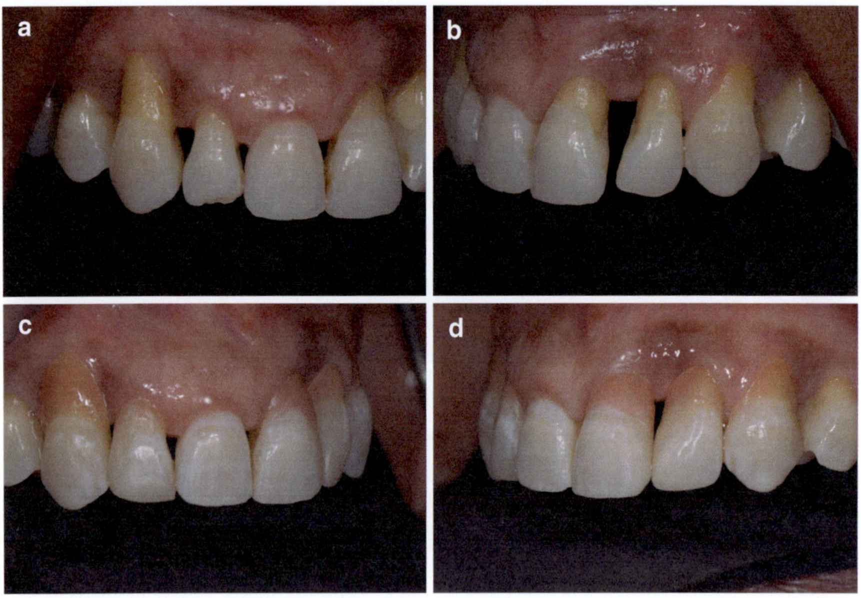

Fig. 4.38 (**a**, **b**) Pre-operative situation (**c**, **d**) Provision of composite resin restorations to teeth 13, 12, 21, 22 & 23 with tooth and gingival coloured materials to give the appearance of natural appearing teeth without root exposure

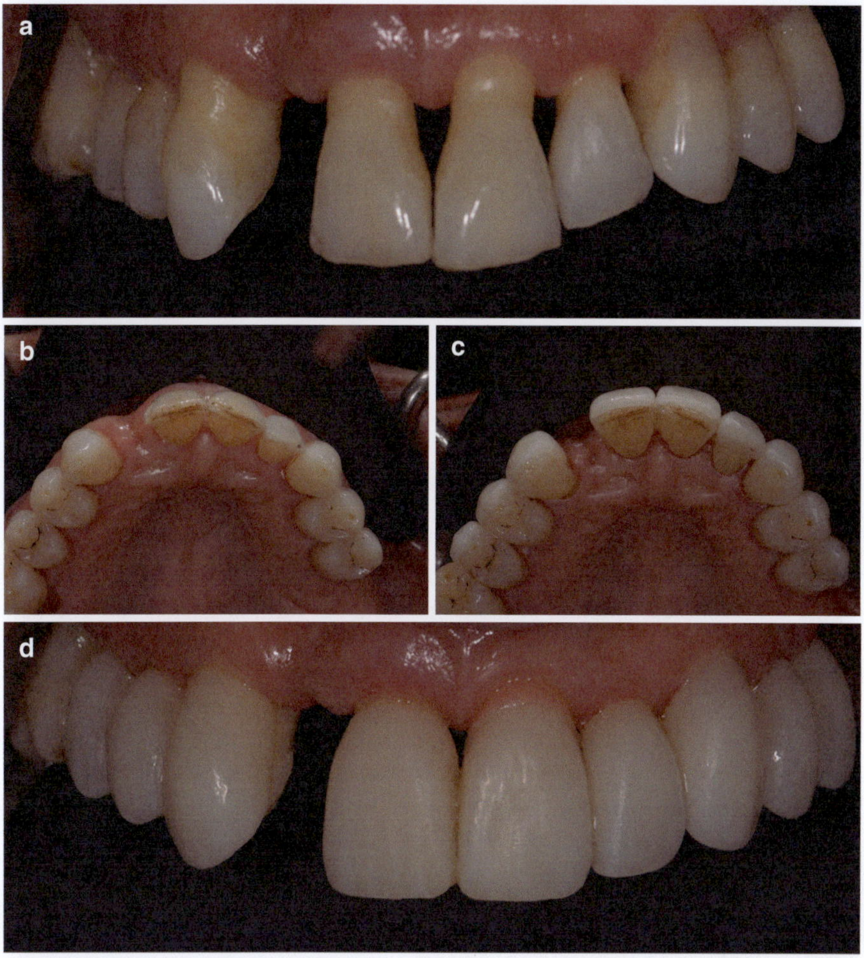

Fig. 4.39 (**a**, **b**) Pre-operative situation of a patient post-periodontal management exhibiting asymmetry and black triangles. (**c**, **d**) Indirect additive no preparation composite resin veneer restorations adhesively bonded on teeth 15–25 to improve upon tooth form, incisal edge profile, embrasure spaces and close black triangles

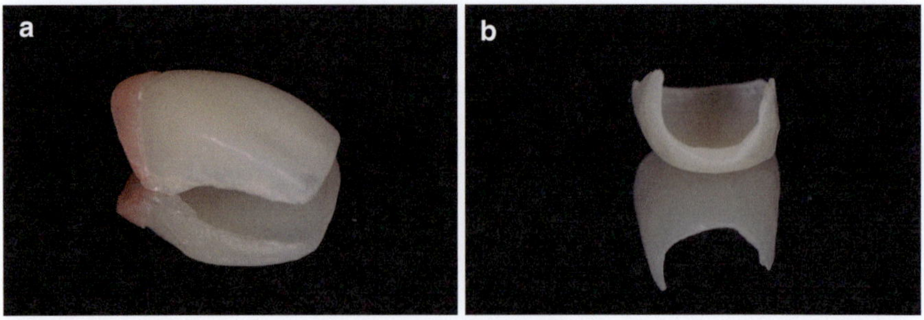

Fig. 4.40 (**a**, **b**) Composite resin veneer restorations showing use of gingival coloured and tooth coloured composite resin materials with interproximal wrap for black triangle closure and embrasure space formation

4.5 Adhesive Technique

To aid treatment planning and visualisation of the planned treatment, analogue or digital diagnostic cast waxing of the proposed tooth form is carried out. The new tooth form offers improvements upon the aesthetic and functional contours of the existing tooth shapes.

The information from the diagnostic wax-up may be transferred or delivered to the teeth in a provisional or definitive way via a PVS stent with the use of either Bis-acryl or restorative composite resin materials. If the latter material is used, a translucent PVS stent is used to allow light curing.

For both methods, the intra-oral transfer as a concept is similar with slight differences being in the detail of application. The methods are further described below.

4.5.1 Prototype Provisional Try-In

This technique allows for the transfer of a Bis-acryl material to the teeth in a provisional manner to trial the aesthetic and functional changes for a short period of time (hours or days). The teeth are not adhesively treated with the material being engaged by 'shrink fit' into embrasure spaces and undercuts.

If a longer trial time is required (up to 8 weeks), the buccal surface of the teeth may be adhesively treated by spot etch and bond application to allow the Bis-acryl material to 'shrink fit' and adhesively bond to the teeth for improved retention and durability. The patient must be warned that the material in non-bonded areas may peel off and is likely to fracture due to the brittle nature of the Bis-acryl material.

The required clinical stages are listed in Table 4.1 and depicted in the following case (Figs. 4.41, 4.42, 4.43, 4.44, 4.45, and 4.46).

Table 4.1 The clinical stages required for the 'Prototype provisional try-in' technique

'Prototype provisional try-in' technique
1. Tooth prophylaxis
2. Selection of impression tray (size, perforated or non-perforated & no adhesive placed)
3. Impression of diagnostic cast wax-up with a PVS putty and light-body wash material
4. Polymerisation of PVS material
5. Separate the impression tray from the PVS stent
6. Trim and adjust PVS stent as required
7. Place PVS stent into impression tray
8. Load PVS stent with Bis-acryl material
9. Locate impression tray and PVS stent—firm axial directed force for stability
10. Remove excess Bis-acryl material
11. Allow polymerisation of Bis-acryl material
12. Remove the impression tray from the PVS stent
13. Remove PVS stent and excess Bis-acryl material
14. Repair any air voids in Bis-acryl with shade-matched flowable composite resin material
15. Finish & Polish

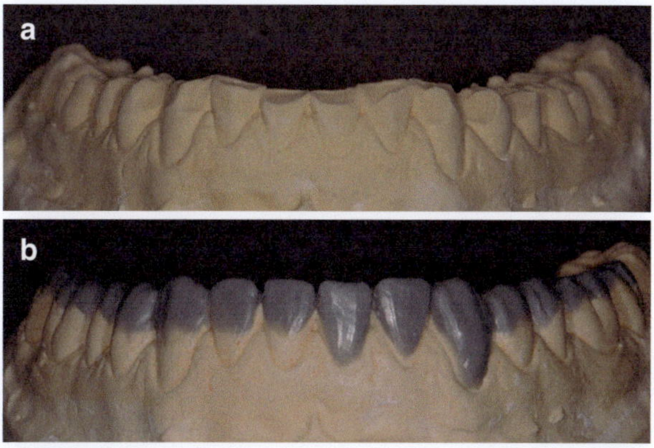

Fig. 4.41 (**a**, **b**) Analogue diagnostic cast waxing of proposed tooth form with improvements upon the aesthetic and functional contours of the existing tooth shapes

4.5.2 Prototype Definitive Restoration

If the tooth trial is to be placed for a longer period of time (6–12 weeks) or the teeth are to be restored in a definitive manner with restorative composite resin material, a translucent PVS stent is used to deliver the material to the teeth to aid in the curing of the material.

The receiving tooth surfaces may be partially or fully adhesively prepared by etching and bonding procedures. The amount of surface coverage for adhesive treatment (bonding area) is dependent upon the amount of time the functional assessment is required. More surface coverage is required for longer time spans, and full surface coverage is required for definitive restoration. It is also advised that for definitive restoration, if multiple adjacent teeth are being treated, then alternate teeth are treated simultaneously to prevent restoration fusion.

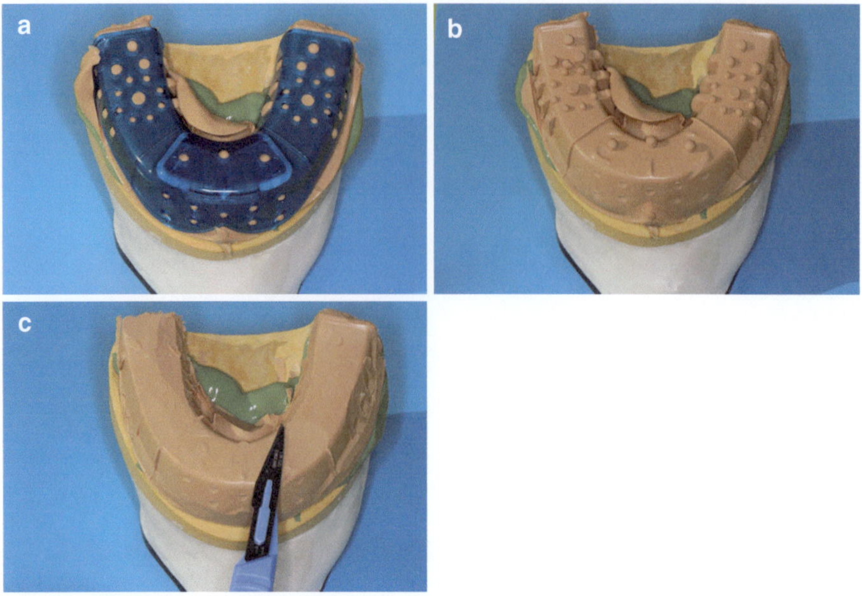

Fig. 4.42 (**a**) Impression of diagnostic cast wax-up with PVS putty and light-body wash material in a perforated impression tray. (**b**) Impression tray separated from PVS stent after polymerisation of PVS material. (**c**) PVS stent trimmed and adjusted

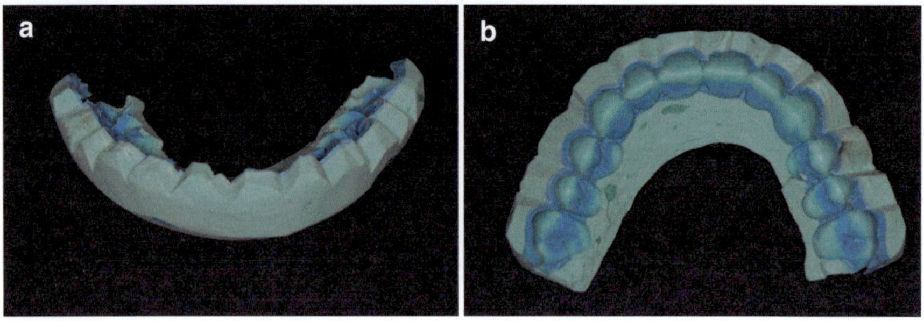

Fig. 4.43 (**a**, **b**) PVS stent trimmed with a gingival scalloped pattern to aid removal of excess material

A case highlighting the definitive restoration of palatal surfaces of multiple maxillary anterior teeth is shown (Figs. 4.47, 4.48, 4.49, 4.50, 4.51, 4.52, and 4.53), and the clinical stages and tips are listed in Table 4.2.

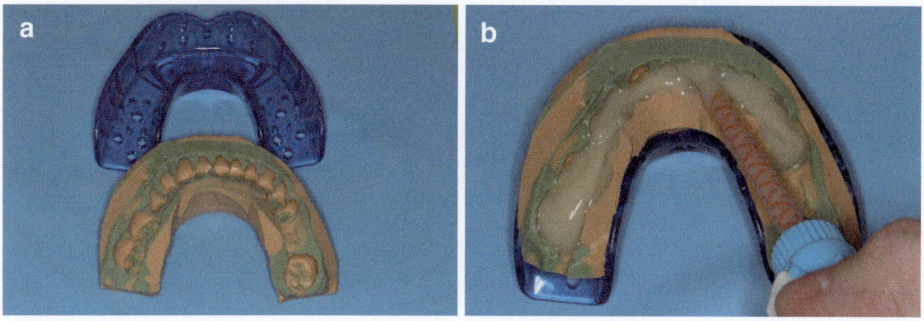

Fig. 4.44 (**a**, **b**) Trimmed PVS stent placed back into impression tray and loaded with Bis-acryl material

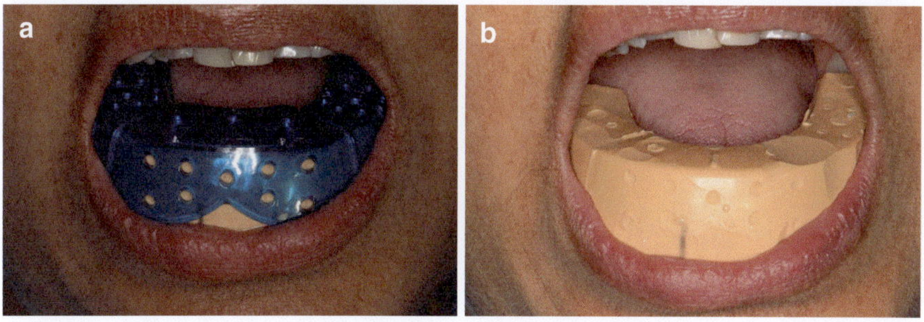

Fig. 4.45 (**a**) Impression tray and PVS stent located. (**b**) Removal of impression tray leaving PVS stent in situ

Fig. 4.46 (**a**) Pre-operative situation. (**b**) Shrink-fit Bis-acryl prototype provisional try-in

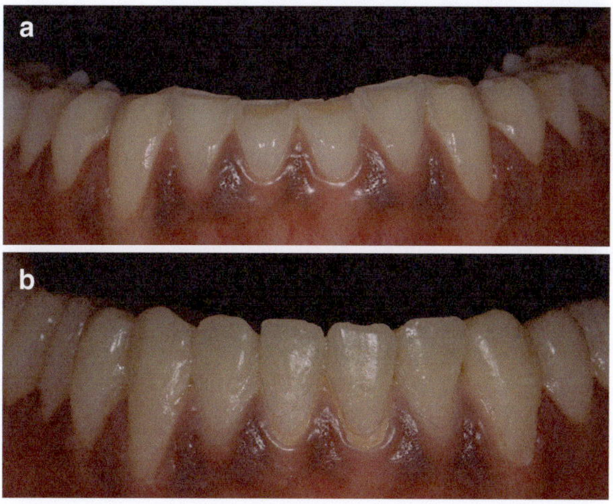

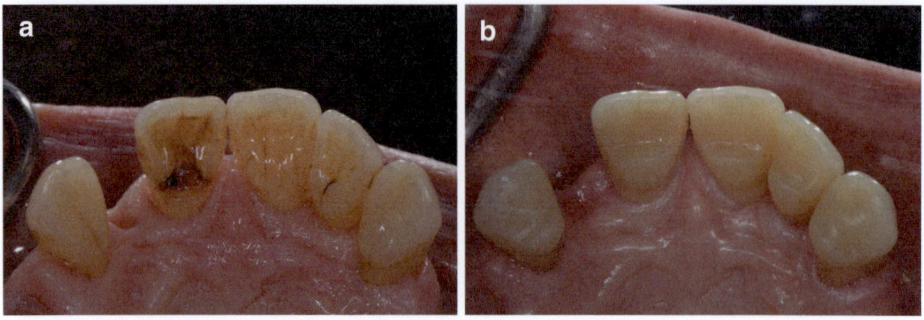

Fig. 4.47 (**a**) Pre-operative palatal surfaces of maxillary anterior teeth. (**b**) Post-operative definitive adhesively bonded composite resin restorations with cingulum rests to allow engagement of a maxillary cobalt chromium removable partial denture prosthesis

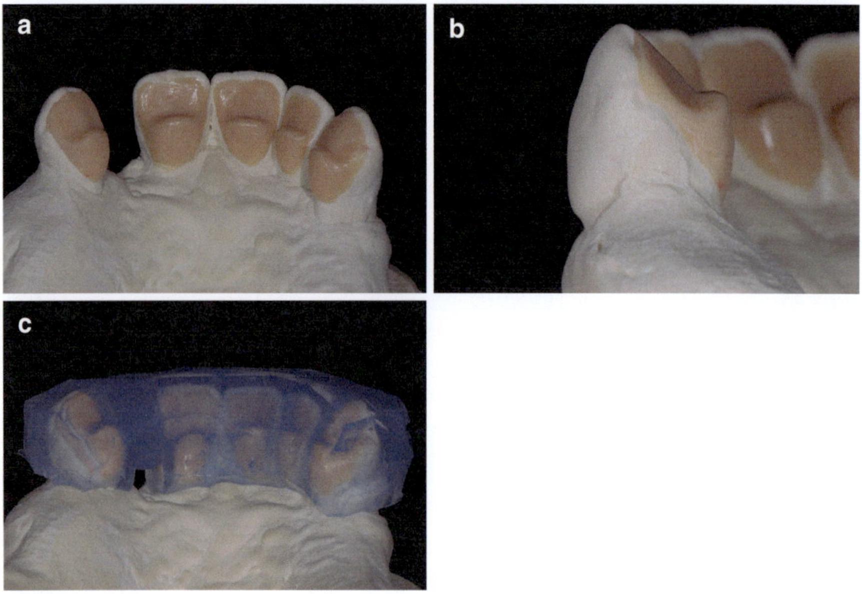

Fig. 4.48 (**a**) Diagnostic cast wax-up of maxillary teeth with sloping palatal surfaces, diagnostically augmented with wax to produce functional surfaces designed with cingulum rest seats to allow engagement of a maxillary cobalt chromium removable partial denture prosthesis. (**b**) Tooth 13 with wax augmentation design details. (**c**) Translucent PVS stent with at least 2 mm of material thickness

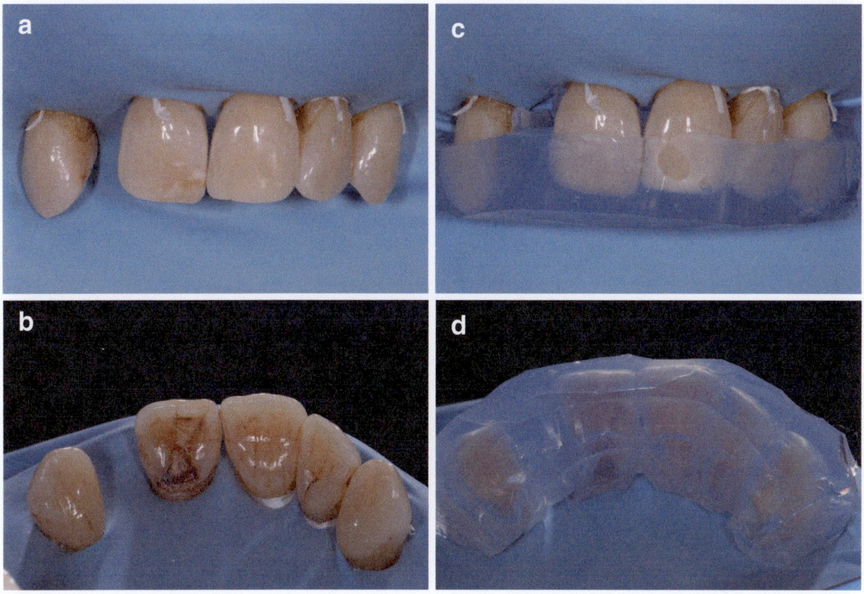

Fig. 4.49 (**a**, **b**) Isolation of anterior maxillary teeth (**c**, **d**) Translucent PVS stent with at least 2 mm of material thickness

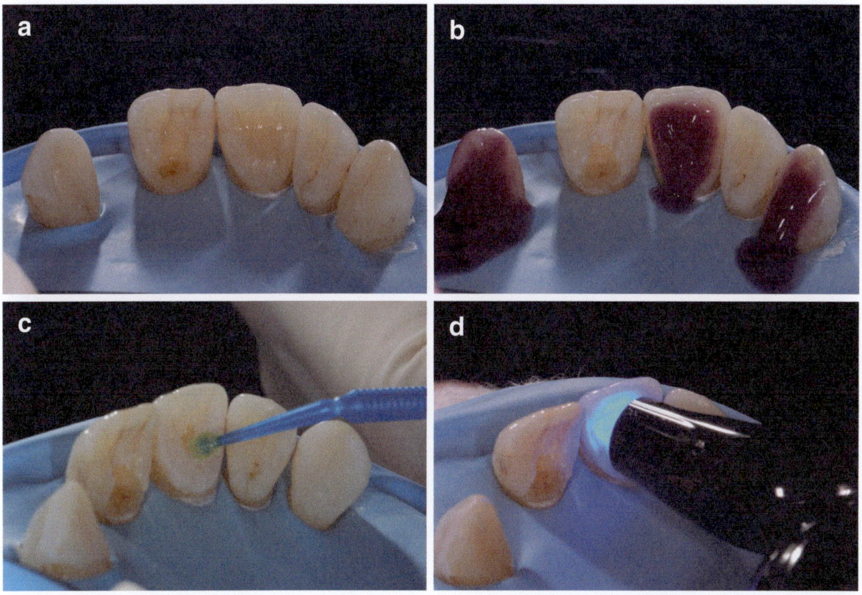

Fig. 4.50 (**a**) Barrier removal of teeth (refer to Fig. 2.13) and adhesive preparation of alternate teeth 13, 21 & 23 with (**b**) 37% phosphoric acid and (**c**) eighth generation bonding agent application, air dry and (**d**) light cure

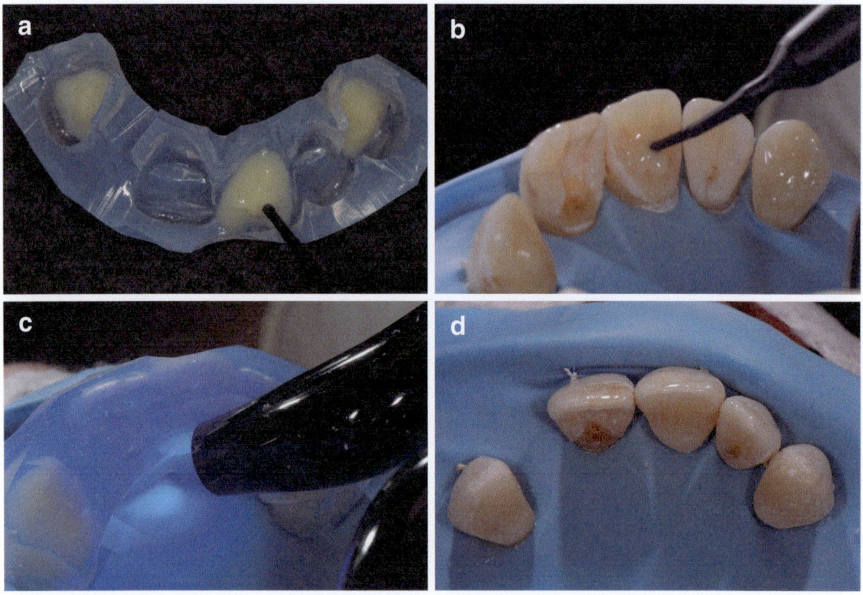

Fig. 4.51 (**a**) Loading of translucent PVS stent and (**b**) teeth with highly filled flowable composite resin material. (**c**) Translucent PVS stent location and light cure through the material. (**d**) Bonded composite resin restorations on teeth 13, 21 & 23 after stent removal

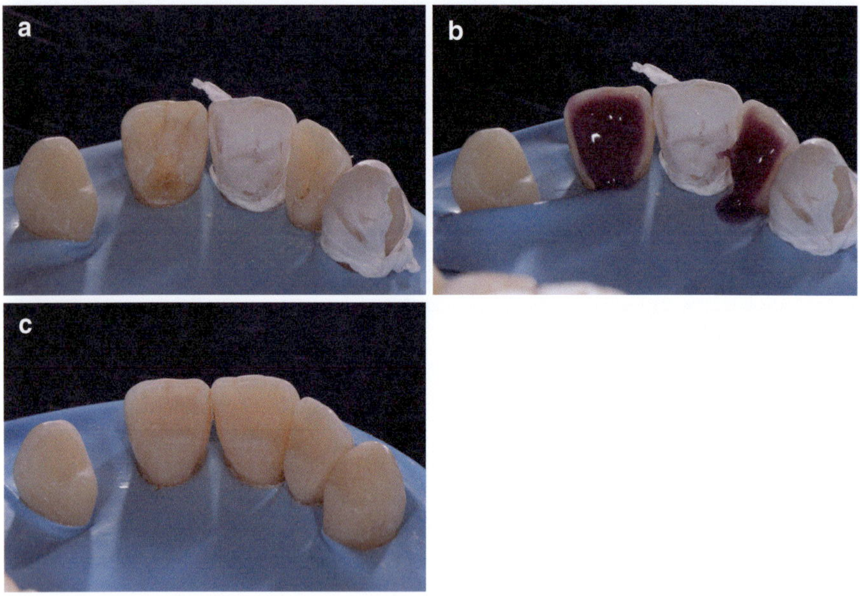

Fig. 4.52 (**a**) PTFE tape placement on restorations of teeth 13, 21 & 24. (**b**) Adhesive preparation of alternate teeth 11 & 22 (**c**) Bonded composite resin restorations on teeth 13, 11 & 22 after stent and PTFE tape removal

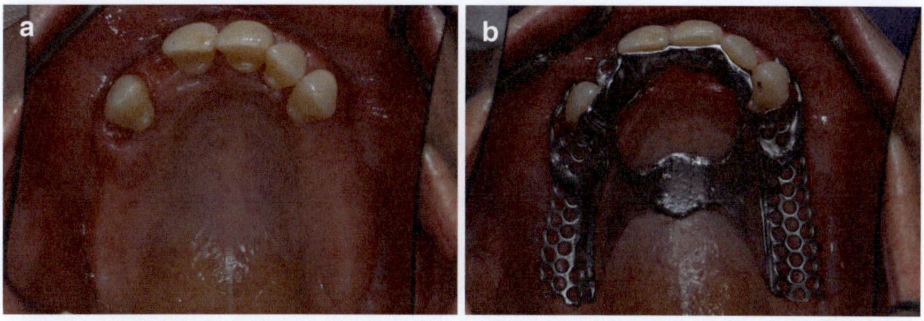

Fig. 4.53 (**a**) Definitive adhesively bonded composite resin restorations on teeth 13, 11, 21, 22 & 24. (**b**) Engagement of a maxillary cobalt chromium removable partial denture prosthesis framework

Table 4.2 The clinical stages and tips required for the 'Prototype definitive restoration' technique

'Prototype definitive restoration' technique	
Stages	Tips
1. Isolation	Rubber dam Floss ligature stabilisation
2. Stent preparation	Impression of diagnostic cast wax-up with a translucent PVS material with at least 2 mm of material thickness. Freehand or with impression tray (translucent, non-perforated & no adhesive placed). Polymerisation of translucent PVS material Separate the impression tray from the translucent PVS stent Trim and adjust translucent PVS stent as required Tested intra-orally for fit and location
3. Barrier removal	Ultrasonic scaler Prophylaxis Sandblast
4. Tooth preparation	Restoration dissection Caries removal Sandblast bonding surfaces
5. Adhesive preparation	Adjacent teeth protection (PTFE tape, metal or acetate strips) Total-etch technique Rinse & dry Fourth or eighth generation bonding agent Indirect air dry Light polymerise
6. Composite resin material placement	Use flowable (highly filled) or paste composite resin material Heat paste composite resin material Load translucent PVS stent with composite resin material (alternate teeth) Load tooth with composite resin material (alternate teeth) Locate translucent PVS stent—firm positive pressure for stability Remove excess composite resin material Light polymerises through translucent PVS stent Remove translucent PVS stent Light polymerise again through oxygen-blocking material
7. Finish & polishing	Finish—Excess resin removed with scalpel blades and pointed fine diamond burs. Abrasive disks at low-speed revolution and interdental strips to define the embrasure spaces and transitional line angles Occlusal check and refinements Polish—Aluminium oxide impregnated points/discs and sequential diamond impregnated polishing pastes with a felt wheel at high-speed revolution

Further Reading

1. Chu SJ. Range and mean distribution frequency of individual tooth width of the maxillary anterior dentition. Pract Proced Aesthet Dent. 2007;19(4):209–15.
2. Dietschi D. Free-hand composite resin restorations: a key to anterior aesthetics. Pract Periodontics Aesthet Dent. 1995;7(7):15–24.
3. Duarte SJ, Schnider P, Lorezon AP. The importance of width/length ratios of maxillary anterior permanent teeth in esthetic rehabilitation. Eur J Esthet Dent. 2008;3(3):224–34.
4. Gurel G, Bichacho N. Permanent diagnostic provisional restorations for predictable results when redesigning the smile. Pract Proced Aesthet Dent. 2006;18(5):281–6.
5. Jefferies SR. The art and science of abrasive finishing and polishing in restorative dentistry. Dent Clin N Am. 1998;42(4):613–27.
6. Lenhard M. Closing diastemas with resin composite restorations. Eur J Esthet Dent. 2008;3(3):258–68.
7. McLaren EA, Schoenbaum TR. The bonded functional esthetic prototype: part 1. Inside Dentistry. 2014;9(1).
8. McLaren EA. The bonded functional esthetic prototype: part 2. Inside Dentistry. 2014;9(5).
9. Sattar M, Patel M, Alani A. Clinical applications of polytetrafluoroethylene (PTFE) tape in restorative dentistry. Br Dent J. 2017;222:151–8.

Direct Adhesive Restorations

5

Contents

Learning Outcomes

- Appreciate planning aspects for the provision of direct composite resin restorations.
- Learn predictable and proficient sequences in providing direct posterior restorations.
- Revise the use and advantages of sectional matrix bands for the provision of Class II restorations.
- Learn generic sequencing of layering Class IV direct anterior restorations.
- Consider the use of alternative adhesive restorative materials for the restoration of Class V defects.

A. Alani, M. Patel, *Adhesive Techniques in Restorative Dentistry*, BDJ Clinician's Guides, https://doi.org/10.1007/978-3-032-07346-4_5

5.1 Introduction

Operative procedures to manage carious cavities or the replacement of restorations that have been previously provided due to caries is a cornerstone of dentistry. The management of the carious lesion has evolved progressively over time, with the approach that less aggressive tissue removal is of greater benefit to the overall scheme of preserving pulp vitality and health. Unlike historical approaches requiring retention form incorporated into the cavity design, modern adhesive techniques aim to optimise the adhesive bond and seal without the need to grossly modify the residual tooth structure.

Tooth type, restoration class and size are significant predictors of difficulty in the provision of treatment, and with most clinical presentations, there often will be variants to the norm. Following a standardised protocol repeatedly will allow a clinician to develop confidence through their experience and will improve clinical efficiency and enjoyment of delivering these procedures.

5.2 General Procedures

Prior to formal instrumentation, an occlusal examination should identify the intercuspal position contacts and any guidance movements that may be encroached upon by the new restoration. These need to be borne in mind during the restoration provision, as the rubber dam application will prevent ongoing assessment during instrumentation (Fig. 5.1). Without appreciation of the baseline static and dynamic occlusion from the outset, a carefully placed and anatomically contoured conformative restoration may need significant adjustment once the rubber dam isolation is removed and the occlusion checked and compared to the baseline record.

Gaining access to the carious lesion should result in the minimal amount of enamel removal to visualise the dentine whilst also eliminating enamel that is

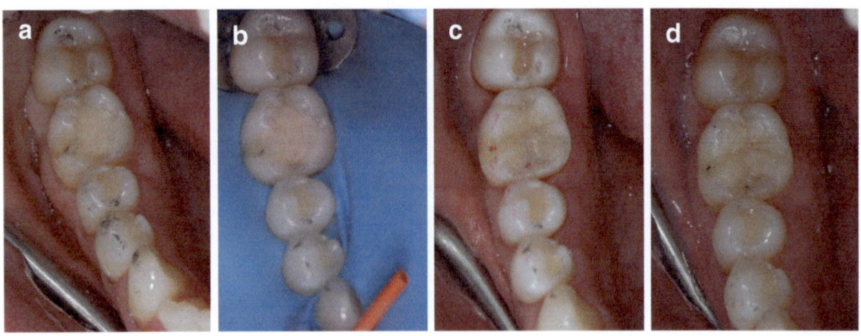

Fig. 5.1 (**a**) Occlusal examination of fourth quadrant to identify quadrant occlusal contacts prior to (**b**) rubber dam isolation and (**c, d**) conformative restoration of tooth 36 with a Class 1 composite resin restoration

stained, debilitated or excessively weakened. Enamel removal can later be revisited if the dentinal extent of the lesion is greater than first envisaged. A sound, definitive enamel margin makes adhesive bonding easier and post-cure finishing neater. Once the enamel margin has been established, the clinician could consider bevelling in non-loading occlusal areas to increase surface area for the adhesive bond.

Once the dentine has been breached, so begins the crucial process of carious tissue removal. The key considerations here are protection of the pulp and achieving an optimal seal at the periphery of the lesion. Where pulpal symptoms are absent and the extent of the lesion is in close proximity to the pulp roof or horns, caries may be left to avoid traumatic exposure. Where the carious margin is remote from the pulp, excavation to sound dentine is advised. With regards to the seal, the important aspect of cavity design is the enamel–dentine junction (EDJ). All infected dentine (damp, soft and darkened) should be removed (Fig. 5.2), especially from the EDJ, as this is likely to jeopardise the peripheral seal of the restoration, the sequelae of which may include post-operative sensitivity, microleakage, secondary caries, pulpitis, loss of pulp vitality and loss of restoration. Once the carious removal process is completed, attention can be diverted towards the need to modify the shape and form of the cavity design, such as the removal of any sharp internal line angles, cavosurface margin correction or further bevelling and flaring of the enamel interdental margins.

Adjuncts to cavity preparation include alumina blasting (using 50 micron alumina particles) the residual tooth tissue once the caries has been removed. Unidentified remnant restorative material may also be removed during this process. The alumina blasting preparation facilitates adhesion by roughening the tooth surface but can also disintegrate any underlying dentine staining that could improve the aesthetics of the final restoration.

The 30-s application of the 37.5% phosphoric acid etchant on enamel margins should extend past the cavity margin to optimise the marginal seal. With certain adhesive systems, the bond can be produced on unetched dentine; therefore, they require selective acid etching of the enamel only. If required, the dentine may be etched for 15 s utilising a total etch approach. The application of the resin bonding agent may require multiple coats and should be scrubbed into the tooth surfaces for 20 s or more, depending upon the manufacturer's instructions. Excessive pooling within areas of the cavity can be addressed by soaking excess material with a new microbrush to leave a shiny tooth surface. Light air drying will evaporate the solvent from the bonding agent and can aid in a consistent thin adhesive film with no pooling present before light polymerisation for 20 s. Care must be taken whilst air drying so that water and oil droplets from the 3:1 syringe do not contaminate the bonded area. It is advised that 'indirect air drying' is undertaken by deflecting the air stream from the 3:1 syringe against an intraoral mirror towards the tooth such that any droplets will contact the mirror and not the tooth surfaces (Fig. 5.3).

There are a range of instruments that can be used to manipulate and model composite resin materials, which may consist of non-stick-coated metal instruments, silicone-tipped instruments, and brushes coated with minimal amounts of modelling resin (Figs. 5.4 and 5.5). The modelling resins are unfilled dimethacrylate light-cure

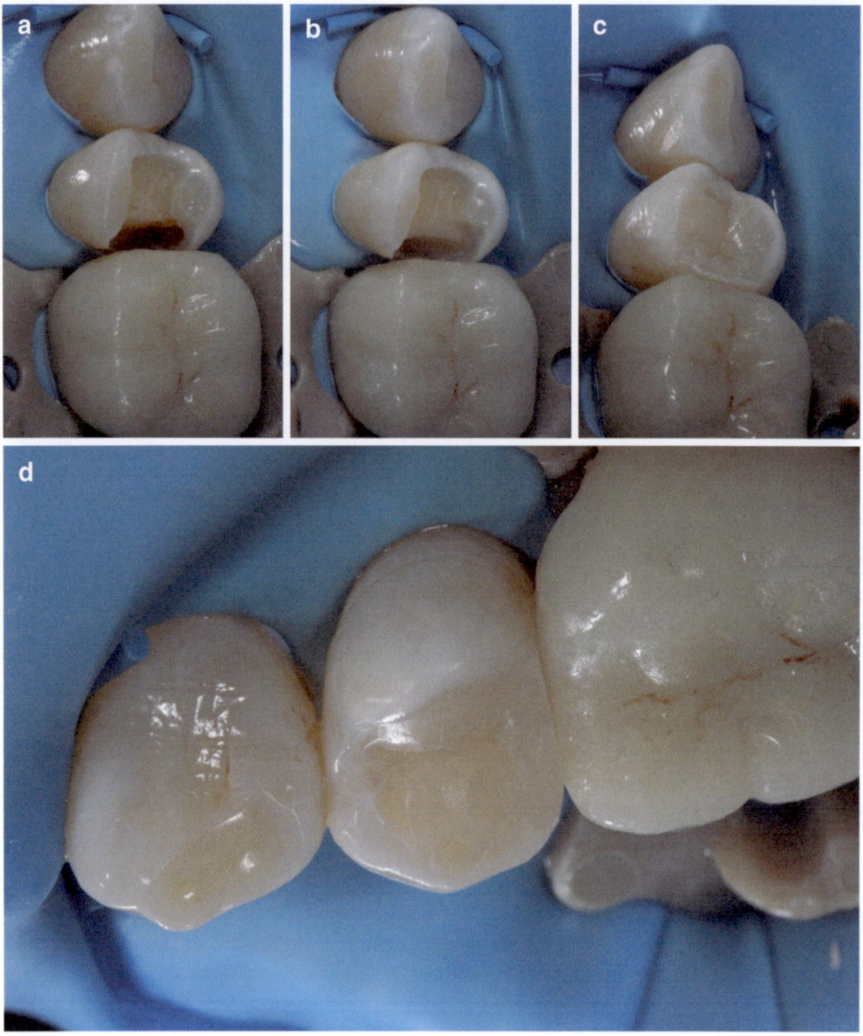

Fig. 5.2 (**a**, **b**) Caries removal from tooth 15 distal box and (**c**, **d**) completed Class II composite resin restoration

products that are indicated for use to lubricate the brush or instrument and also to reactivate the inhibited dispersion bonding surface between composite layers prior to repair procedures of old composite resin restorations (Fig. 5.5). Straight probe instruments are good at delivering the composite resin material increments to the tooth and manipulating the resin contours for cusp shape, mapping fissures and primary anatomy. After light polymerisation, scalpel blades (Nos. 11, 12 & 15) may be used to remove excess resin material and flash from tooth structure and interdental areas to prevent plaque aggregation, marginal staining and gingival irritation (Fig. 5.6).

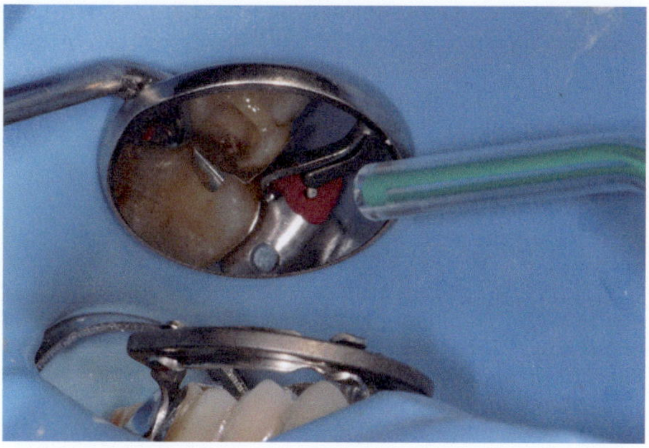

Fig. 5.3 Indirect air drying allows deflecting the air stream from the 3:1 syringe against an intraoral mirror directed towards the tooth surfaces

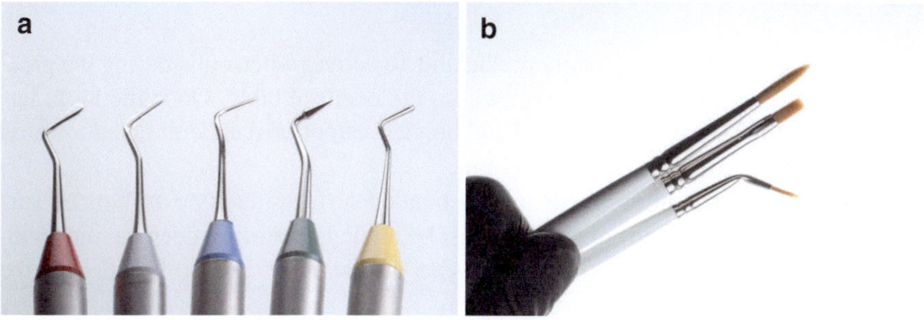

Fig. 5.4 Examples of a (**a**) non-stick metal instruments and (**b**) modelling brushes. (Images courtesy of Dr. Minesh Patel)

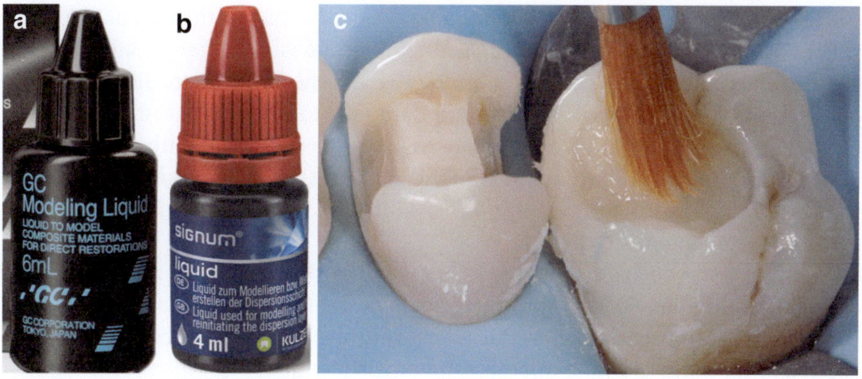

Fig. 5.5 (**a**, **b**) Modelling resin can be used to (**c**) lubricate brush for modelling composite resin material during its placement. (Image (**a**) courtesy of GC U.K and image (**b**) courtesy of Kulzer Ltd.)

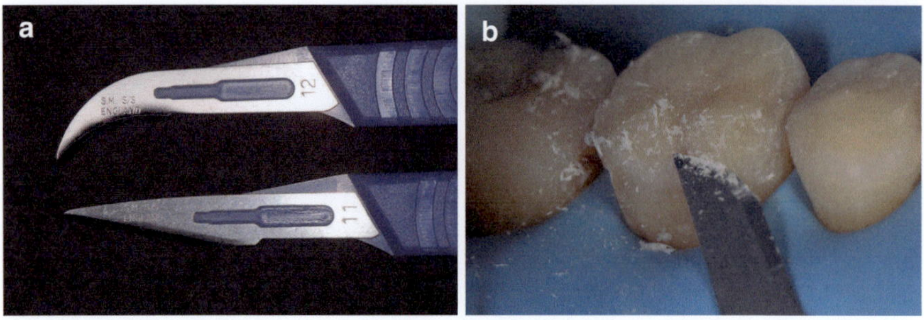

Fig. 5.6 (**a**, **b**) Scalpel blades (No. 11,12 & 15) used to remove excess resin material and flash

5.3 Class I Restoration

The Class I restoration is relatively predictable to deliver when considering the presence of an accessible enamel margin within the occlusal table. Once the tooth has been isolated and the cavity prepared and bonded, attention can be directed towards restoration placement and occlusal design.

In the Class I restoration, there are five bonded surfaces and one un-bonded surface, resulting in a C-factor of 5. Care must be made in restoring deep cavities with thin peripheral walls that shrinkage stresses do not have any profound negative effect upon the residual tooth structure.

Incremental application and curing of the composite resin material to reduce shrinkage stresses can be considered here. A flowable composite resin gingival base layer (up to 4 mm thickness) is placed to adapt to the cavity floor and block out the underlying dentine colour and light polymerised. Subsequent occlusal cuspal build-up of the cavity is undertaken as each cuspal increment is placed and light polymerised for 10 s. Final tints and intensities may be added to the cuspal ridges and colour staining placed into the fissure pattern to allow harmonious aesthetic integration of the restoration into the tooth and the rest of the dentition (Figs. 5.7 and 5.8). As the restoration process is additive, with careful study of the static and dynamic occlusion and adjacent tooth anatomical form, the shape and contour of the restoration is built up with minimal occlusal adjustments and refinements required.

If the original occlusal anatomy of the tooth is still intact and not cavitated, a recording of this can be made prior to cavity cutting and caries access with a transparent silicone material or flowable composite material. The chosen material is applied to the surface with a microbrush immersed within prior to polymerising or curing. This is then later applied to the uncured final composite increment to shape the surface and recreate the previous anatomy prior to the final light polymerisation. This 'occlusal stamp' technique will aid in the recreation of the original occlusal table anatomy within the composite restoration, with minimal occlusal adjustments required. It is described and depicted in Sect. 5.9.1.

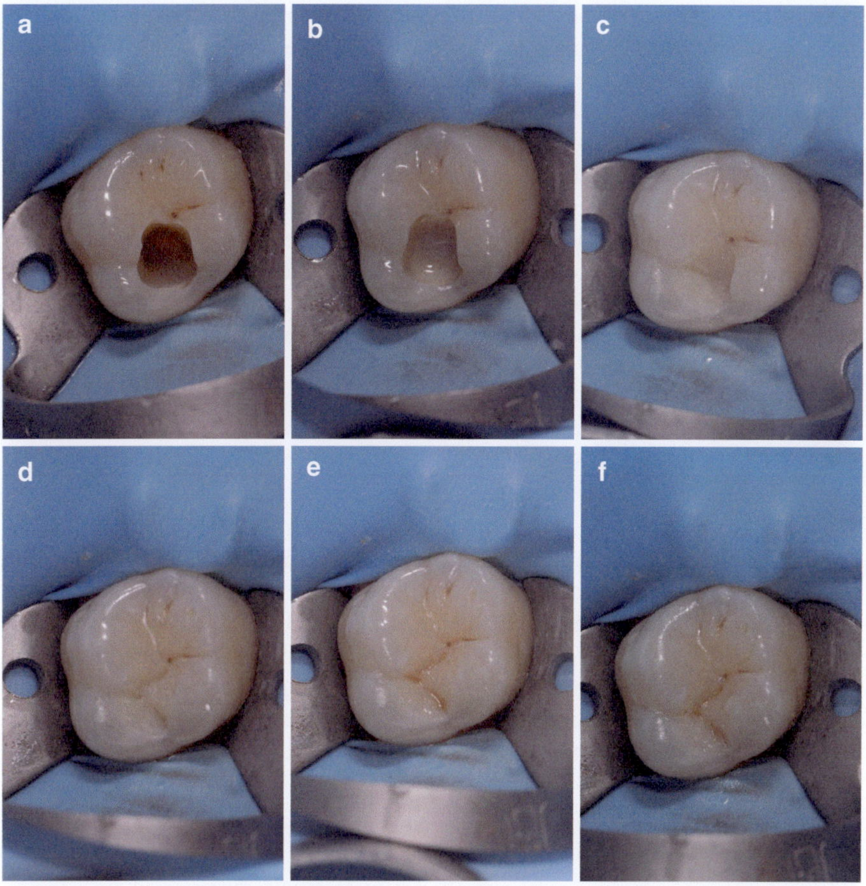

Fig. 5.7 Tooth 26 Class 1 composite resin restoration incremental build-up. (**a**) Completed occlusal cavity preparation. (**b**) Flowable composite resin base. (**c**, **d**) Cuspal incremental build-up. (**e**, **f**) additions of fissure stain and cusp highlights

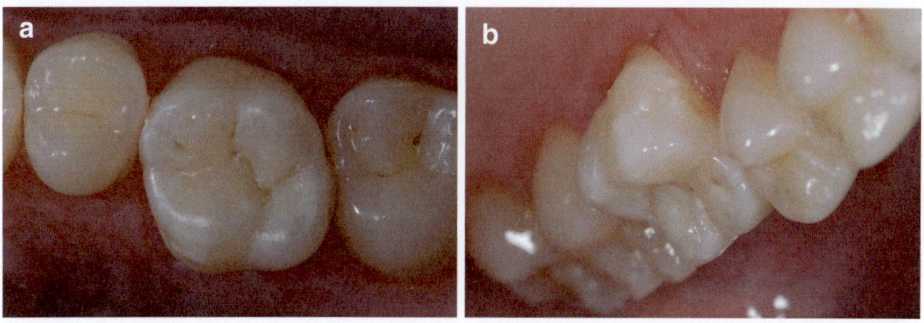

Fig. 5.8 (**a**, **b**) Tooth 26 Class 1 composite resin restoration showing aesthetic integration

Once the composite is placed, attention can be diverted to finishing and polishing. The majority of finishing a restoration should take place with the rubber dam isolation still in place. The retraction provided will allow protection of oral soft tissues, especially if scalpel blades are used (Fig. 5.6). After rubber dam removal, the occlusion can be checked and refinements made to the restoration's functional surfaces. Thereafter, polishing procedures can be carried out to ensure a void and defect-free lustrous restoration surface. This can take the form by use of aluminium oxide or diamond impregnated abrasive rubber burs to ensure adequate smoothness of the main body of the restoration and the marginal interface between the composite restoration and the enamel. The burs are available in a variety of shapes and sizes and can be used in conjunction with fine diamond abrasive pastes for enhanced polishing.

5.4 Class II Restoration

The Class II restoration is significantly more demanding on the clinician than the Class I due to the proximal component of the cavity. Interdental pre-wedging with wooden or plastic interdental wedges can prise open the interdental contact to allow easier instrumentation in the interdental areas and protect the adjacent teeth from iatrogenic damage (Fig. 5.9). Wedges also serve to protect the rubber dam from tearing during cavity preparation (Fig. 5.10). The wedge placement should be just cervical to the deepest portion of the proximal box area. Where the interproximal contact is tight, the area can be relieved with an interproximal strip.

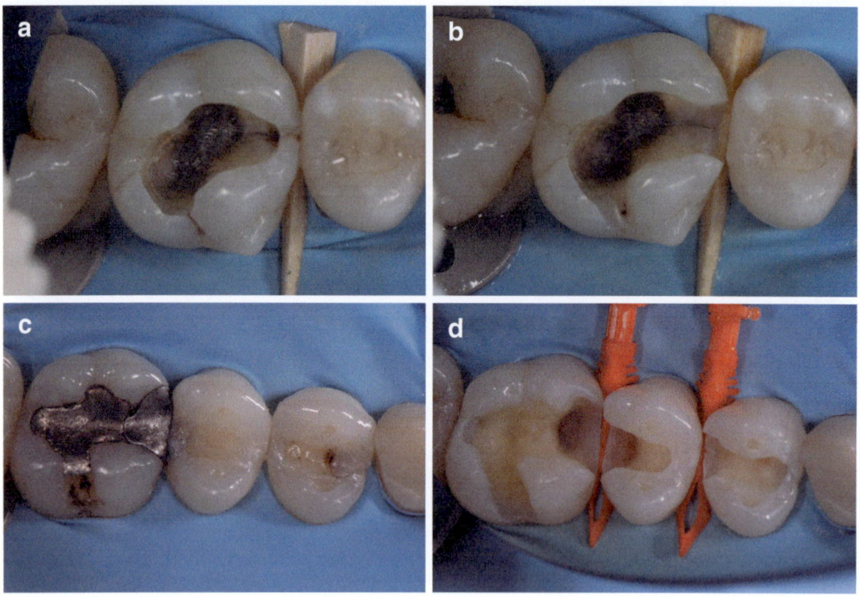

Fig. 5.9 Pre-wedging with (**a**, **b**) wooden or (**c**, **d**) plastic interdental wedges to allow easier access and instrumentation in the interdental areas

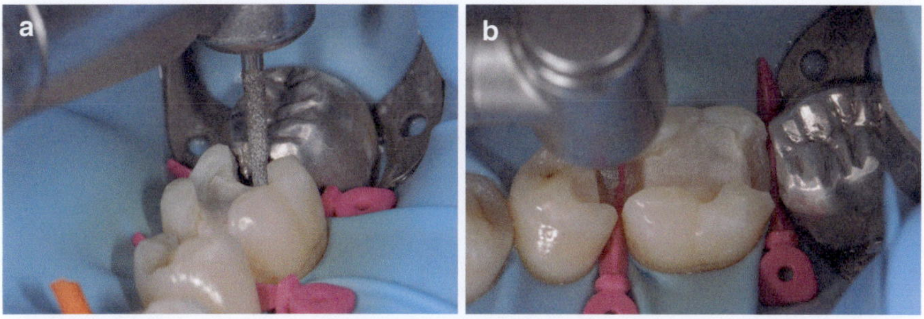

Fig. 5.10 (**a**, **b**) Interdental wedges protecting the rubber dam during proximal surface cavity preparation

The interdental contact area of the affected surfaces needs to be identified prior to instrumentation. The cavity is initially cut in the fossa area and then is extended into the proximal area towards the interdental contact point. The outline form and base of the proximal box need to be smooth without any ledges. The contact point is to be fully broken in both buccal-palatal/lingual and occluso-gingival directions, and the enamel interdental box margins flared (Fig. 5.11). This will aid to place a matrix band with ease and, in addition, allows the convenient form of the final restoration for margin inspection in the long term.

The crucial aspect of restoration delivery is the management of the matrix band and ensuring fabrication of an adequate interdental contact point to the adjacent tooth, whilst ensuring the cavity is optimally restored.

Sectional matrix systems may have the advantage over traditional matrix bands and strips in that they are designed to allow delivery of anatomical restoration shapes. The metal matrix foils used are available in different sizes and are convex in form to allow for a natural anatomical contour of the restoration (Fig. 5.12). The size of the matrix foil should be chosen on the premise that it will be placed at the same height as the marginal ridge of the adjacent tooth and extends adequately to cover the base of the cavity in the gingival aspect. To avoid restoration gingival overhangs, the use of anatomically shaped plastic wedges approximates the matrix to the base of the tooth in the cervical area. A plastic wedge is optimally shaped to sit over the natural shape of the interdental papillae without over compression as is found with the triangular cross-sectional shape of wooden wedges (Figs. 5.9, 5.10, and 5.11). Plastic wedges also have the ability to be stacked upon one another to aid in the optimal seal of the foil to the tooth and to allow minimal finishing to the restoration. If it is found that the wedge compresses the matrix foil into the cavity and distorts its shape, it is possible to delay the placement of the wedge ('delayed wedging') and restore the first 2 mm at the base of the box first to allow the metal foil to then stabilise against the base restoration without shape distortion that will affect the interdental contour.

Finally, the sectional metal matrix ring when engaged into the interdental embrasure spaces, allows separation of adjacent teeth to accommodate the thickness of the metal matrix foil used to allow formation of a tight interproximal contact. The tines of

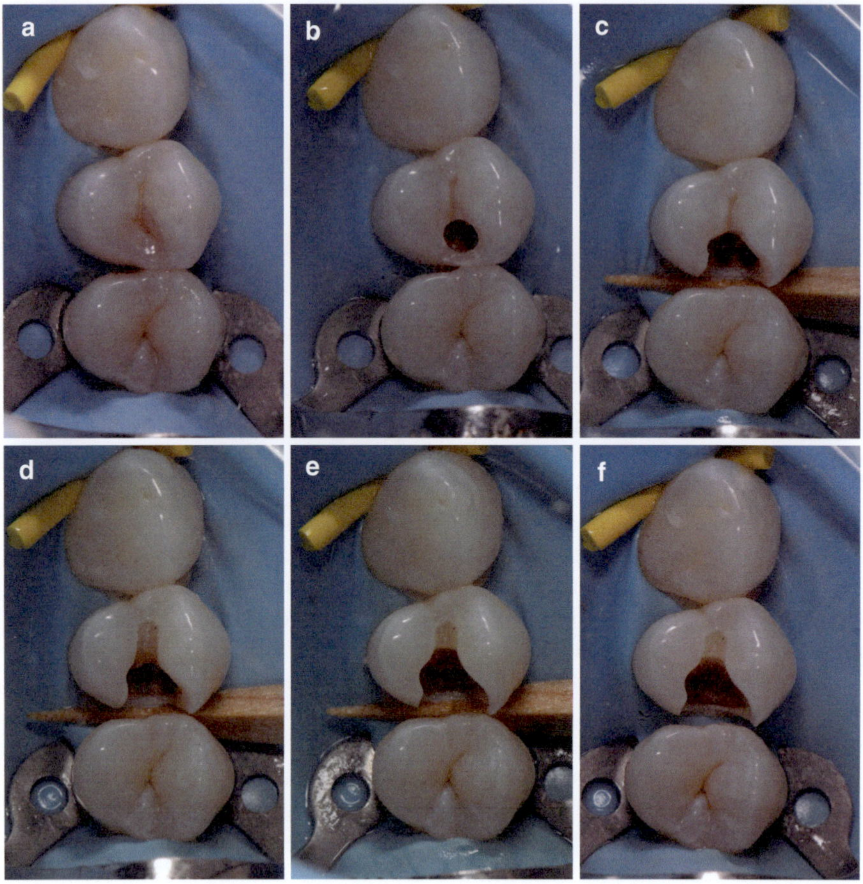

Fig. 5.11 Cavity preparation evolution for tooth 24 distal occlusal cavity. (**a**) Pre-operative situation. (**b**) Occlusal cavity access. (**c**) Wedge and interdental extension. (**d**) Occlusal fissure cavity extension. (**e**) Rounding and flaring of outline form. (**f**) Completed cavity preparation

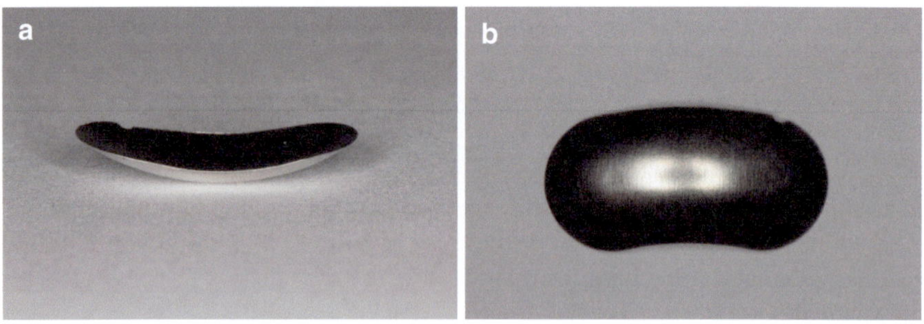

Fig. 5.12 (**a**, **b**) Convex form of posterior sectional matrix metal foil

the sectional ring (system dependent) are shaped to allow approximation of the interdental wedge; they secure and adapt the metal foil matrix to the interdental embrasure spaces (Figs. 5.13 and 5.14). Attention must be made as the rubber dam clamp can interfere with the engagement of the tines into the embrasure space, which may affect the ability of the ring to separate the teeth, as shown previously (Fig. 2.10).

Adjunctive measures to ensure matrix adaptation include the placement of materials to push the matrix foil to ensure adequate adaptation between the matrix and the tooth. Materials such as polytetrafluoroethylene (PTFE) tape could be utilised in

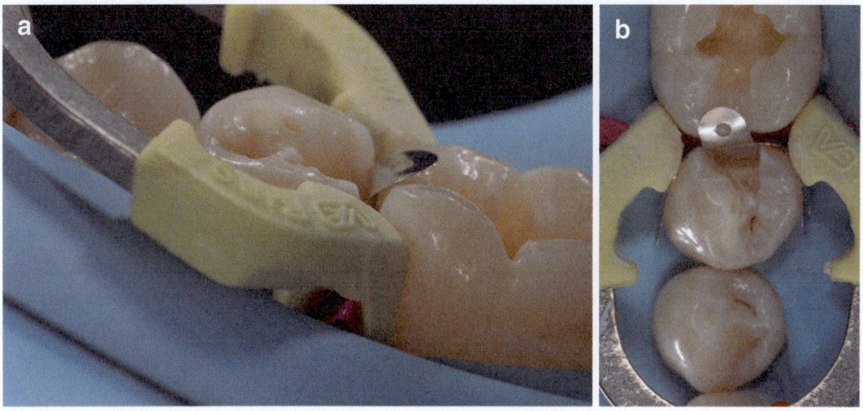

Fig. 5.13 (**a**) Lingual and (**b**) occlusal views of mandibular teeth 45 & 46 with sectional matrix system assembly comprising of a metal matrix foil, plastic interdental wedge and sectional metal ring. The sectional ring secures and adapts the metal foil matrix, the tines allow approximation of the interdental wedge

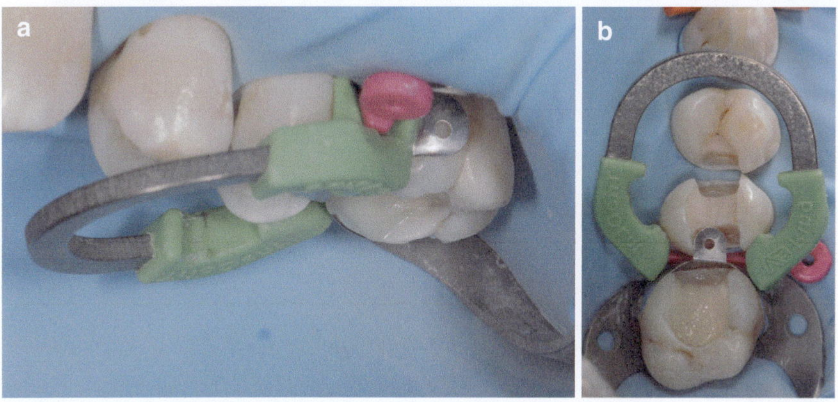

Fig. 5.14 (**a**) Buccal and (**b**) occlusal views of maxillary teeth 24, 25 & 26 with sectional matrix system assembly comprising of a metal matrix foil, plastic interdental wedge and sectional metal ring. The sectional ring secures and adapts the metal foil matrix, the tines allow approximation of the interdental wedge

this manner (Fig. 5.15). Another advantage of the sectional matrix system is the ability of the ring to separate adjacent tooth units to accommodate the matrix thickness for contact point creation. The tines of the ring may also be customised to allow improved adaptation of the matrix foil to the tooth; however, this may interfere with wedge placement. From here, the matrix foil is contoured and burnished to the adjacent tooth to create an appropriate contact area and marginal ridge.

Once assembled, the matrix system will contain the 37% phosphoric acid etch and selected bonding agent within the cavity to prevent fusion of excess material to the adjacent tooth. Efforts can now focus on restoration placement. The deepest portion of the proximal box and base of the cavity can be restored with a bulk fill flowable composite material, allowing optimum void-free material adaptation to the cavity floor. This gingival base layer should be no more than 4 mm in thickness. Placement of an increment of composite resin paste material against the metal matrix foil forms the proximal wall marginal ridge; this can be adapted with a microbrush lubricated with a modelling resin. Before light polymerisation of this increment, the ridge area should be rolled with a probe instrument to allow formation of the marginal ridge and to aid the passing of dental floss through the contact. As a general guide, the thickness of the material placed should match the adjacent tooth's ridge for height and contour. The Class II cavity has now been converted to a Class I in a modified 'centripetal build-up' technique. The sectional matrix assembly may be carefully removed at this stage if required (Fig. 5.16). There may be a risk of gingival bleeding through the rubber dam. The rest of the cavity may now be

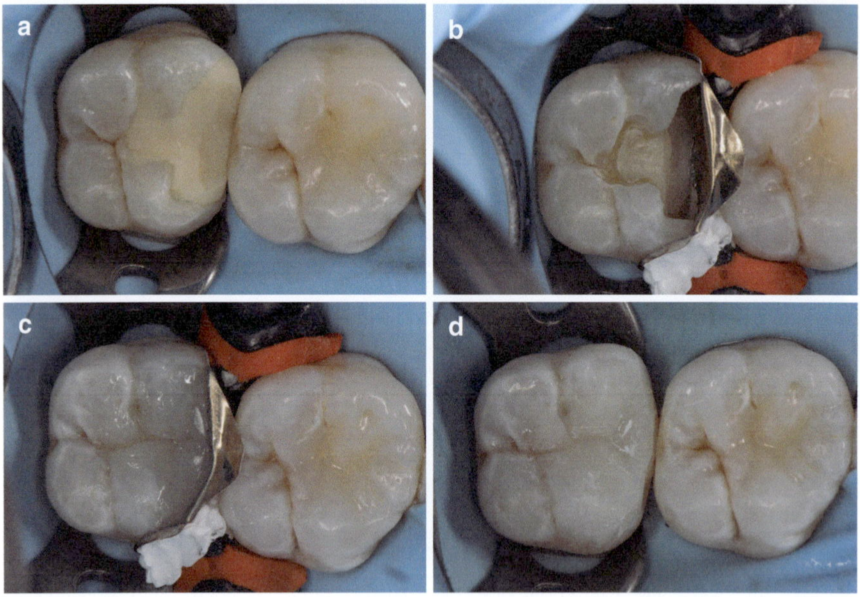

Fig. 5.15 Tooth 17 MO Class II composite resin restoration. (**a**) Pre-operative situation. (**b**) Cavity preparation and PTFE tape used in the palatal embrasure area to adapt the metal matrix foil to the tooth to allow (**c**, **d**) recreation of adequate palatal embrasure shape of the restoration

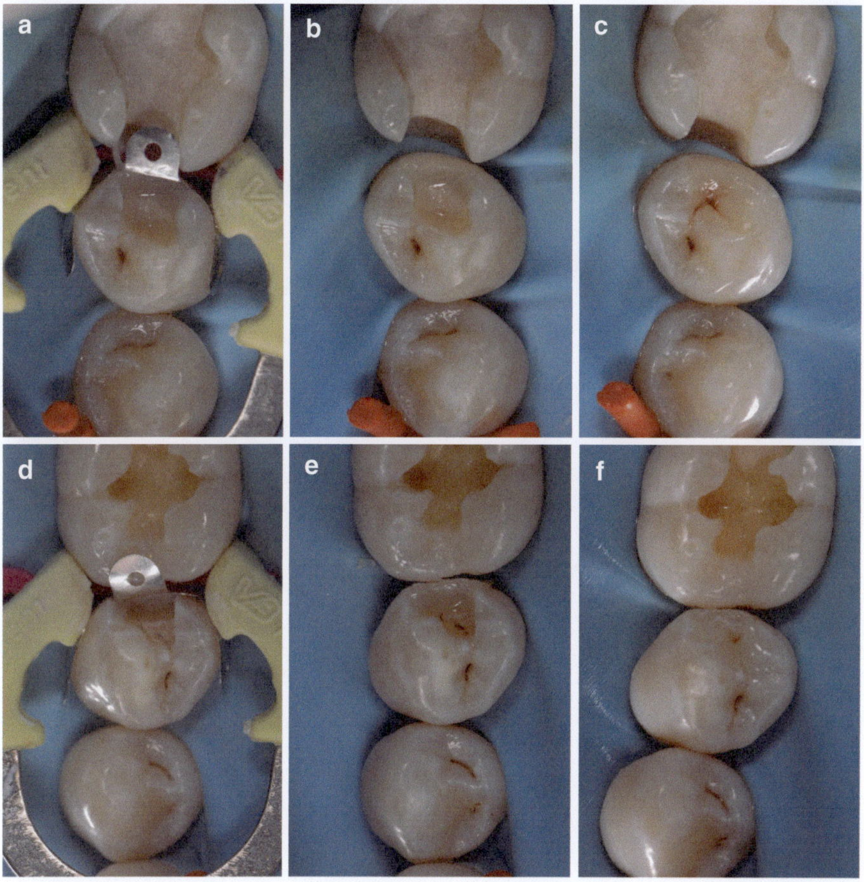

Fig. 5.16 Class II to Class I cavity conversion (**a**–**c**) Tooth 35 DO & (**d**–**f**) Tooth 45 DO by placement of proximal wall marginal ridge, removal of the sectional matrix assembly and subsequent composite resin restoration

restored in a similar manner to that described for the Class I restoration. In deep cavities, free hand application of composite resin material increments involves the segmental layering of the restoration in 2 mm oblique, horizontal or vertical increments to ensure completeness of cure and minimising shrinkage stresses whilst also constructing cuspal inclines and anatomy (Fig. 5.17).

Where the Class II cavity defect affects both marginal ridges of the tooth (i.e. mesial-occlusal-distal cavity), the author's preference is to restore each interproximal area separately, utilising the sectional matrix assembly prior to incremental restoration build-up of the occlusal table (Figs. 5.18 and 5.19).

The main challenge with finishing and polishing the restoration stems from the interproximal area and ensuring no plaque-retentive features are introduced cervically. The clinician can probe these areas to gain tactile feedback in order to identify

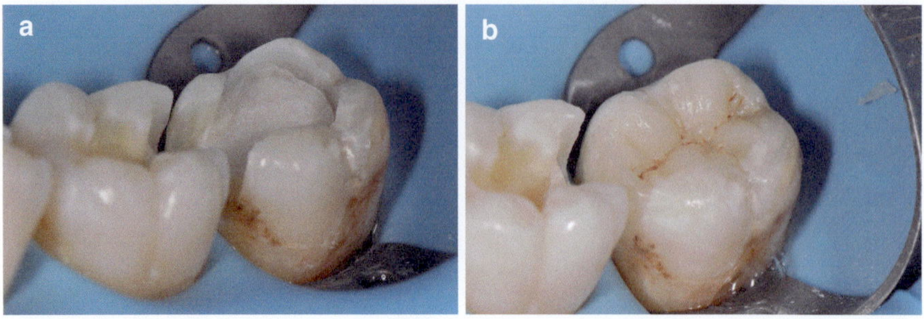

Fig. 5.17 (**a**) Tooth 37 MO Class II cavity and (**b**) restoration highlighting cuspal inclines and anatomy

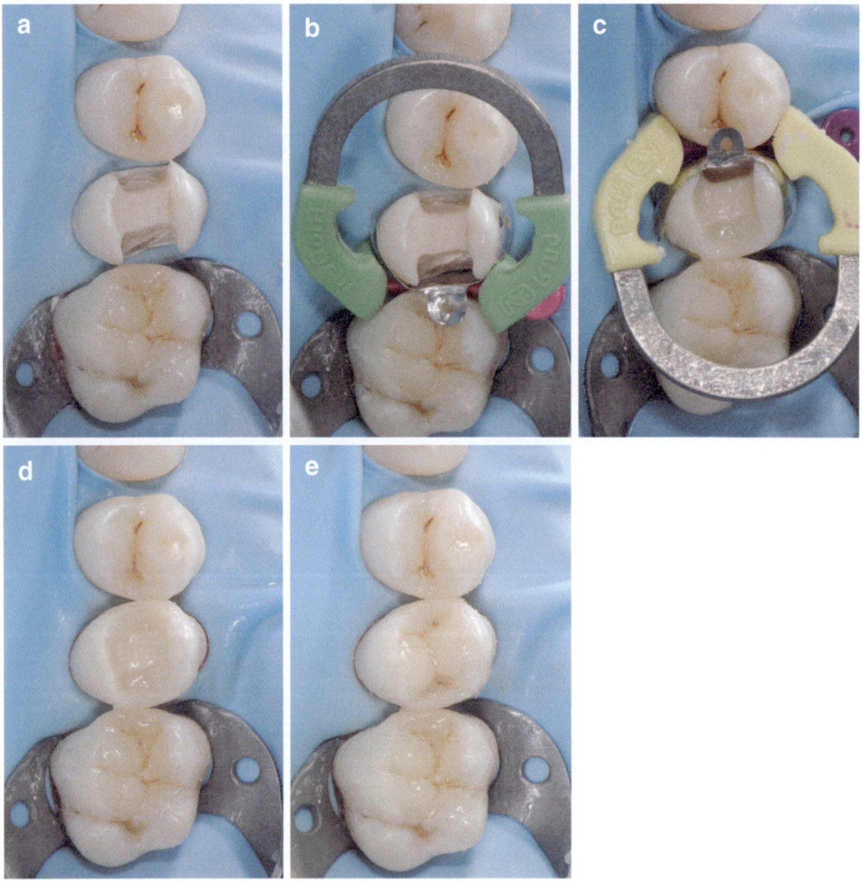

Fig. 5.18 Tooth 25 MOD Class II to Class I cavity conversion by (**a**–**c**) placement of individual proximal wall marginal ridges. (**d**, **e**) Removal of the sectional matrix assembly and subsequent composite resin restoration

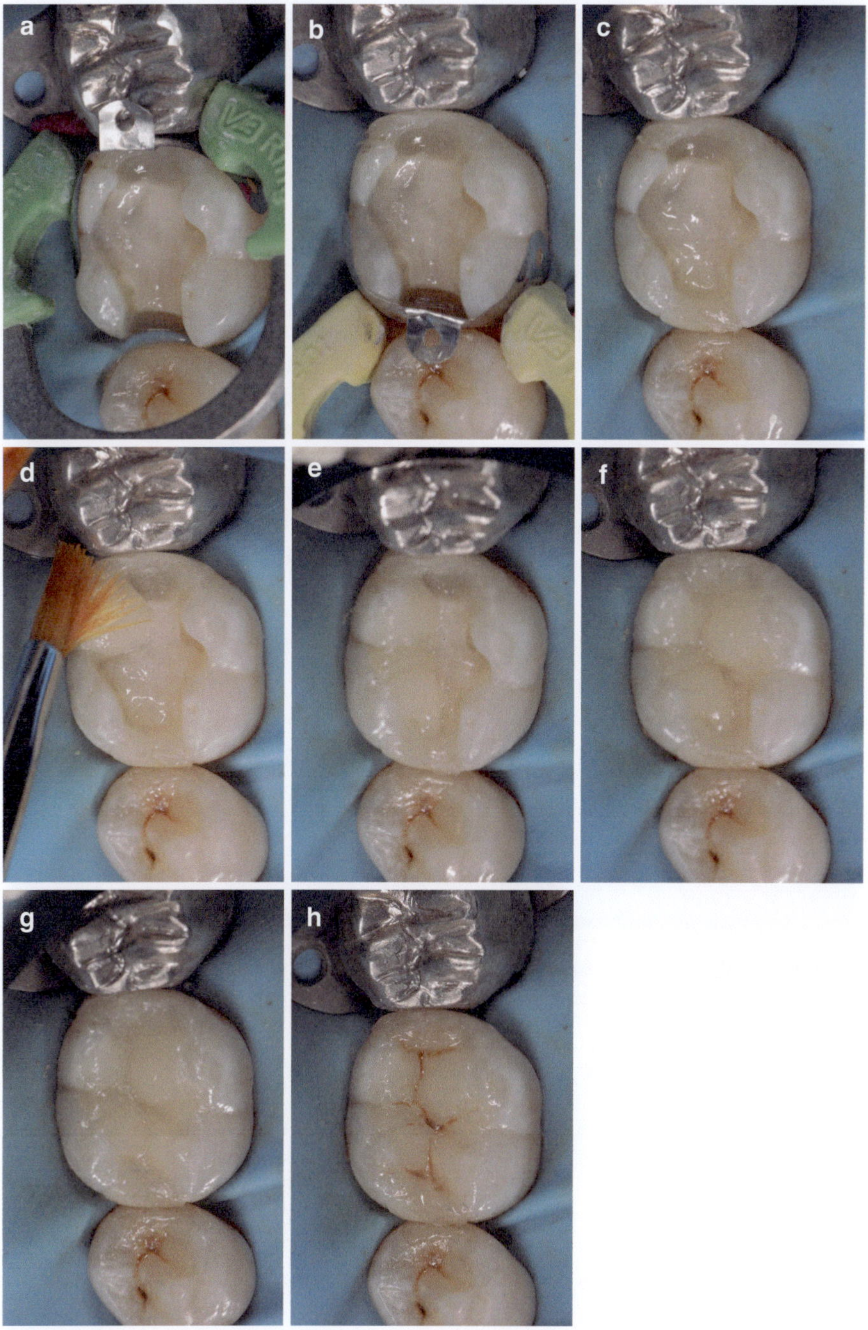

Fig. 5.19 Tooth 36 MOD Class II to Class I cavity conversion by (**a**–**c**) placement of individual proximal wall marginal ridges and removal of the sectional matrix assembly. (**d**–**h**) Subsequent composite resin restoration incremental occlusal build-up

areas of roughness or overhang. A No. 12 scalpel blade can also remove any resin bond flash due to its rake-like shape, getting in between the teeth. Furthermore, one-sided diamond abrasive strips can be utilised to remove any catches or smoothen the restoration-tooth interface. Interdental contact point testing with floss and gauging the size of the embrasure space with an interproximal brush is recommended to advise the patient on future restoration maintenance.

5.5 Class III Restoration

The Class III cavity on anterior teeth is preferably managed wholly from the palatal aspect to prevent breach of the buccal enamel (Fig. 5.20). This may not always be possible due to the extent of the lesion and the potential need to access the caries from both the buccal and palatal aspects (Fig. 5.21). Once caries removal has been completed (Figs. 5.20 and 5.21), attention can be drawn to the enamel margins.

If the cavity is 'through and through', presenting on both buccal and palatal surfaces, the need to blend the restoration into the surrounding tooth tissue is

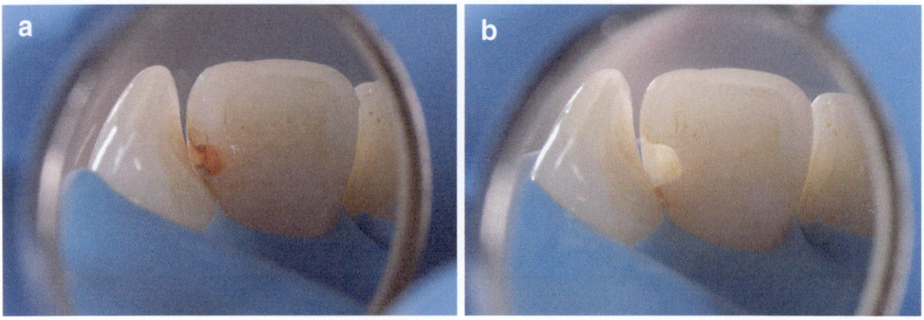

Fig. 5.20 (**a**) Tooth 21 with Class III caries on mesial surface. (**b**) Caries removal and palatal cavity preparation with intact buccal surface enamel

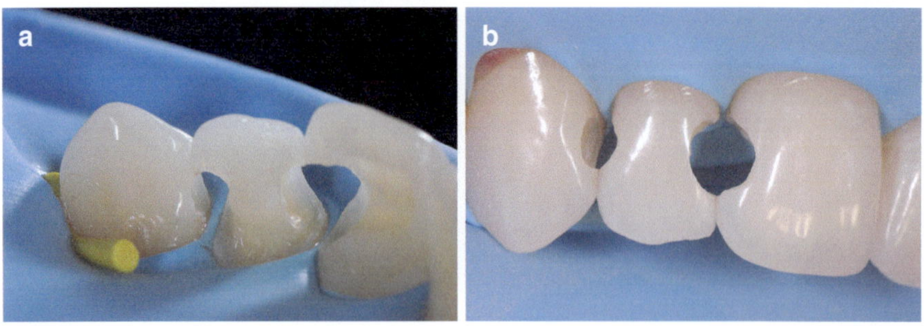

Fig. 5.21 (**a**, **b**) Extensive Class III cavities on teeth 13, 12 & 11 extending to palatal and buccal surfaces

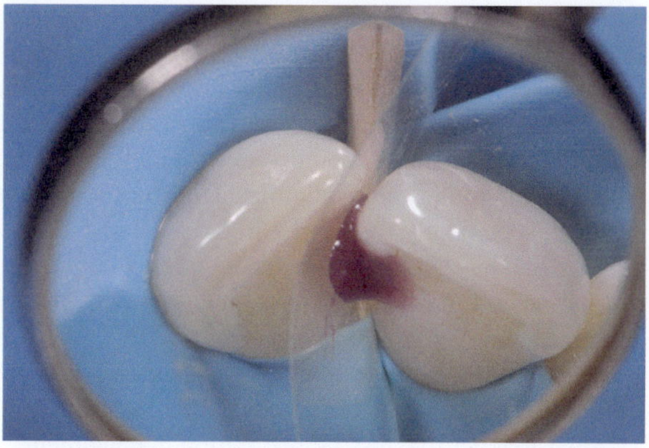

Fig. 5.22 Translucent acetate Mylar strip supported by an interdental wedge contains etching and bonding procedures to the cavity. The strip without manipulation is not secure and is of an incorrect contour to guide restoration form

important. One aspect is the optical properties, where there is a need to incorporate some opacity into the restoration to prevent a significant mismatch in colour and shade with the natural tooth tissue. This can also be aided by bevelling the buccal enamel margin to help blend the restoration.

Similar to Class II cavities, management of the matrix is important for restoration delivery. The most common technique is to utilise a translucent acetate strip supported by an interdental wedge. The strip will adequately contain etching and bonding procedures to the cavity; however, the strip requires continuous manipulation to secure it to hold the correct contour to guide restoration form (Fig. 5.22). The challenge of recreating the contour of the restoration is twofold with the Class III restoration. The buccal outline of the tooth needs to be maintained, whilst the contour of the restoration in the interproximal and palatal area needs to be appropriately shaped to avoid plaque stagnation or inadequate contact point design for interdental cleaning. Under-contouring or over-contouring the restoration may result in stagnant areas.

The translucent acetate strip can be recontoured by wrapping around a circular object such as a mirror handle to ensure better adaptation around the tooth. Once the shape is adequate, the matrix can be placed and supported by the insertion of a wedge. The wedge also serves to separate the teeth to allow the formation of a contact point. Care must be taken not to tear the rubber dam or injure the gingiva or during these stages as bleeding may result in haemorrhage and the need to abort the treatment if uncontrolled.

The composite placement stage requires support for the translucent strip against the palatal surface, but open in the facial area to allow insertion of the composite resin material. The initial increment can be made in an opaque dentine shade and light polymerised. Further increments are added but are not fully extended to the interdental area and are light polymerised. Once the cavity is adequately filled, the final enamel increments are packed against the strip in the interdental area and added to the buccal surface. The translucent strip is then folded against the interdental wall towards the buccal surface to shape the material, and light-curing is carried out through it. On removal of the wedge and interdental strip, finishing and polishing procedures extend from buccal to palatal and interdental surfaces. Interdental abrasive strips may be used for the latter.

Posterior sectional matrix metal foils may also be used as an alternative to the translucent acetate strip. These have the advantage that they are adequately contoured and have shape memory to provide an anatomic shape to the restoration without continuous manipulation. Translucent anatomical anterior matrices are designed specifically for the use in Class III and Class IV situations with occlusal-gingival and buccal-palatal/lingual contours that provide a favourable contour to the restoration and may be used in conjunction with anatomically shaped plastic interdental wedges (Fig. 5.23).

In addition, where the cavity form is extensive, a putty matrix can be fabricated prior to caries or restoration removal, then utilised for new restoration placement in a similar manner to Class IV restoration management.

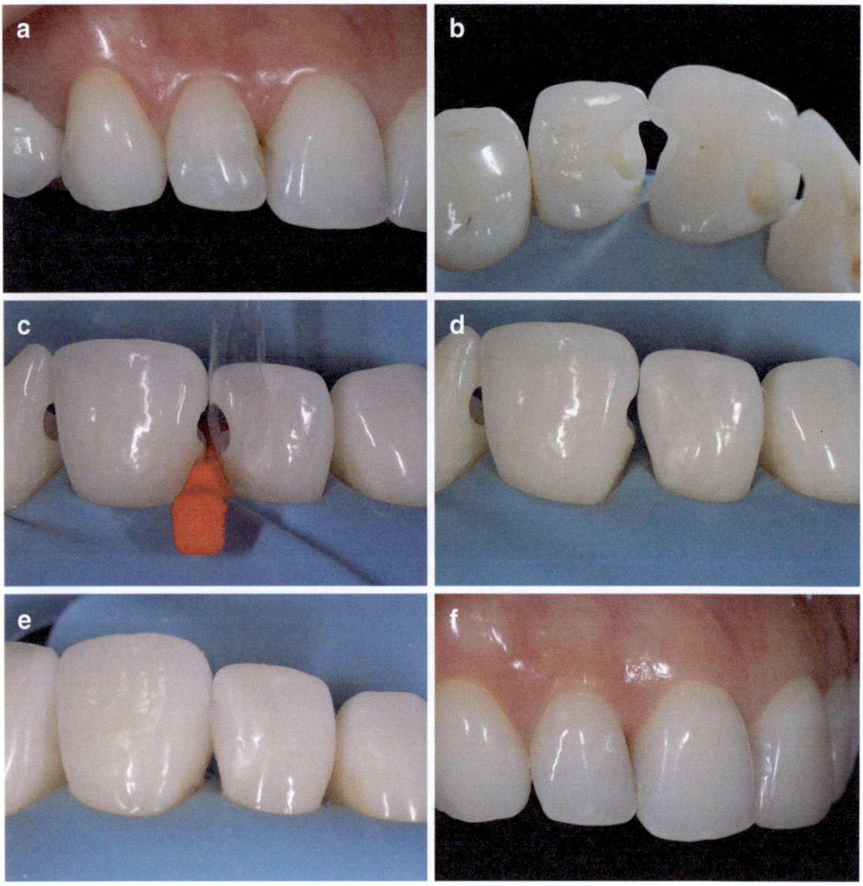

Fig. 5.23 (**a**) Teeth 12,11 & 21 with defective Class III composite resin restorations, (**b**) cavity preparation and (**c–f**) subsequent composite resin restorations using anatomically shaped translucent matrices and plastic interdental wedges

5.6 Class IV Restoration

The Class IV restoration is a common restoration provided for anterior teeth due to trauma resulting in an enamel dentine fracture or tooth surface loss, providing shortening of a unit. Depending on the presentation of dental trauma and the patient retaining the fragment, the fractured fragment may be adhesively re-bonded back into place utilising a flowable composite resin material (Fig. 5.24). If the fragment is not located, artificial replacement is indicated via restoration build-up.

The solitary Class IV defect on a maxillary anterior tooth is the most challenging of direct resin restoration even for a highly skilled experienced clinician for a variety of reasons. The task of mimicking and recreating shade, shape and the translucency with a synthetic material to the adjacent unit is demanding, especially in the high smile line or the aesthetically aware patient. This may provide a considerable test to the clinician, less so from being able to shape the restoration to resemble the correct morphology and more so, how the restoration will transmit light (Fig. 5.25).

There are numerous commercially available composite resin systems that allow material layering for the clinician to mimic natural tooth tissue as closely as possible to provide a seamless transition from natural tooth tissue. Resin systems offer a number of dentine and enamel shades of varying opacities and translucencies, and colour effects that the clinician has at their disposal. The points expressed here are

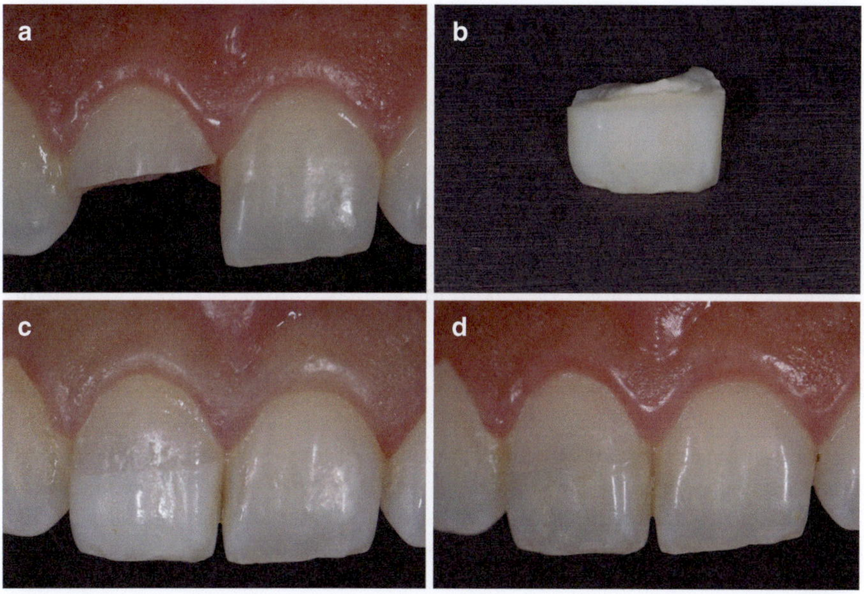

Fig. 5.24 (**a**) Traumatic injury to tooth 11 where (**b**) the retrieved dehydrated tooth fragment (**c**) is adhesively bonded back to the coronal portion. (**d**) Full aesthetic integration after rehydration of the fragment 10 days after rebonding it

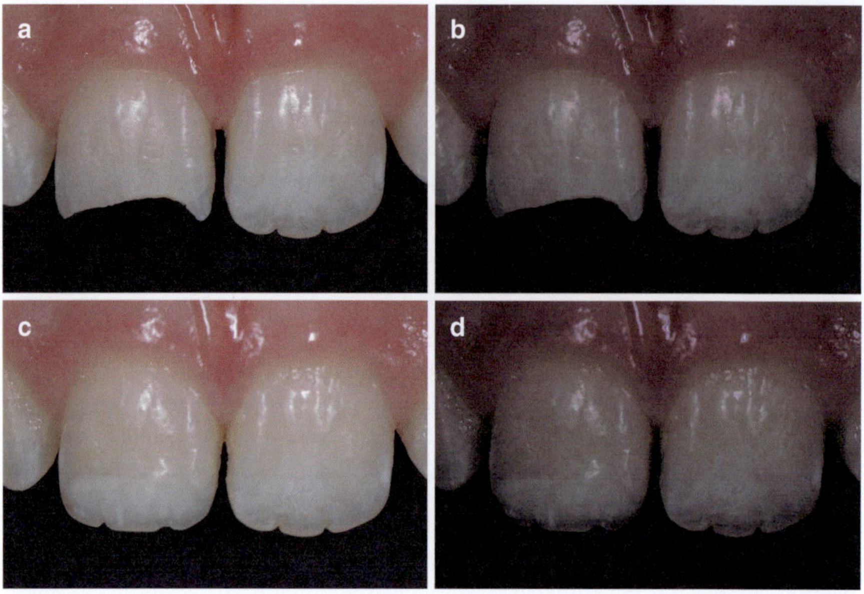

Fig. 5.25 (**a**, **b**) Tooth 11 Class IV defect is a challenging case to replicate morphology, shade, effects and translucency to allow restoration will transmit light. This cannot be done successfully with a monoshade application of composite resin material. (**c**, **d**) A layered composite resin material system must be used for an optimal aesthetic outcome

generic to the management of Class IV restorations but not specific to the plethora of systems available.

Planning for restoration provision can be conducted through a diagnostic wax-up of aesthetic and functional surfaces on articulated study casts. This is especially relevant for situations where the tooth unit is extensively fractured, or the current restoration is inadequately shaped and contoured and needs replacing. Using a contrasting colour of wax to the colour of the gypsum model allows the clinician to adequately identify what areas and surfaces are proposed to change (Figs. 5.26 and 5.27). Using similar colours of wax to model makes distinction very challenging and can limit diagnostic use (Fig. 5.28).

The diagnostic wax-up can be utilised to construct a palatal silicone matrix through which the initial palatal increment of enamel composite resin material can be placed to form the outline palatal shell to support further layers. The silicone matrix is made from a dual consistency putty and light-body wash 'addition reaction' polyvinyl–siloxane (PVS) material. The light-body wash consistency allows the capture of detail of the palatal embrasures and incisal edge without air voids, which can distort the recording of the shape of the functional surfaces. The PVS matrix needs to be extended at least one tooth or more adjacent to the tooth being treated for positional stability (Fig. 5.29). It is required to be trimmed away from areas that may impede its full seating (e.g. stabilising rubber dam clamps). It also is required to be made in thick section such that there is no distortion in its shape

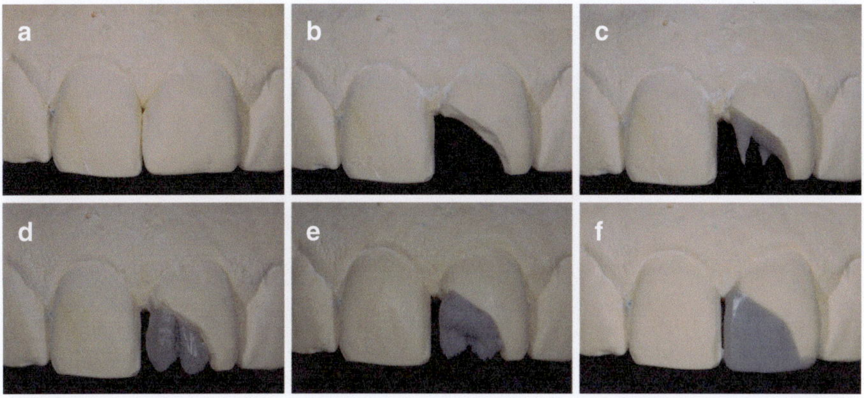

Fig. 5.26 Tooth 21 diagnostic wax-up sequence of aesthetic and functional surfaces. (**a**–**d**) The gypsum cast is sectioned, and a dentine core waxed-up. (**e**, **f**) The enamel component is subsequently added. Note the contrasting colour of the wax to the gypsum model

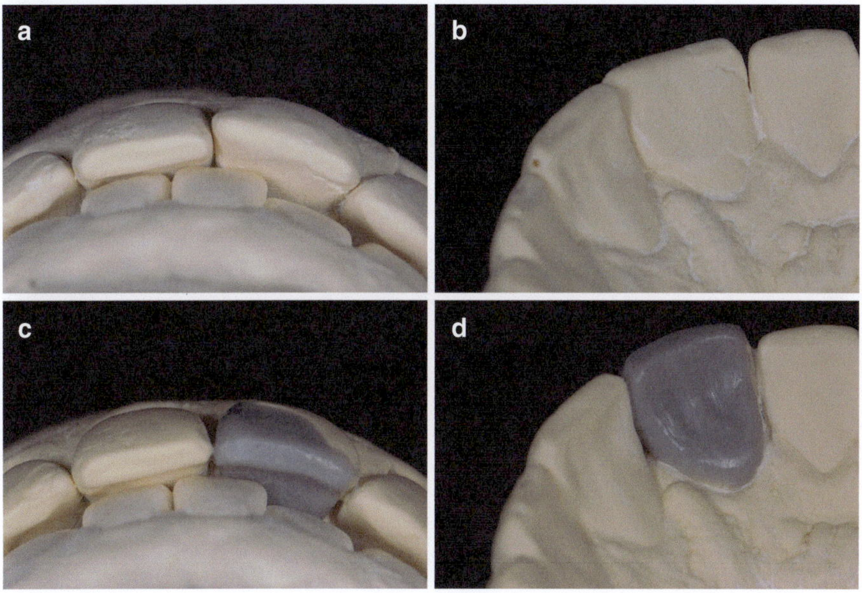

Fig. 5.27 Tooth 21 diagnostic wax-up (**a**, **b**) before and (**c**, **d**) after of functional incisal-edge and palatal surfaces. Note the contrasting colour of the wax to the gypsum model

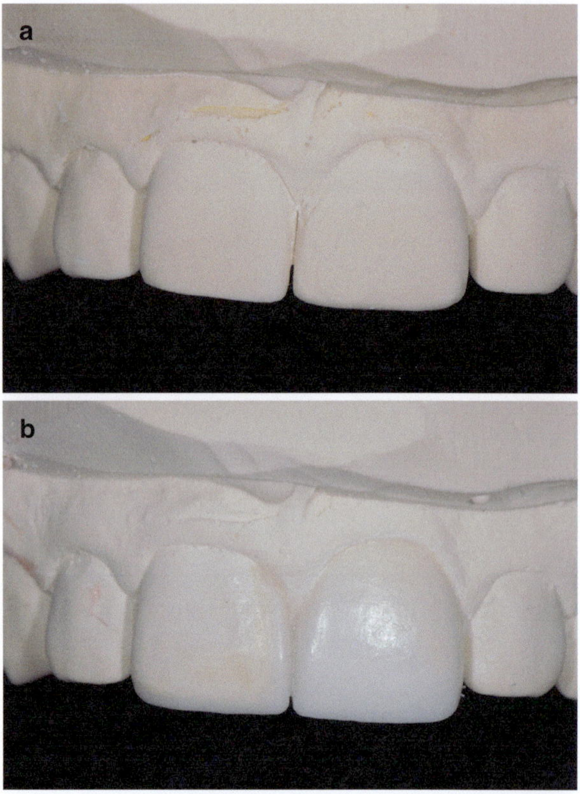

Fig. 5.28 (**a**) Asymmetry of teeth 11 & 21. (**b**) Diagnostic wax-up, the similar wax and gypsum model colours make proposed changes challenging to identify

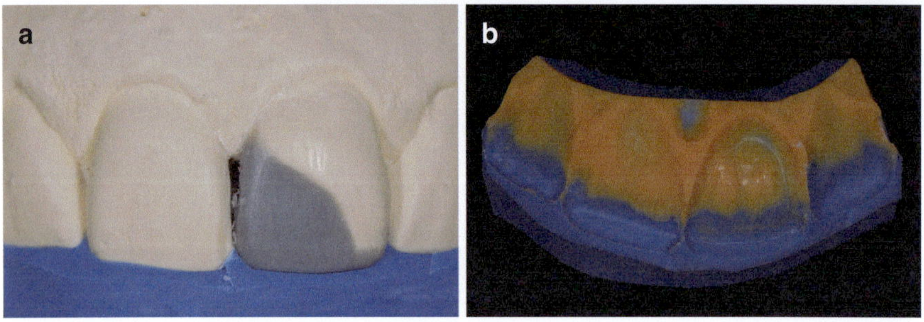

Fig. 5.29 (**a**, **b**) PVS matrix made from the diagnostic wax-up in a dual consistency PVS material

whilst being used which can extrapolate error to the final shape and incisal edge position of the composite resin restoration.

Alternatively, a palatal PVS matrix to form the palatal shell can be constructed chairside from a direct intra-oral mock-up of the ideal definitive restoration shape to be delivered to the tooth (Figs. 5.30 and 5.31). The matrix may also be made without the mock-up, instead a PVS putty impression is made of the defect and the ideal outline form of the fractured tooth is drawn in pencil on the matrix and trimmed

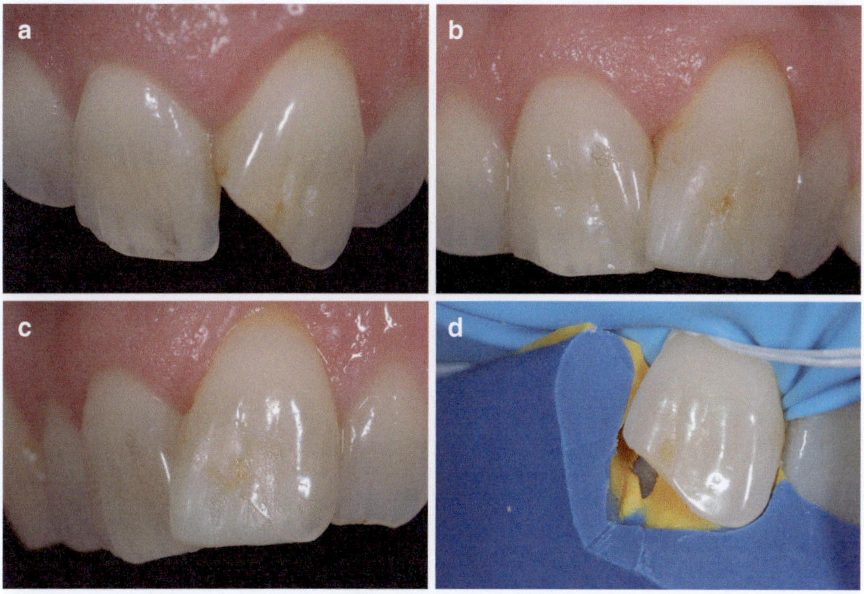

Fig. 5.30 (**a–c**) Fractured tooth 21 and intra-oral mock-up of the proposed definitive shape. (**d**) Chairside construction of palatal PVS matrix fitted to isolated tooth to help guide Class IV composite resin restoration provision

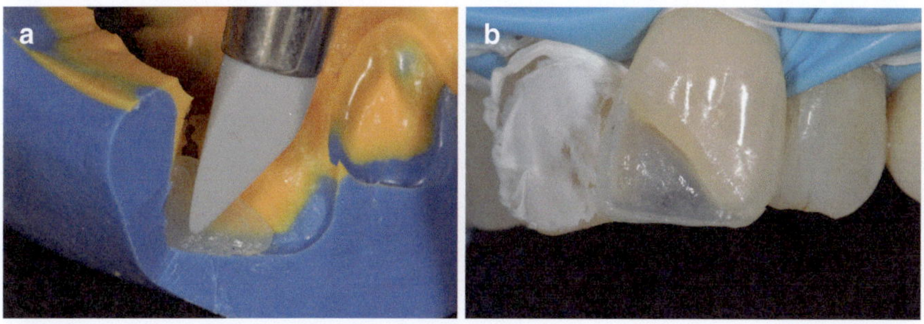

Fig. 5.31 (**a**, **b**) Enamel material increment application to PVS matrix with a silicone tipped instrument transferred to tooth 21 to form the restoration palatal shell

against the palatal surface using a No. 11 scalpel blade to create the space required for the placement of the composite resin material increment for the palatal shell (Figs. 5.32, 5.33, 5.34, and 5.35).

If the fabrication of a PVS index is not possible, the use of a translucent acetate strip with finger manipulated can be used (Figs. 5.36 and 5.37). This technique requires additional time and effort due to the lack of positional stability of the acetate strip. The disadvantage of utilising this technique is that the incisal edge position has to be estimated in height and level, the palatal contour is also subject to continual stable finger manipulation of the acetate strip.

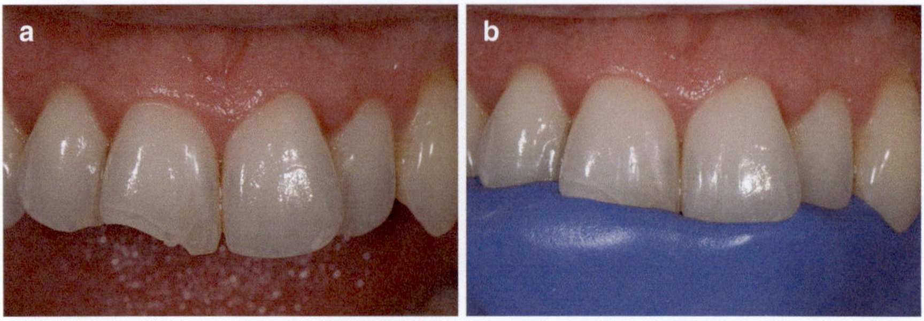

Fig. 5.32 (**a**) Tooth 11 Class IV fracture. (**b**) PVS putty impression taken of the defect

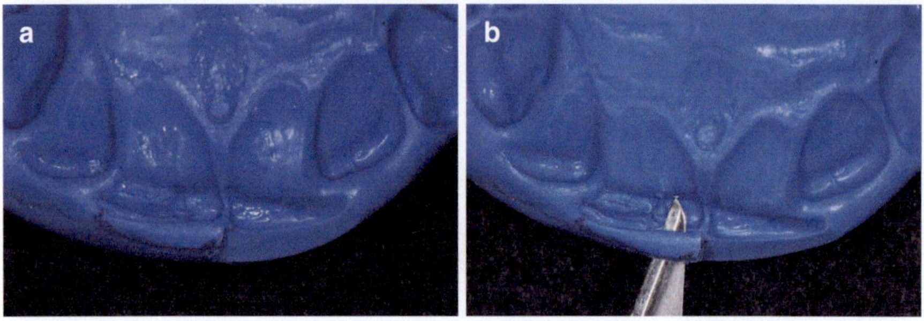

Fig. 5.33 PVS matrix. (**a**) Ideal tooth 11 outline form drawn in pencil and (**b**) trimmed against the palatal surface using a No. 11 scalpel blade

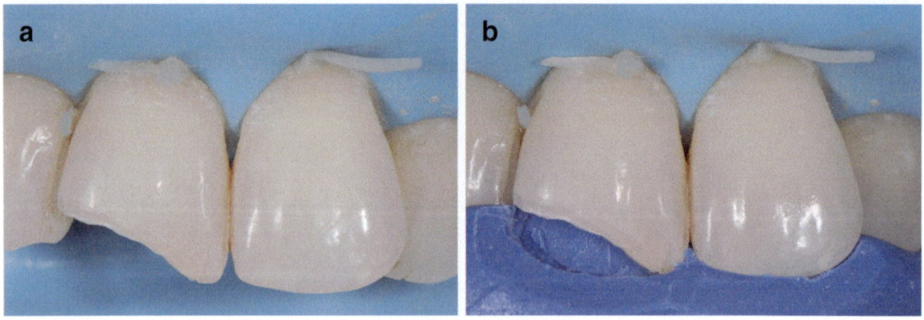

Fig. 5.34 (**a**) Isolation of tooth 11 (**b**) Seating of the PVS matrix with the space required for the placement of the composite resin material increment to form the palatal shell for tooth 11

Prior to the provision of Class IV restorations, the need to shade map the adjacent tooth to be matched comprehensively is important. The shade take procedure needs to be conducted on the day of treatment under natural light with the teeth fully hydrated before the rubber dam isolation. Dehydration of the teeth can change their refractive index leading to alteration in their shade appearance (increased value/brightness). Bleaching procedures should be carried out in advance of this and adequate time (2–4 weeks) allowed for shade settling. A shade map of a tooth can be

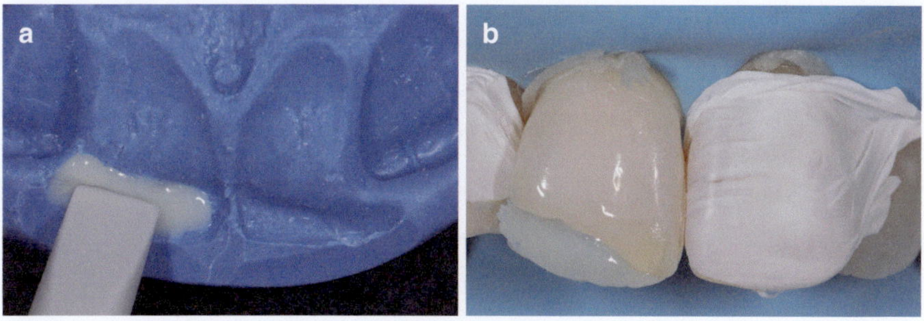

Fig. 5.35 (**a**) Enamel material increment application to PVS matrix with a silicone tipped instrument (**b**) transferred to tooth 11 to form the restoration palatal shell

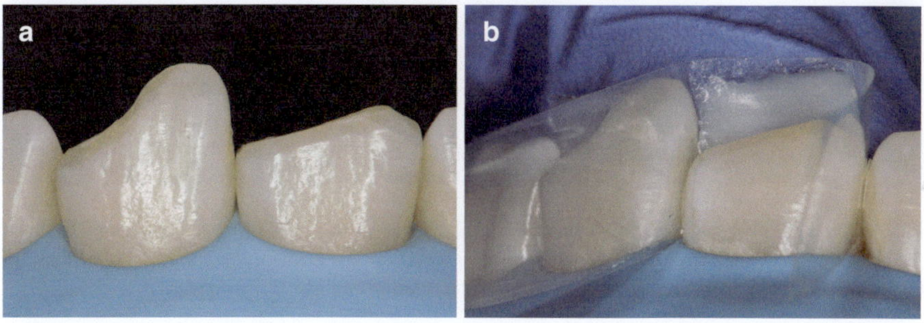

Fig. 5.36 (**a**) Isolation of teeth 11 & 21. (**b**) Finger manipulation of Mylar acetate translucent strip required for the placement of the composite resin material increment to form the palatal shell for tooth 11

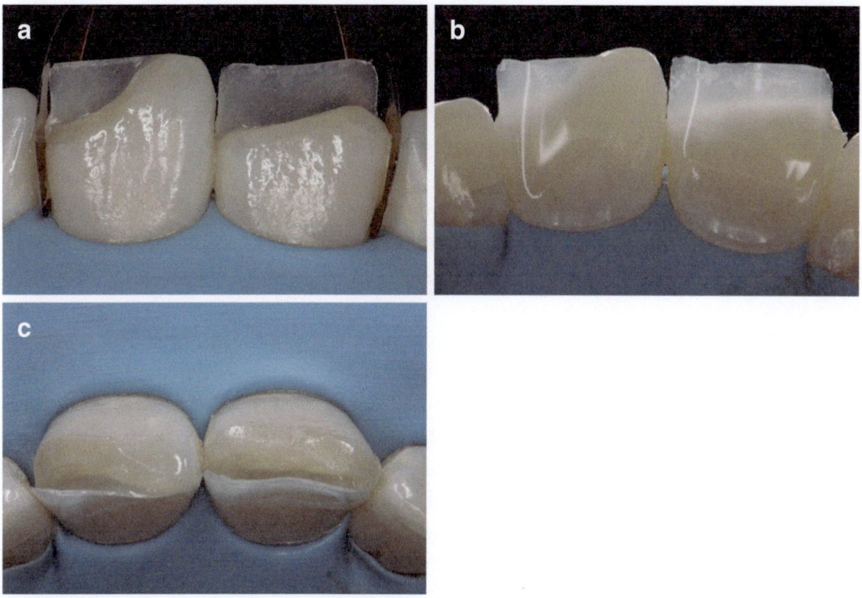

Fig. 5.37 Teeth 11 & 21 enamel palatal shells. (**a**) Buccal, (**b**) palatal and (**c**) occlusal views

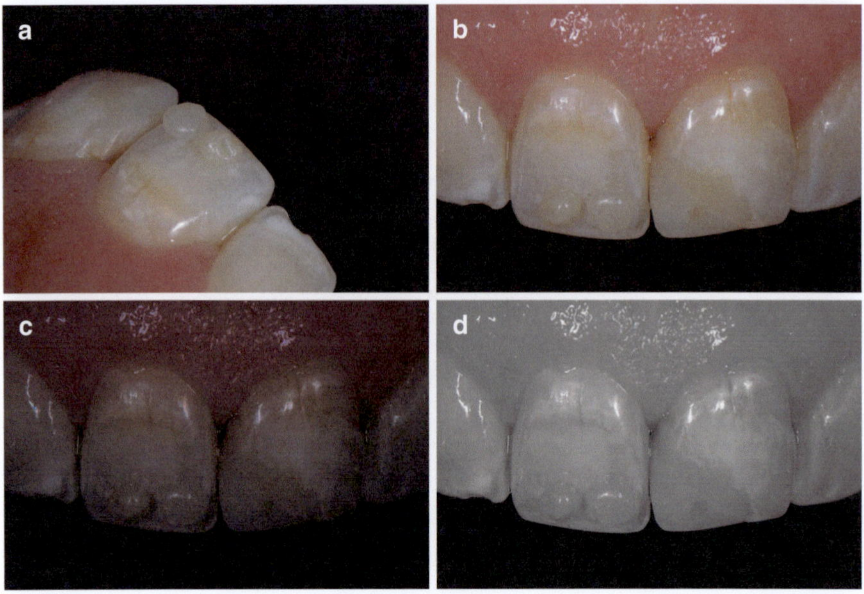

Fig. 5.38 The 'composite bead' technique for shade selection. (**a**, **b**) Enamel and dentine shade polymerised beads of composite resin material placed on the assessment tooth. (**c**, **d**) Digitally edited photographs to assess shade, chroma, characteristics and value

included in the notes for records. Clinical photographs can be taken with a cross-polarisation filter and computer software editing are useful adjuncts. Both colour and black and white photographs may be used to assess shade, value, chroma and characteristics of the tooth. Customised composite resin material shade tabs may be used for comparison. In addition, the 'composite bead' technique allows to place a small, polymerised bead of the proposed enamel and dentine shades of composite resin material to be used on the assessment tooth. The tooth with the bead can then be photographed and the photographs digitally edited to aid shade selection (Fig. 5.38). From here, the shade chosen is agreed with the patient prior to the treatment commencing.

Rubber dam isolation may be augmented by the use of floss ligatures for further gingival retraction, tooth exposure and stabilisation. Stabilisation clamps close to the operative area may not be used as they may prohibit the complete seating of a PVS index.

Dissection of the existing restorative material must be carefully carried out under water spray to ensure that the integrity of the existing tooth is respected. In the case of existing dentine pin restorations, these can be readily removed utilising agitation from an ultrasonic scaler tip. Functional and aesthetic finish lines of choice are placed, and the tooth structure is alumina blasted to receive the adhesive bonding procedures required for the restoration (Fig. 5.39).

Interdental matrices are secured with an interdental wedge aid replication of an appropriately contoured interdental surface and embrasure spaces, allowing contour

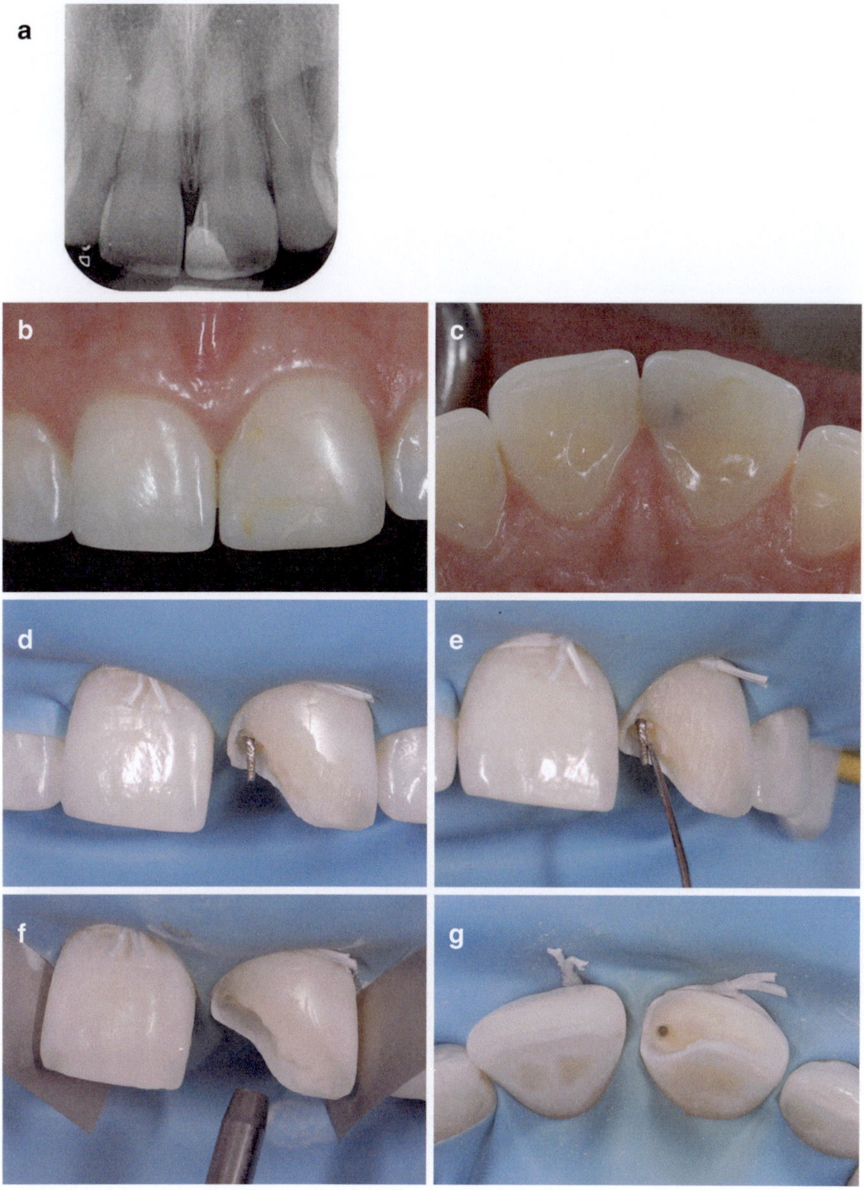

Fig. 5.39 Asymmetry of teeth 11 & 21 (see Fig. 5.28). (**a–c**) Tooth 21 with dentine pin retaining a defective Class IV restoration. (**d**) Dissection of the existing restorative material and placement of finish lines. (**e**) Dentine pin removed with an ultrasonic scaler. (**f**, **g**) Teeth further prepared by sand blasting

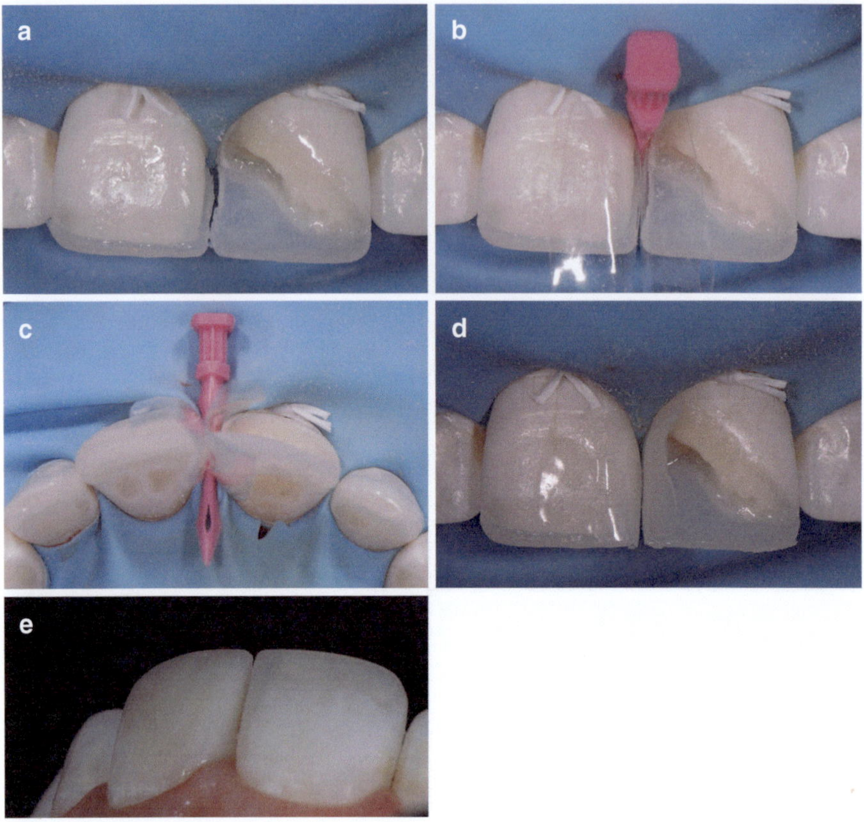

Fig. 5.40 Palatal shells of teeth 11 & 21. (**a–d**) Use of plastic interdental wedge to support anatomical contoured acetate matrices for replication of appropriate contour of interproximal surfaces and embrasure spaces and (**e**) subsequent composite resin restorations

from both an occlusal–gingival and buccal–palatal perspectives. Anatomically contoured acetate matrices may be used for this (Fig. 5.40). Alternatively, a posterior sectional metal matrix may be turned to 180° and seated in between the teeth with the concave surface facing the area to be built up (Fig. 5.41). A clinical case depicting the Class IV restoration protocol is described in Sect. 5.9.3.

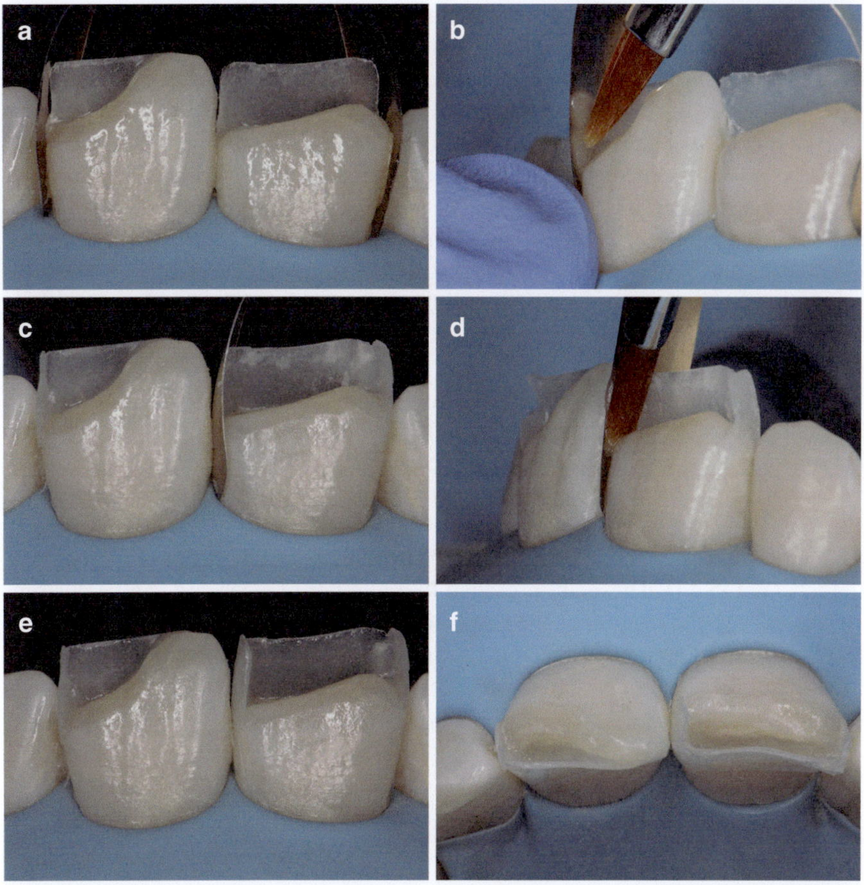

Fig. 5.41 Palatal shells of teeth 11 & 21. (**a**, **c**) Use of posterior sectional metal matrix for replication of appropriate contour of interproximal surfaces and embrasure spaces. (**b**, **d**, **e**) Application of composite resin material with a brush lubricated with modelling resin. (**f**) Occlusal view of view of palatal shells and interdental walls of restorations

5.7 Class V Restoration

The clinical reasoning for restoring Class V cavities is likely to be multiple in nature, ranging from unsightly aesthetics of tooth surface loss lesions to frank caries and physiological symptoms of hypersensitivity. In minor cases, where the cavity is shallow, the clinician should consider the use of desensitising toothpaste in the first instance.

As the cavity is in close vicinity to the gingival crevice, rubber dam application in combination with gingival retraction may be required. Where this does not reveal the extent or the cavity, then gingivectomy may have to be considered prior to the restorative phase. Once isolated, the need for cavity preparation is minimal, especially where root caries is not present. The enamel margin can be bevelled to improve available surface area for bonding and aid blending with the surrounding tooth tissue. Alumina blasting allows a roughened high-energy surface required for adhesive bonding, self, selective or total-etch techniques may be used. A shade selected highly filled flowable composite resin material may be used to restore the Class V cavity as these materials exhibit favourable properties such as high strength, excellent wear resistance and optimal polishing potential (Figs. 5.42 and 5.43). If the lesion is large and progresses cervically, the restoration may transition from enamel bonding to dentine bonding-this is more likely in the periodontal patient. In such cases, self or selective acid etching are conditioning options.

The emergence profile of the restoration should be contoured appropriately. The temptation to make the restoration flat lacking anatomical shape needs to be balanced against creating an emergence profile that blends with adjacent teeth without creating an area for plaque stagnation and consequently further gingival recession.

There are a number of commercially available matrix systems for Class V defects (Fig. 5.44). These are provided in a number of sizes and can be customised to be applied to fit over the uncured resin. They may also be used for contouring glass-ionomer cement (GIC) restorations and left in situ until the GIC material is fully polymerised and protected from water sorption over a 24–48-h period (Fig. 5.45).

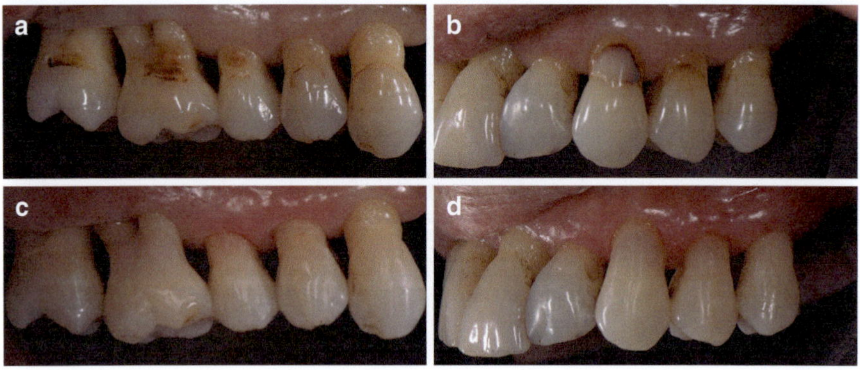

Fig. 5.42 (**a**, **b**) 1st & second quadrant Class V cavities from tooth surface loss and caries. (**c**, **d**) Subsequent restoration of teeth 17–13 & 23–25 with highly filled flowable composite resin material

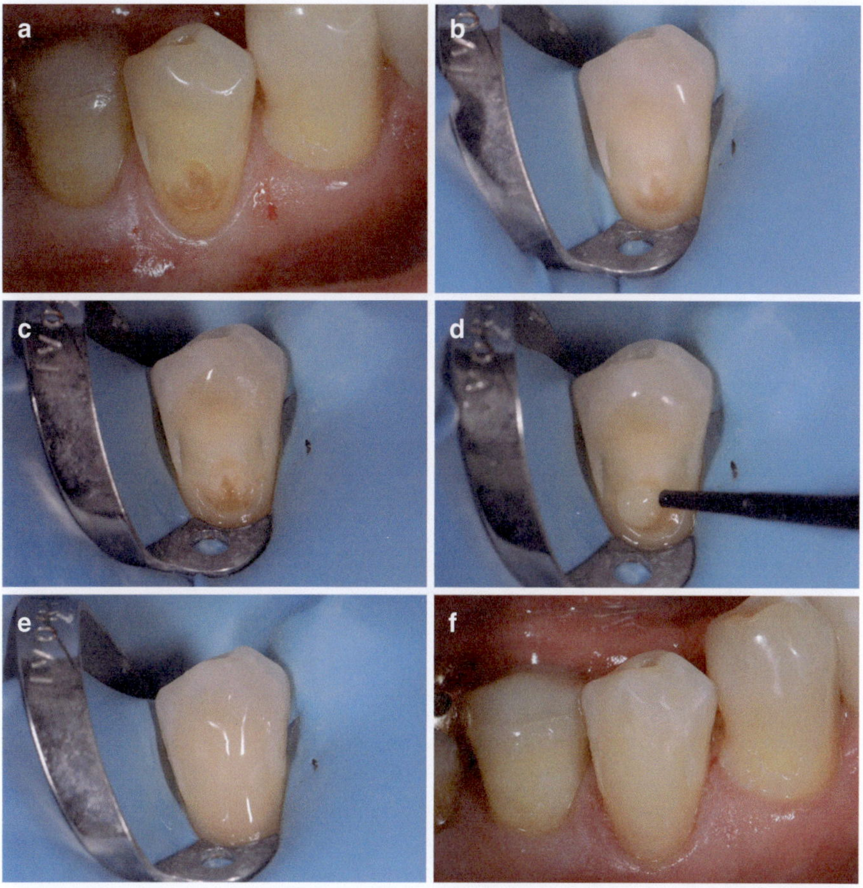

Fig. 5.43 (**a**, **b**) Tooth 34 Class V cavity and isolation. (**c**) Cavity margin bevelling and sand blasting preparation. (**d–f**) Restoration of cavity with highly filled flowable composite resin material

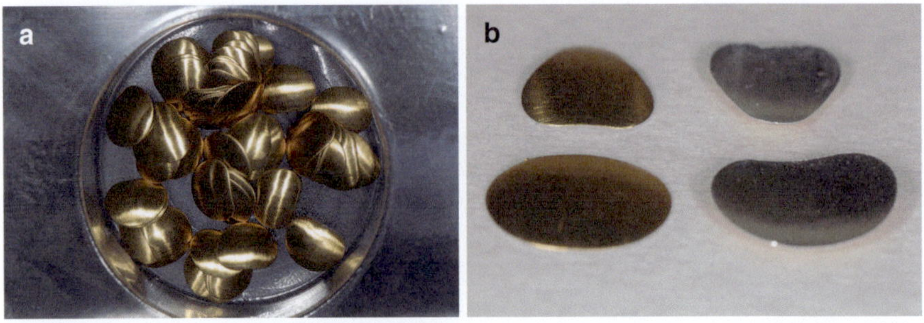

Fig. 5.44 (**a**, **b**) Gold foil contoured matrix system for Class V defects

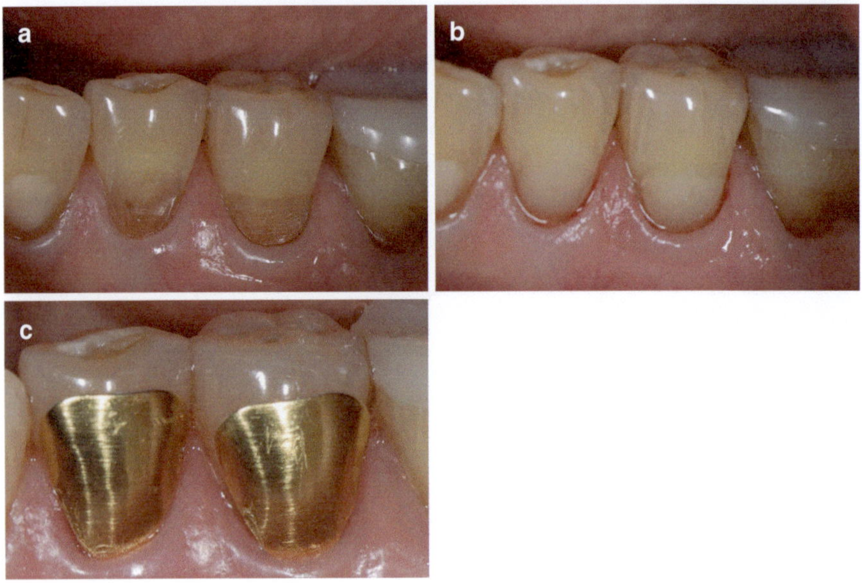

Fig. 5.45 (**a**, **b**) Teeth 35 & 34 Class V defects and provision of GIC restorations. (**c**) Use of gold foil contoured matrices for contouring and protecting GIC restorations

5.8 Maintenance

Refurbishment or restoration, replacement of direct resin restorations is an unfortunate inevitability. Due to the inherent nature of adhesive techniques being less invasive, their future management is also of minimal harm. One important aspect that the clinician needs to take special note of at the time of replacement is the aetiology of failure or the source of need for replacement. Where restorations are worn, marginally compromised or discoloured, this may be readily apparent. If the reason behind restoration failure is less apparent further investigation, such as occlusal analysis may reveal factors unapparent from the outset. Issues such as anterior or lateral guidance issues should not be replicated in the new restoration. Such problems may require further occlusal analysis using study casts and articulation.

Where restorations may present with partial fracture of the residual composite, the clinician will need to decide as to the benefit of replacing the entire restoration and utilising the superior enamel bond or bonding to the remaining composite resin. The latter has an inferior bond and is likely to result in an obvious junction between the old and new resin in addition to a difference in shade. If the clinician has a choice, where resources are available, the replacement of the entire restoration would be most favourable.

Removal of the residual restoration can be challenging to achieve, especially where the previous restoration's margin was seamless with the tooth surface or is similar in shade to the tooth itself. One beneficial resource to have at hand is any previous diagnostic wax-up or the accompanying PVS matrix. This can make restoration replacement much easier and quicker, as a new diagnostic wax-up will not be required, with replacement being provided in one clinical visit. Delineation between tooth and composite resin can be achieved through a number of techniques. Composite removal burs or instruments, those commonly utilised for the removal of resin retaining orthodontic brackets, are also very useful in this respect. One further characteristic property is that composite will tend to mark if scraped with a probe which doesn't not occur so readily with hard dental tissue. 'Black light' torches allow remnant composite resin material to be highlighted when exposed to specific light emitted from the torch (Fig. 5.46). Alternatively, etching enamel will give the tooth tissue a chalky appearance.

Once the clinician is confident that the majority of restoration has been removed, treating the surface of the dental tissue by alumina blasting further optimises the substrate for repeat adhesive bonding. Once fully cleaned, the tooth surface can be adhesively treated and the new restoration placed in the most appropriate manner.

If a repair is chosen over wholesale restoration replacement, the surface of the resin restoration should be roughened by way of diamond bur and alumina blasting. The surface of the composite resin is reactivated by applying a thin coat of resin primer to allow adhesive bonding of the repair increment to the freshly activated surface (Fig. 5.47).

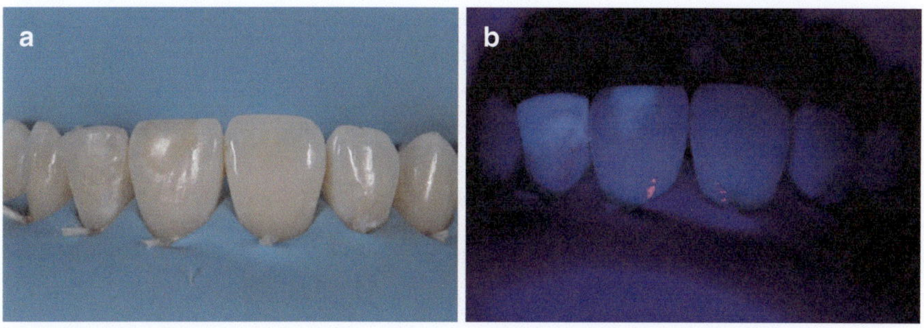

Fig. 5.46 (**a**) Teeth 21 & 22 existing composite resin restorations (**b**) highlighted by the use of a 'black light' torch. (Images courtesy of Dr. Monik Vasant)

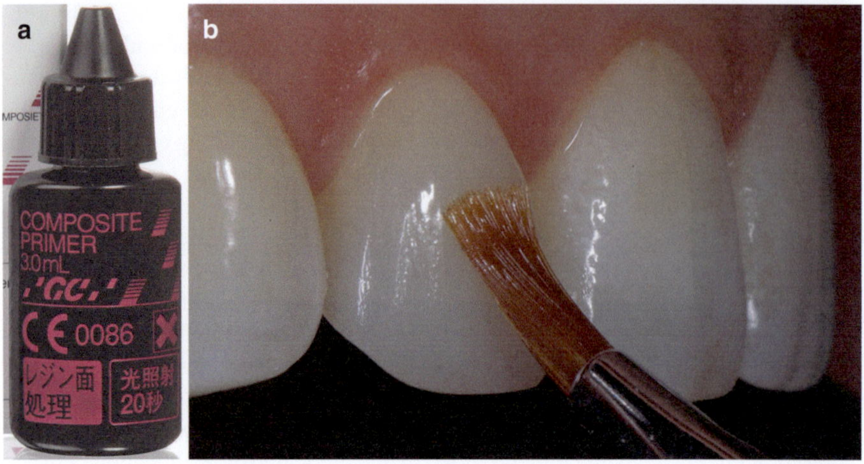

Fig. 5.47 (**a**) Composite primer used on (**b**) a modelling brush for repair of defective composite resin restoration. (Image (**a**) courtesy of GC UK)

5.9 Adhesive Technique

The following adhesive techniques can aid the operator in certain clinical cases where the presentation of the cavity defect allows.

5.9.1 Class I Restoration Occlusal Stamp

This technique allows for replication of the preoperative anatomical occlusal surface of the tooth to aid in delivering an occlusal restoration requiring minimal occlusal adjustment. The 'occlusal stamp' may be made from various materials, which are depicted in the following cases where a translucent PVS material (Figs. 5.48, 5.49, 5.50, 5.51, and 5.52) or flowable composite resin material (Figs. 5.53, 5.54, and 5.55) is used. The required clinical stages are listed in Table 5.1.

5.9.2 Class II Restoration Axial Shield

Where the Class II defect extends beyond the embrasure space onto the buccal or palatal/lingual axial surface, the tines of the sectional ring may compress against and collapse the sectional metal foil matrix into the cavity defect, where the supporting wall is lost. This will deform the shape of the restoration. Much like the

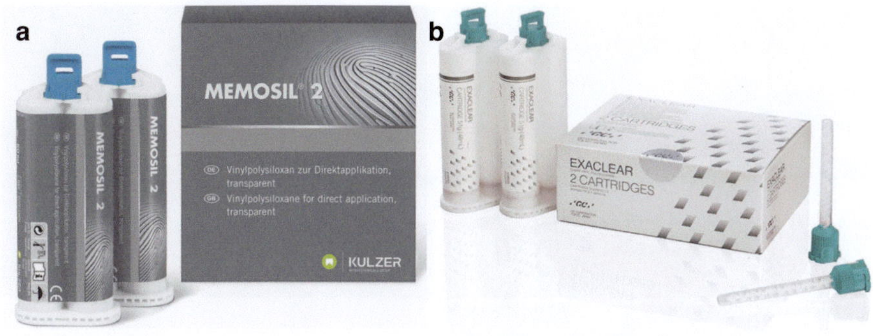

Fig. 5.48 (**a**, **b**) Examples of translucent PVS materials used for production of stamps or stents. (Image (**a**) courtesy of GC U.K and image (**b**) courtesy of Kulzer Ltd.)

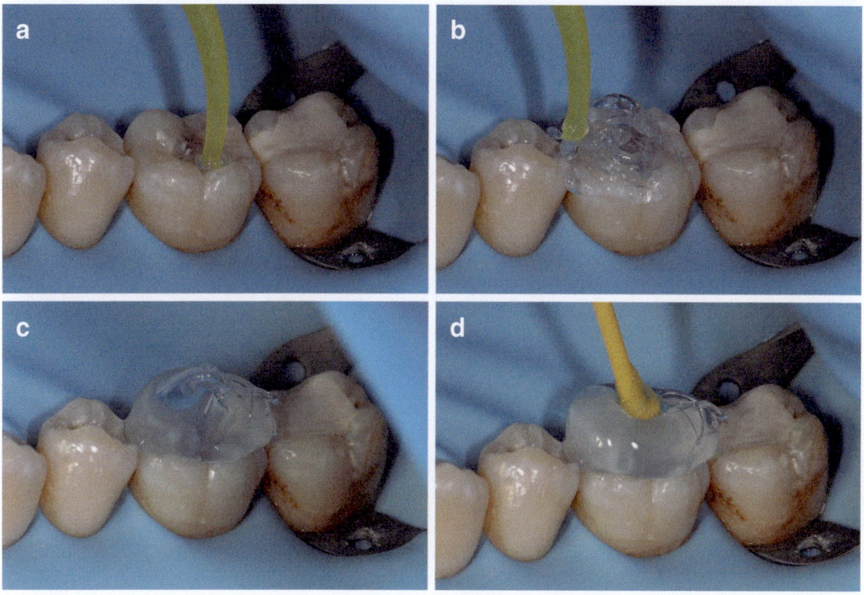

Fig. 5.49 (**a**, **b**) Pre-operative recording of the occlusal surface of tooth 36 and (**c**, **d**) handle attachment into the unpolymerised translucent PVS stamp material

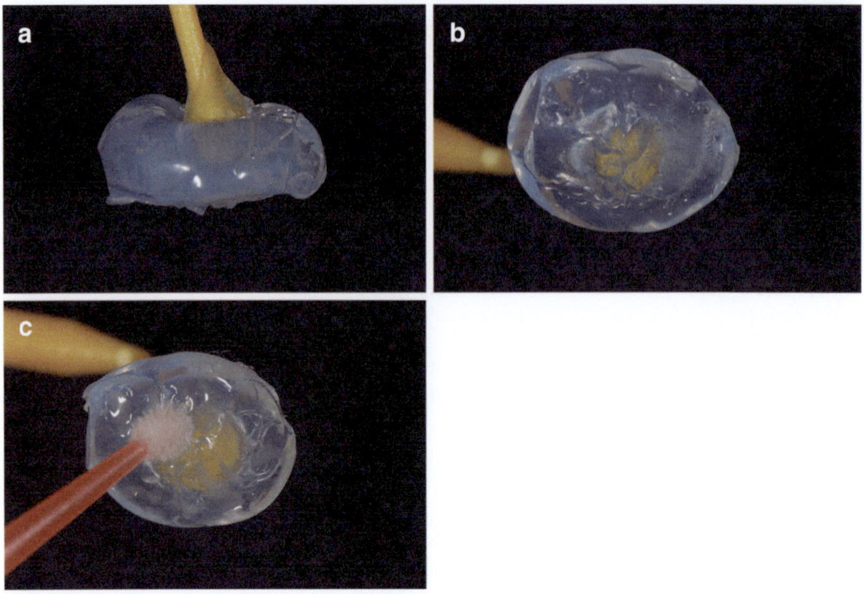

Fig. 5.50 (**a**, **b**) Polymerised translucent PVS 'occlusal stamp' and (**c**) glycerine separator application to the intaglio surface

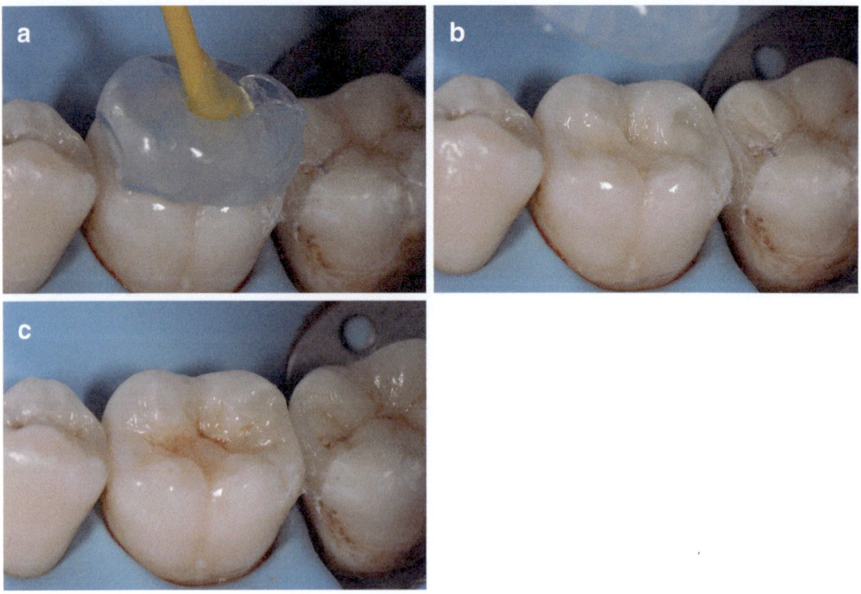

Fig. 5.51 (**a**) Tooth 36 occlusal stamp location, (**b**) excess composite resin material removal and (**c**) modelling and characterisation of composite resin material

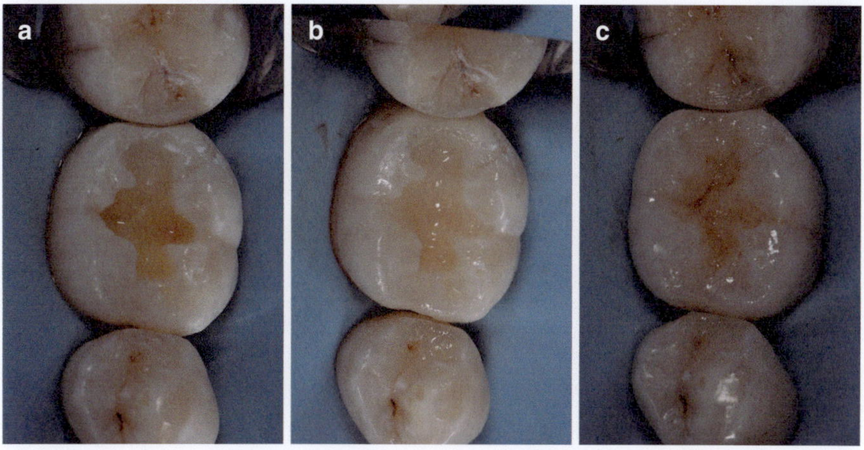

Fig. 5.52 (**a**) Tooth 36 cavity, (**b**) base restoration and (**c**) definitive 'occlusal stamp' Class 1 restoration

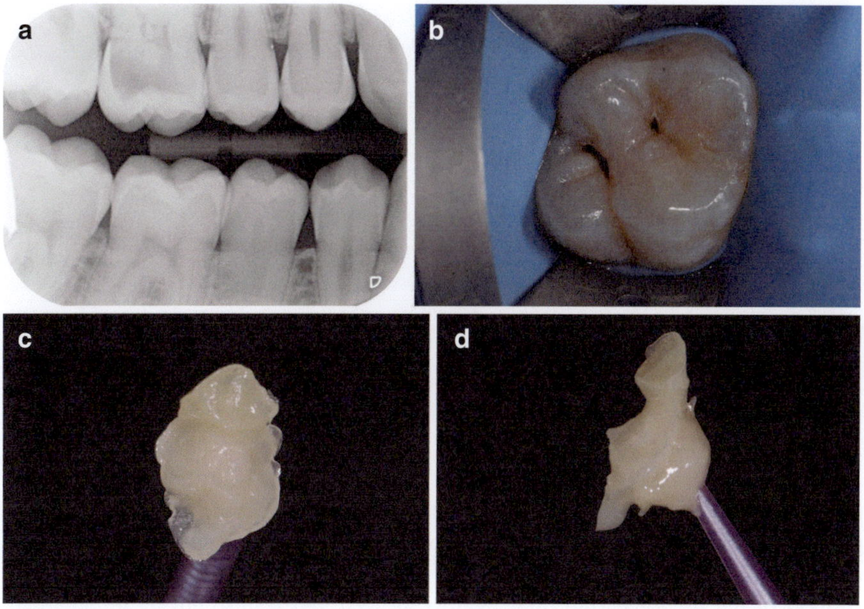

Fig. 5.53 (**a**, **b**) Tooth 16 with a deep occult carious lesion and intact occlusal table showing enamel demineralisation. (**c**, **d**) Flowable composite resin 'occlusal stamp' with handle

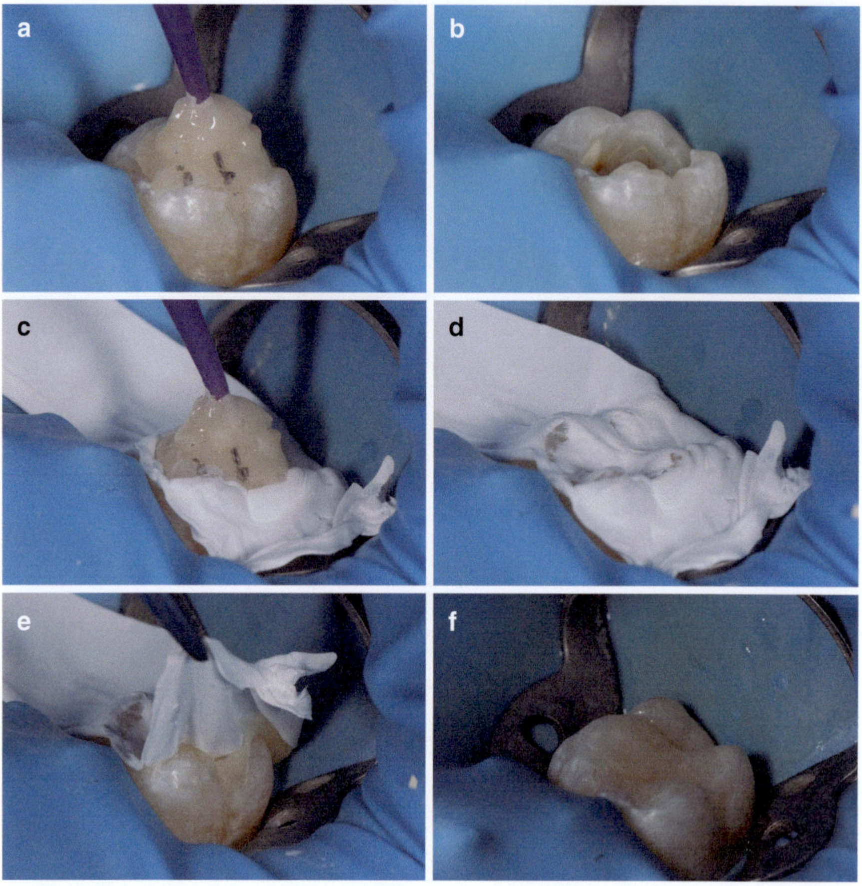

Fig. 5.54 (**a**) Tooth 16 (buccal view) pre-operative recording of the occlusal surface with stamp material and handle attachment. (**b**) Occlusal cavity preparation. (**c**) PTFE tape separator and occlusal stamp location. (**d–f**) Removal of stamp, PTFE tape separator and excess composite resin material

capture of an ideal palatal surface in PVS putty for a Class III or Class IV situation, the 'axial shield' technique uses a PVS impression to capture the preoperative shape of the affected wall before it is lost as part of the Class II cavity preparation. The defective wall is first restored first using the PVS matrix and therefore allows the support of the sectional ring tines against the restored wall to ensure an adequate adaptation of the metal foil matrix and subsequent shape of restoration. This technique is shown in a clinical case (Figs. 5.56 and 5.57), and the required clinical stages are listed in Table 5.2.

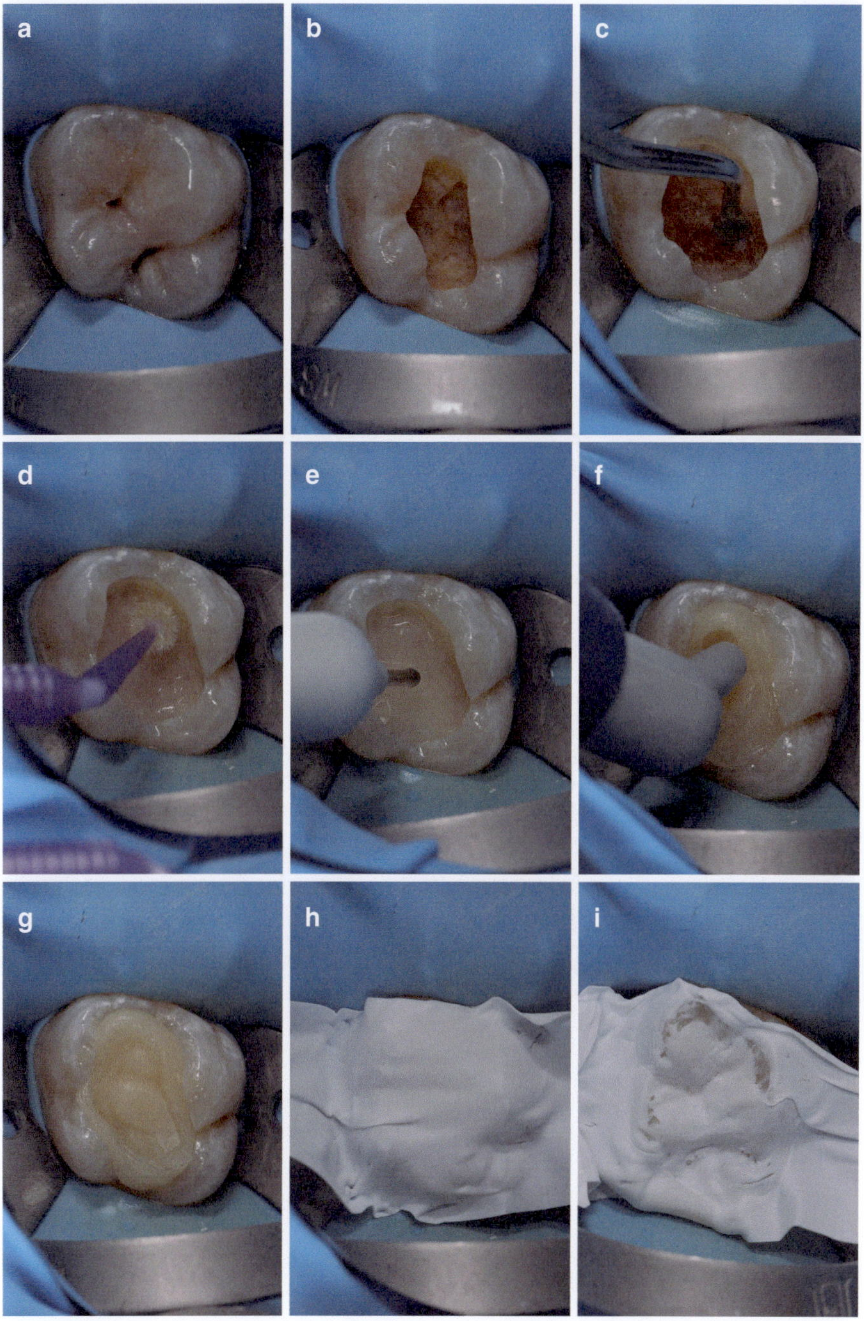

Fig. 5.55 (**a**) Tooth 16 (occlusal view) (**b**, **c**) deep occlusal caries removal. (**d**) After enamel etching, rinse and drying, application of self-adhesive eighth generation bonding agent. (**e**) Placement of flowable bulk-fill composite resin base restoration. (**f**, **g**) Placement of composite resin paste capping material into cavity. (**h**, **i**) PTFE tape separator, occlusal stamp location and removal of stamp. (**j**) Removal of PTFE tape separator and excess composite resin material. (**k**, **l**) Polishing of light polymerised restoration with an aluminium oxide impregnated rubber point

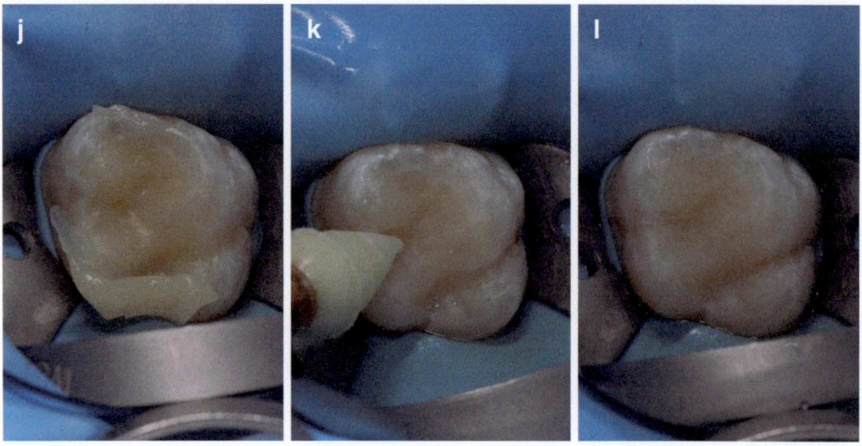

Fig. 5.55 (continued)

Table 5.1 The clinical stages required for the 'occlusal stamp' technique

'Occlusal stamp' technique
1. Tooth prophylaxis/alumina blasting
2. Preoperative recording of the tooth occlusal surface with stamp material
3. Handle attachment to the uncured stamp material
4. Polymerisation of stamp material (self or light polymerised)
5. Prepare cavity and place composite resin base restoration
6. Apply composite resin paste capping material into the cavity (<2 mm thickness)
7. Apply separator to intaglio surface of stamp or occlusal surface of tooth—Glycerine or PTFE tape
8. Locate stamp—Firm axial directed force for stability
9. Remove excess composite resin material
10. Light polymerises through the stamp material if translucent PVS is used
11. Remove stamp, PTFE separator and excess composite resin material
12. Model and characterise composite resin material
13. Light polymerises composite resin material
14. Finish & Polish

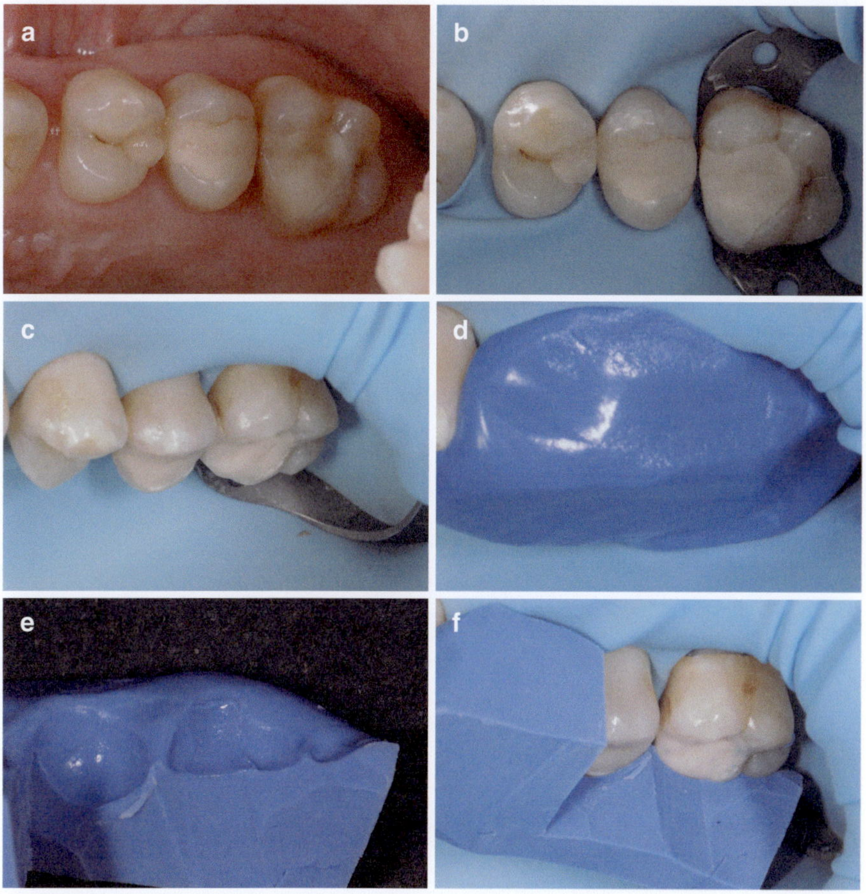

Fig. 5.56 (**a**–**c**) Tooth 26 existing GIC restoration with extension onto palatal axial wall and second quadrant isolation. (**d**–**f**) PVS putty pre-operative impression taken and sectioned through cusp tips forming 'axial shield' reseated on teeth to check stability

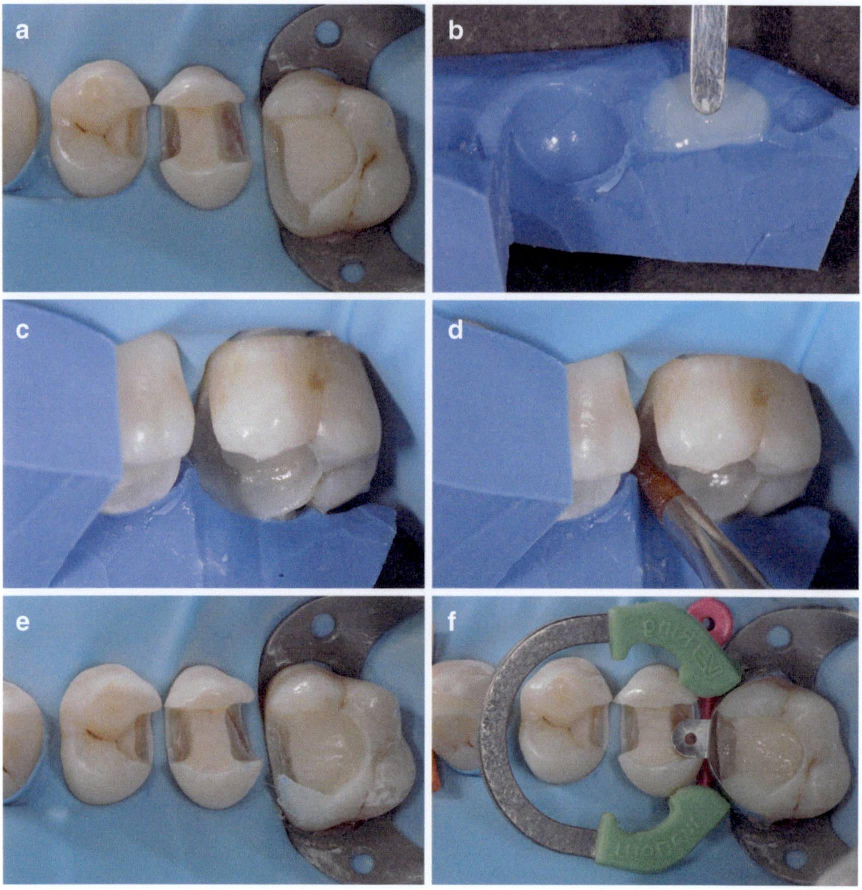

Fig. 5.57 (**a**) second quadrant Class II cavity preparations. (**b**) Composite resin material applied onto PVS shield. (**c**, **d**) Location of shield and adaptation of composite resin material to mesial-palatal wall of tooth 26 with a brush lubricated with modelling resin. (**e**) Material light polymerised and shield removed. (**f**) The restored mesial-palatal wall allows the support of the sectional matrix ring tines to allow provision of Class II restoration without collapse of the metal foil matrix by compression for the sectional ring tine

Table 5.2 The clinical stages required for the 'axial shield' technique

'Axial shield' technique
1. Tooth prophylaxis/alumina blasting
2. Preoperative recording of the buccal/palatal/lingual surface with PVS putty
3. Prepare tooth cavity
4. Section through the cusp tips of PVS impression recording
5. Apply composite resin material and model with brush or metal–/silicone-tipped instrument onto PVS shield
6. Locate PVS shield—Firm lateral directed force for stability
7. Adapt composite resin material to tooth with a brush
8. Light polymerise
9. Remove axial shield
10. Assemble sectional matrix
11. Continue with the provision of class II restoration

5.9.3 Class IV Restoration Full Protocol

A case highlighting the full Class IV restoration protocol is shown (Figs. 5.58, 5.59, 5.60, 5.61, 5.62, 5.63, 5.64, 5.65, 5.66, 5.67, and 5.68) and the clinical stages and tips are listed in Table 5.3.

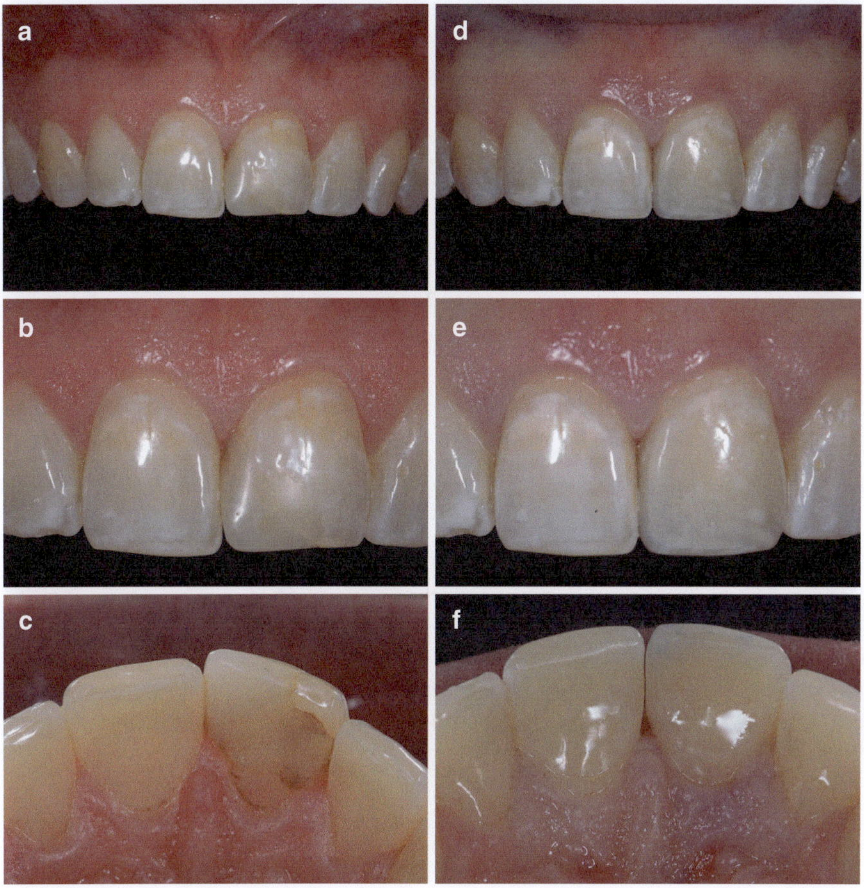

Fig. 5.58 (**a–c**) Tooth 21 pre-operative situation. (**d–f**) Provision of Class IV, V & III composite resin restorations showing aesthetic and functional integration

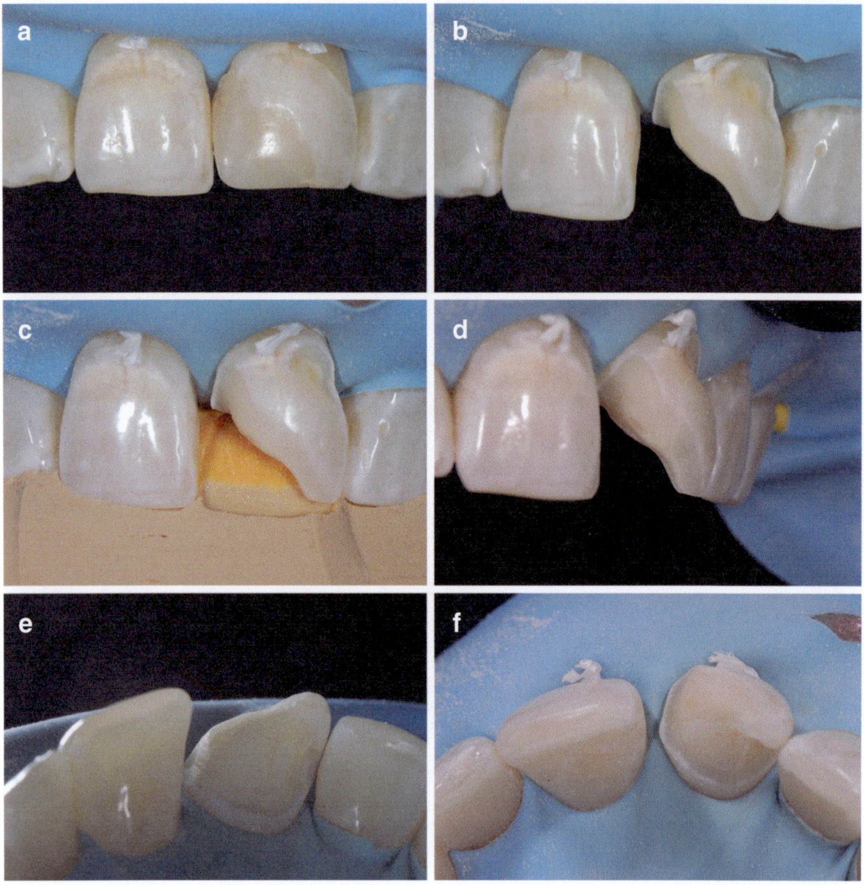

Fig. 5.59 (**a**, **b**) Tooth 21 tooth preparation with dissection of exiting restorative resin material and Class IV, V & III cavity preparations. (**c**) Seating and stability of PVS matrix. (**d**–**f**) Aesthetic bevel and functional chamfer finish lines placed, and tooth sandblasted

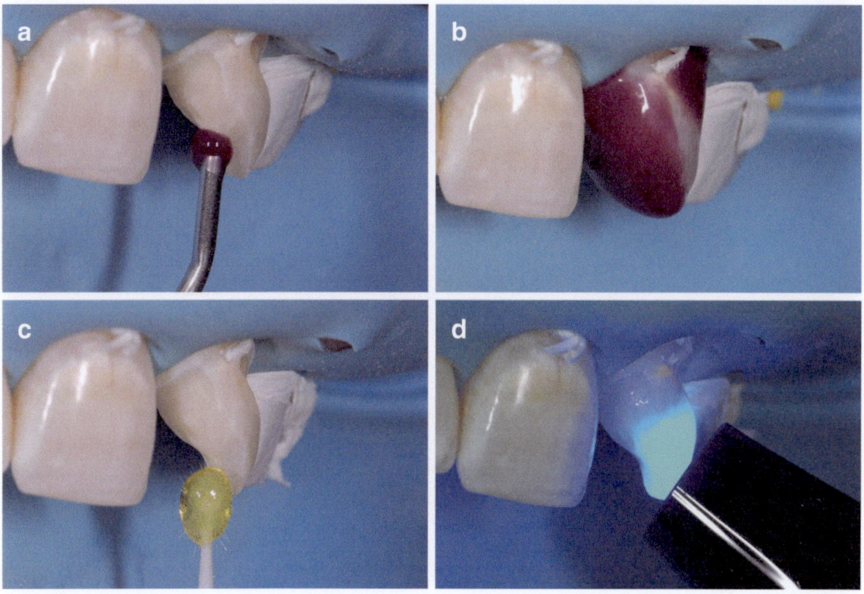

Fig. 5.60 Tooth 21 adhesive preparation of tooth surface with (**a**, **b**) application of 37.5% phosphoric acid total-etch, (**c**) eighth generation bonding agent, (**d**) air dry and light cure

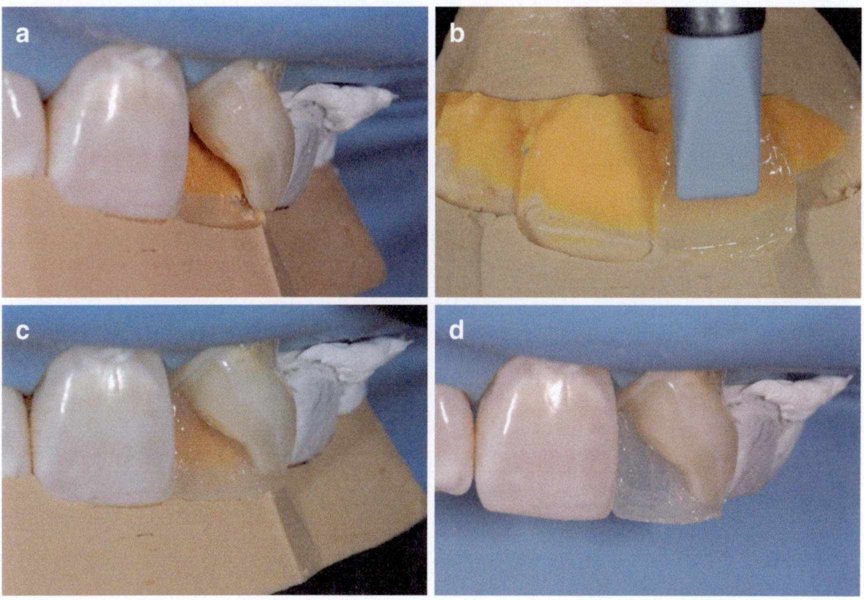

Fig. 5.61 (**a**) Tooth 21 seating of PVS matrix. (**b**) Enamel material increment application to PVS matrix with a silicone tipped instrument, (**c**, **d**) transferred to tooth to form the restoration palatal shell

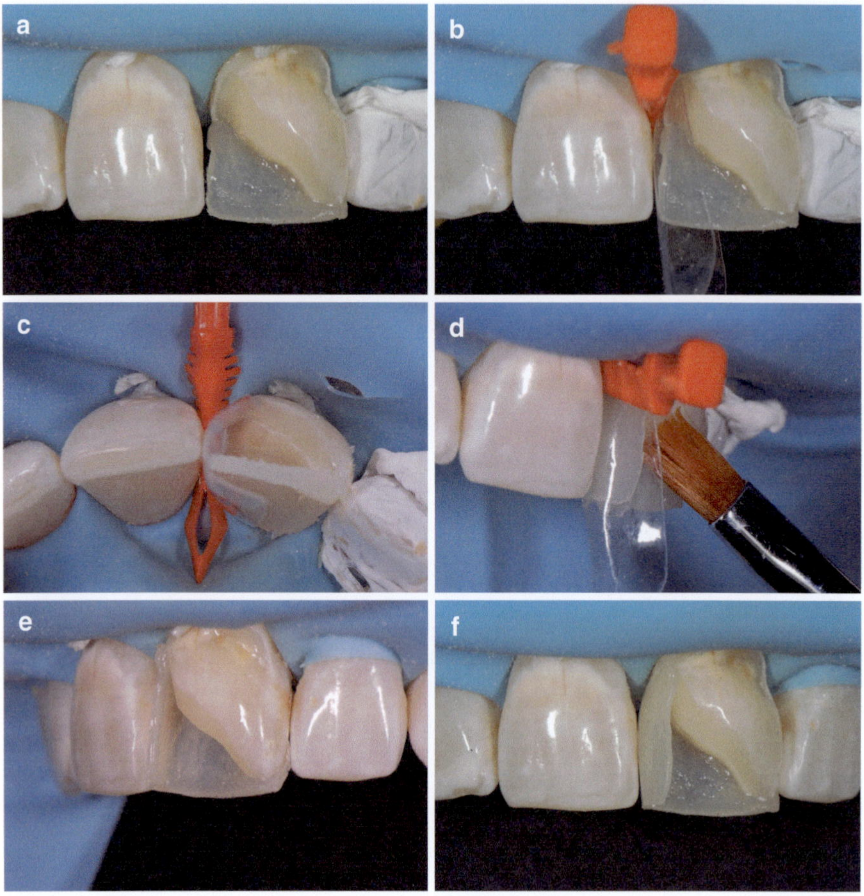

Fig. 5.62 (**a**) Tooth 21 palatal shell and (**b**, **c**) use of plastic interdental wedge to support anatomical contoured acetate matrix for replication of appropriate contour of interproximal surface and embrasure space. (**d**) Application of composite resin material with a modelling brush lubricated with modelling resin (**e**, **f**) forming mesial interdental surface

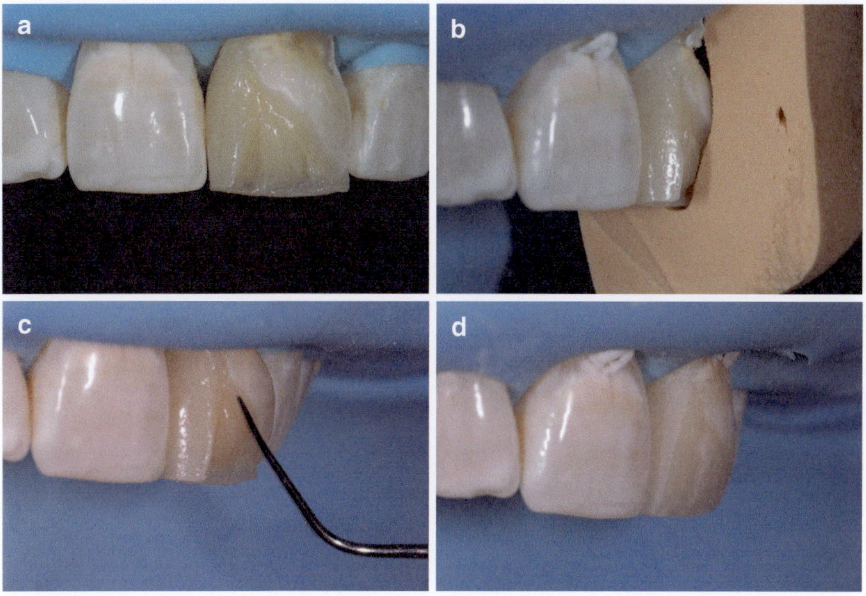

Fig. 5.63 (**a**) Tooth 21 application of dentine body mass and formation of mammellon lobes adapted to bevel. (**b**) Space checked with a sectional putty matrix. (**c**) Application of tints and effects with a straight probe. (**d**) Addition of final outer enamel layer primary anatomy

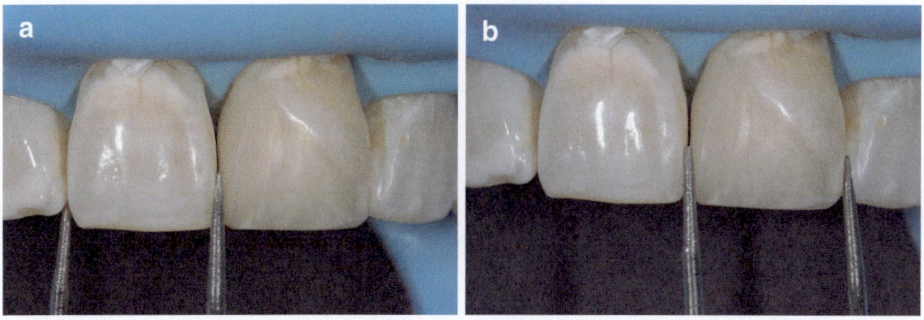

Fig. 5.64 (**a**, **b**) Tooth 21 symmetry check with callipers compared to baseline tooth 11

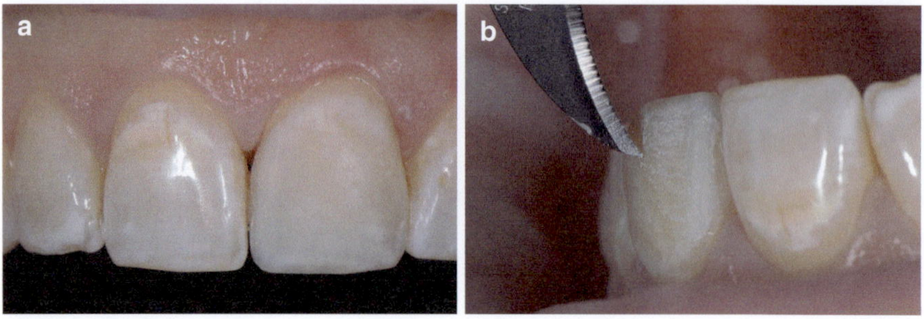

Fig. 5.65 (**a**, **b**) Tooth 21 finishing of restoration to remove resin flash and perikymata texture application with No. 12 scalpel blade

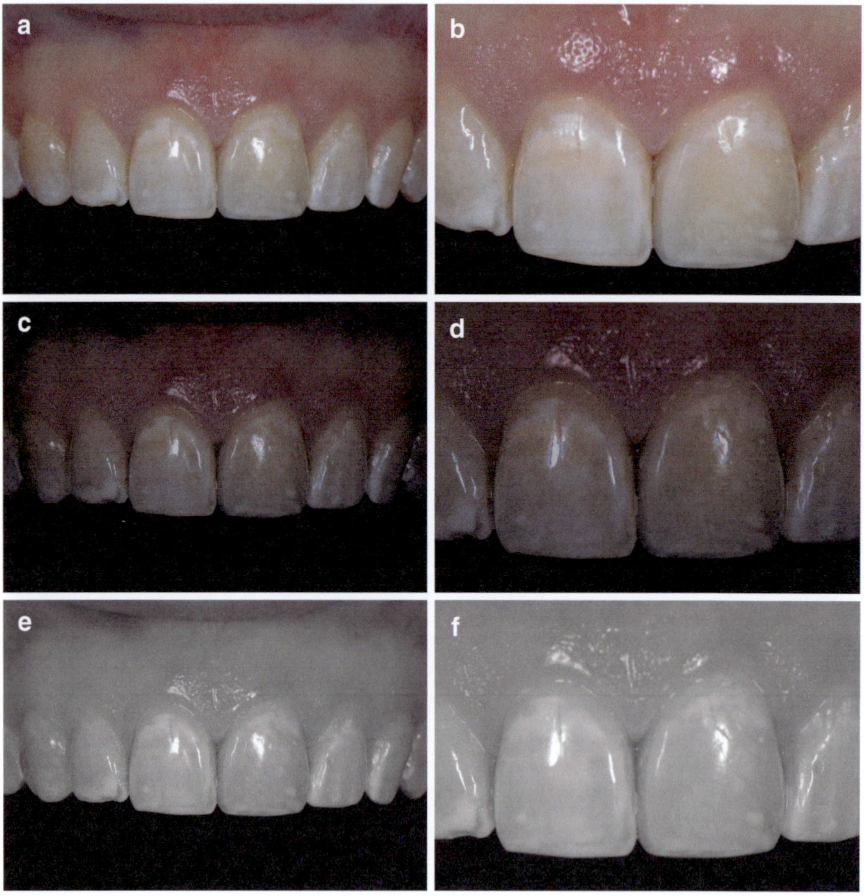

Fig. 5.66 (**a**, **b**) Tooth 21 completed composite resin restorations after polishing. (**c**–**f**) Digitally edited photographs to assess shade, value, chroma and characteristics of the restoration compared to adjacent baseline tooth

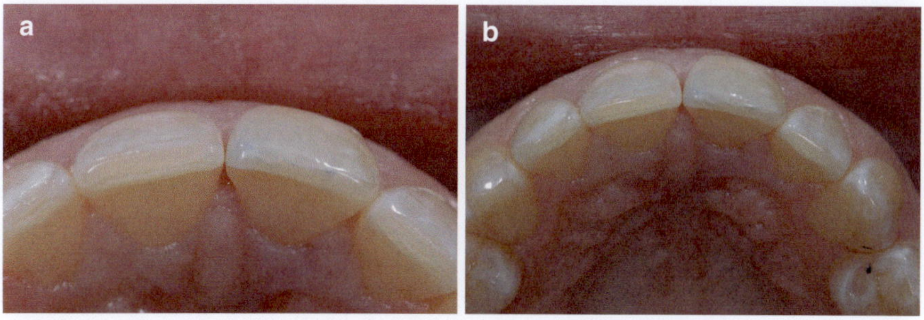

Fig. 5.67 (**a**, **b**) Tooth 21 completed composite resin restorations. Incisal edge view highlighting incisal edge thickness, interdental embrasure shapes and facial transitions

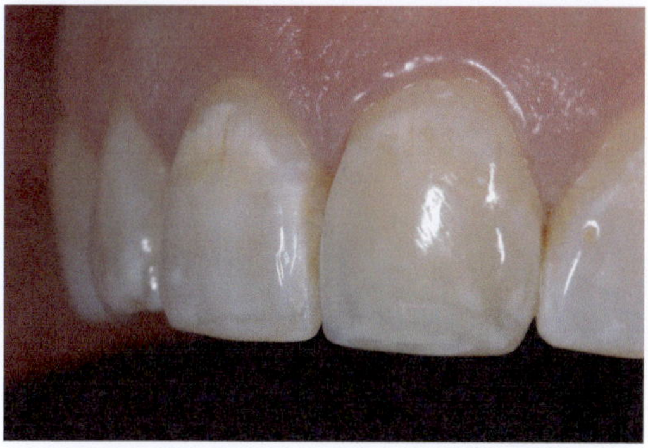

Fig. 5.68 Tooth 21 completed Class IV, V & III composite resin restorations showing harmonious integration of restorations into tooth and with adjacent intra-oral surroundings

Table 5.3 The clinical stages and tips for class IV restoration

Class IV restoration	
Stages	Tips
1. Isolation	Rubber dam—Dry teeth with air to invert Floss ligature stabilisation
2. Barrier removal	Ultrasonic scaler Prophylaxis Alumina blast
3. Tooth preparation	Restoration dissection Caries & dentine pin removal Finish line placement (aesthetic & functional) Alumina blast bonding surfaces
4. Adhesive preparation	Total-etch technique Rinse & dry Fourth or eighth generation bonding agent Indirect air-dry Light polymerise
5. Composite resin layering	PVS matrix—Defect margin scribed with probe to guide loading with composite resin enamel increment Palatal shell—Enamel resin layer adapt with brush lubricated with modelling resin, <0.3 mm thick Interproximal wall—Anatomical contoured acetate matrix and wedge. Adapt interdental enamel increments with a brush Dentine body—Apply as one mass and sculpt lobes and primary anatomy. Check thickness against sectioned matrix. Apply effects and tints Enamel layer—Apply as one mass and sculpt with a large flat plastic instrument, manipulate and blend with a brush
6. Finish & polishing	Callipers—Check tooth width and length Pencil—Highlight transitional line angle and grooves for primary contouring Finish—Excess resin removed with scalpel blades. Abrasive disks at low speed revolution to define the incisal edge, embrasure space and transitional line angles Texture—Secondary and tertiary surface anatomy. Horizontal lines, acute curvature cervically with coarse diamond bur or No. 12 scalpel Polish—Multistep dry protocol with Aluminium oxide impregnated points/discs and sequential diamond impregnated polishing pastes with a felt wheel at high-speed revolution

Further Reading

Bichacho N. The centripetal build-up for composite resin posterior restoration. Pract Periodontics Aesthet Dent. 1994;6:17–23; quiz 24.

Devoto W, Saracinelli M, Manauta J. Composite in everyday practice: how to choose the right material and simplify application techniques in the anterior teeth. Eur J Esthet Dent. 2010;5(1):102–24.

Dietschi D. Optimising aesthetics and facilitating clinical application of free-hand bonding using the 'natural layering concept'. Br Dent J. 2008;204:181–5.

Dietschi D. Optimizing smile composition and esthetics with resin composites and other conservative esthetic procedures. Eur J Esthet Dent. 2008;3(1):14–29.

Fahl N. Achieving life-like anterior composite restorations. Considerations and technique concepts. J Cos Dent. 2013;28:60–72.

Giachetti L, Scaminaci Russo D, Bambi C, Grandini R. A review of polymerization shrinkage stress: current techniques for posterior direct resin restorations. J Contemp Dent Pract. 2006;7:79–88.

Gönülol N, Yilmaz F. The effects of finishing and polishing techniques on surface roughness and color stability of nanocomposites. J Dent. 2012;40(Suppl):2.

Manhart J, Chen H, Hamm G, Hickel R. Buonocore memorial lecture. Review of the clinical survival of direct and indirect restorations in posterior teeth of the permanent dentition. Oper Dent. 2004;29:481–508.

Opdam NJ, Roeters FJ, Feilzer AJ, Verdonschot EH. Marginal integrity and postoperative sensitivity in Class 2 resin composite restorations in vivo. J Dent. 1998;26:555–62.

Sattar MM, Patel M, Alani A. Clinical applications of polytetrafluoroethylene (PTFE) tape in restorative dentistry. Br Dent J. 2017;222(3):151–8.

Sundfeld RH, Croll TP, Briso AL, de Alexandre RS, Sundfeld Neto D. Considerations about enamel microabrasion after 18 years. Am J Dent. 2007;20:67–72.

Szep S, Frank H, Kenzel B, Gerhardt T, Heidemann D. Comparative study of composite resin placement: centripetal buildup versus incremental technique. Pract Proced Aesthet Dent. 2001;13:243–50.

Vanini L. Light and color in anterior composite restorations. Pract Periodontics Aesthet Dent. 1996;8:673–82.

Restoring Root-Canal-Treated Teeth

6

Contents

Learning Outcomes

- Improve upon treatment planning for the restoration of RCT teeth
- Understand clinical justification for restoration approaches
- Gain an understanding of adhesive methods that allow the clinician to provide direct restoration of non-vital teeth

6.1 Introduction

Root-canal-treated teeth represent a significant challenge to the clinician that differs from that of teeth otherwise vital with significant tooth tissue remaining. By virtue of their vitality loss and need for root canal treatment, the tooth is highly likely to have reduced volumetric mass or acquired structural defects. The tooth itself, having been accessed, will be more hollow and hence physically more vulnerable to mechanical functional forces imparted. The loss in mass needs to be considered not only through numerical amount but also strategic position. For example, a 30%

A. Alani, M. Patel, *Adhesive Techniques in Restorative Dentistry*, BDJ Clinician's Guides, https://doi.org/10.1007/978-3-032-07346-4_6

reduction in volume by way of removal of occlusal tissue mass is biomechanically more favourable than 30% removal via a mesio-occlusal or disto-occlusal restoration that has breached the pulp chamber and undermined the adjacent cusps. The concern for undermined adjacent cusps is compounded once the tooth has been accessed for root canal treatment. The removal of the pulp roof results in a loss of structural resilience due to the bracing role of the occluso-pulpal portion of the coronal dentine. This process of access actually makes already weakened cusp structures weaker and undermined as the cusp height increases once the pulp chamber is exposed.

Anterior teeth may be more likely to have suffered trauma resulting in tissue loss and loss of vitality. These units may be intact but harbouring weak points such as underlying fractures or cracks. In other cases, teeth may have suffered Class IV fractures resulting in the need for re-bonding fragments, direct or indirect composite resin restorations or extra-coronal restorations. At its most severe, an absence of any supragingival tooth tissue presents a challenge due to a lack of coronal tooth structure and absence of any substantial enamel bonding substrate (Fig. 6.1).

As a result of root canal treatment and tissue loss, the remaining tooth structure is weaker and less able to manage functional loading. Hence, restorations have a greater responsibility to redistribute load to the remaining tooth tissue and periodontal ligament evenly through the axial portion of the tooth. This may be even more fraught or challenging where patients have lost vitality as a result of non-axial forces due to habitual parafunction, a significant factor to consider which the clinician may find difficult to remove, mitigate against or even reduce when providing a future restoration. Cracked teeth that have lost vitality are also likely to have been weakened due to the presence of residual restorations, making cracks even more likely (Fig. 6.2).

Physiologically, root-canal-treated teeth are less able to manage changes in loading due to the absence of proprioceptive feedback the pulp provides. Patients may

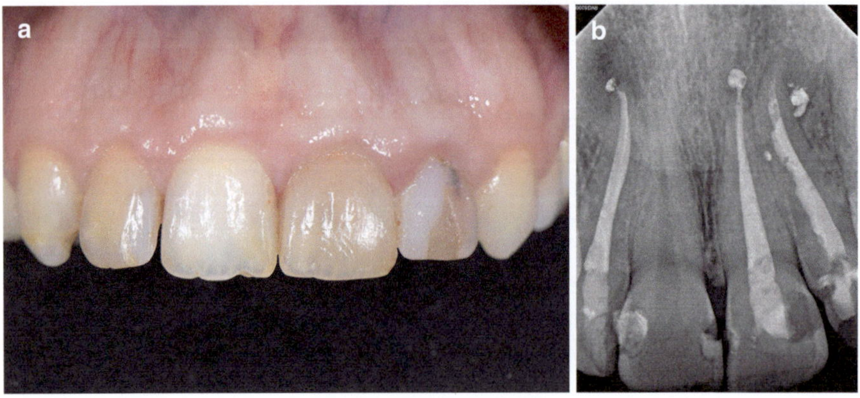

Fig. 6.1 (**a, b**) Heavily restored RCT incisor teeth that present with significant restorative challenges to allow long-term predictable biological, functional and aesthetic integration

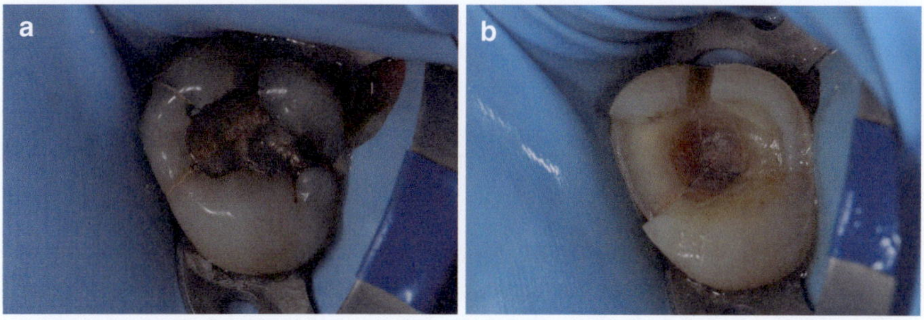

Fig. 6.2 (**a, b**) Extensive cracking within a maxillary second molar tooth highlighted after removal of amalgam restoration

expect, however unreasonable that may be, to chew and utilise root-canal-treated teeth to the same level that they did previously. This is unfortunately not possible, and communicating that in a salient way to the patient can be difficult. Managing patient expectations through the process of the time and resource required for root canal treatment and ensuring that there is an awareness that the definitive coronal restoration is just as vitally important as the root canal treatment itself can be challenging.

Other than volume and distribution the tooth tissue the process of root canal treatment changes the physical properties of the tooth. This stems from the effect that root canal disinfection irrigants and antibacterial dressing materials confer on the residual dentine. A good example of this is the long-term dressing of traumatised teeth with non-setting calcium hydroxide that coincided with root fractures. This observation resulted in changes in protocol for immature non-vital incisors. The dehydration of dentine through the loss of the pulp as a source of moisture has been cited as a cause for brittleness and, subsequently, a greater risk of fracture. The evidence for this is as yet inconclusive. Other factors may include iatrogenic weakening of the tooth through over-preparation of the canal system. Aggressive orifice opening and poor negotiation of canal curvatures further compromise the remaining tooth tissue.

In essence, the provision of the definitive coronal restoration is the last of many crucial stages that need to be observed when providing root canal treatment. A poor or compromised restoration overlying an expertly provided root canal treatment is still suboptimal treatment. The coronal restoration not only protects the remaining underlying tooth tissue but also continues the process of preventing further bacterial ingress to the apex or entombing bacteria that may remain within the root canal system post-endodontics. Unlike restorations placed solely for aesthetic or functional reasons, coronal restorations have a greater anti-bacterial obligation when considering the survival of the tooth. The seal is vitally important. Similar to the strength of teeth being associated with the remaining tooth structure, the volume and the topography of remaining tooth tissue also play a role in the ability to seal. The superior bonding to enamel is a marker of the potential for optimal seal. The greater the enamel present the improved prognosis for restorability. The margin and position of the tooth tissue also play a role. A deep carious margin is more difficult to predictably seal than a definitive, visually apparent and readily isolated supragingival margin.

6.2 Tooth Restorability

Published methods have been proposed to quantify the restorability of a tooth unit and thereby suggest a restoration management strategy. However, the assessment of tooth restorability can be highly subjective. Any tooth that can be 'restored' is based upon operator skill level and their experience, but the essential component that makes any treatment option realistic is longevity. Survival of both tooth and restoration is symbiotic and is a significant factor for any patient embarking on treatment. The question of 'How long will this last ?' can only be partially supported by quality evidence-based research that is applicable to the individual presenting clinical situation. The assessment of a tooth for restorability should not be conducted in isolation from the general clinical presentation. General plaque control and susceptibility to caries and periodontal disease may weigh against the provision of endodontics and restoration, especially if further teeth are likely to deteriorate in the meantime. Patients with parafunction and bruxism place unfavourable occlusal functional loads on teeth, and as such, may be best treated with less aesthetic but more resilient restorations such as gold or non-precious metal alloys. This may not be aesthetically appealing to the patient, and a compromise may have to be accepted. The role the tooth will play in the future needs to be considered. The functional and aesthetic needs of a discoloured, optimally root-canal-treated and otherwise intact central incisor in a patient with a high smile line will differ significantly from a mandibular second molar with difficult root canal anatomy and a large MOD restoration.

The assessment of the remaining tooth begins with radiographic assessment of the root canal treatment and migrates to the coronal tooth tissue. Ideally, prior to the provision of root canal treatment, an assessment of restorability should be conducted but may not always have occurred. Removal of all existing restorative material and an appraisal of the remaining tooth tissue prior to deciding the definitive strategy aids the identification of opportunities, strengths and weaknesses of a tooth for the subsequent restoration. Unlike vital teeth, the surface area available for adhesive bonding is practically greater in non-vital teeth due to the exposure of the pulp chamber. This greater availability needs to be tempered against the unfortunate poorer bonding ability of dentine and the likely reduced enamel substrates. Engagement of the pulp chamber may load the floor of the pulp unfavourably, especially where this is thin or anatomically unfavourable. The topography of the remaining tooth is also a source of deliberation. A deep, subgingival distal or mesial box can result in the absence of an avenue for predictable restoration outside of crown lengthening or orthodontic extrusion.

One other important consideration is whether or not an intermediate restoration or 'core' is applied to the tooth prior to the overlying restoration, or the intra-pulpal area is filled with the overlying restoration in a one-piece arrangement. One needs to be wary that the 'core' material is not part of the tooth but another portion of the restoration, and failure of the core may automatically confer failure or debond on the overlying restoration.

6.3 Bonding Issues

Dentine and root canal dentine differ in their bonding capacity in comparison to enamel. Outside of the differences in the effect of etching between enamel and dentine, root canal dentine provides a further challenge. Root canal dentine has inherently less dentinal tubules and as such the potential for micromechanical retention is reduced. The shape of the canal does not lend itself to optimal bonding. A tapering canal shape as the space progresses to the residual gutta-percha is likely to result in unfavourable polymerisation shrinkage away from the canal walls and so jeopardise the seal and attachment of the restoration. The bond within the canal system may be compromised by the materials present as a result of the endodontic treatment. At the macro level, the remnants of obturation, such as gutta-percha and cement sealer, hamper the bonding process purely through preventing contact with the canal surface. Optical magnification to remove materials to ensure a debris-free bonding surface is advisable, especially where gutta-percha is removed from within 4–5 mm of the apex of the tooth. This is unlikely to be achieved without good visualisation. The root surface can be cleansed by gentle ultrasonic instrumentation without significant contact with the root canal walls. Ultrasonic wave agitation is likely to disrupt any residual remaining biofilm in addition dental material. Concerns with regard to the effect that eugenol-containing cement sealers have on bonding due to their effect on composite initiators have not been fully proven in the literature, regardless, this effect can be theoretically mitigated against through flushing with ethanol once the root dentine is visibly clean and material-free. The canal space itself presents some practical challenges to the bonding process. In contrast to bonding to a smooth surface, the process of acid etching and applying the adhesive resin is likely to be more difficult due to inability to assure acid etch coverage throughout the length of the root canal and preventing the pooling of the bonding agent at the bottom of the canal.

6.4 Anterior Teeth

The otherwise intact anterior tooth that has undergone root canal treatment may not require any special considerations when restoring other than ensuring optimal sealing not only to prevent bacterial re-infection but also to limit the ingress of substances that may discolour the tooth. The provision of a subseal of IRM, followed by a glass-ionomer cement layer replacing the dentine and a final capping layer of composite resin on the outer extremity of the cavity may fulfil the required role of the restoration (Fig. 6.3). If the patient is unfortunate enough to need future revision of the root canal retreatment, then relocating the canal without iatrogenic damage to

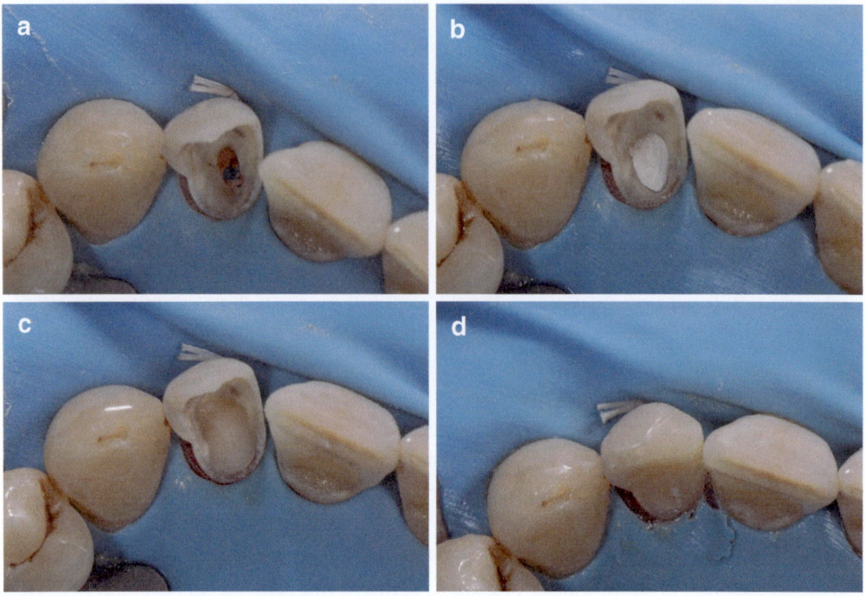

Fig. 6.3 Restoration of RCT tooth 12 with; (**a, b**) a subseal of IRM, (**c**) a glass-ionomer cement base and (**d**) a capping layer of composite resin

the residual dentine is easier utilising materials easily recognisable and distinctive from tooth tissue.

Where anterior teeth present with a significant Class IV pattern of tooth loss, the clinician may consider various options for management. By virtue of the traumatic injury suffered in the unit, the pulp may have been exposed and severely compromised, hence the need for root canal treatment. It may be intuitive to consider such extensive Class IV defects as requiring a post-retained direct or indirect restoration or at the more severe end of the spectrum needing extraction. These approaches are likely to be fuelled by concerns at both the functional and aesthetic qualities of direct composite resin restorations. If a direct composite resin restoration is provided, anterior guidance on protrusion is likely to migrate from the tooth surface onto the restoration. This transition can put the interface between tooth and restoration under strain and tension, making failure more likely. From an aesthetic point of view, due to the differing optical properties between the enamel and composite resin, the mismatch in light absorbance and reflection may be apparent (Fig. 6.4). These are realistic considerations for clinicians and patients. These aspects of direct restoration provision can be tempered by the manner in which the restoration is provided. Bleaching the residual tooth tissue can lighten and reduce variation in colour to aid shade match with the subsequent restoration. To maximise adhesive bonding capacity, the clinician can consider encasing the tooth within a composite resin restoration in its entirety on buccal and palatal surfaces to the cervical margin. This is advantageous in that it makes the restoration margin less conspicuous and

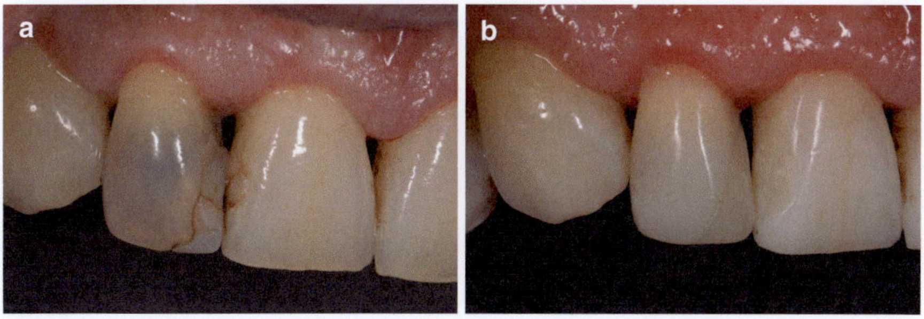

Fig. 6.4 (**a, b**) Before and after restoration of RCT tooth 12 showing aesthetic differentiation of tooth and composite resin restoration

essentially blurs the interface between the tooth and the restoration. This is also beneficial in that the Class IV restoration margin may pick up stain and be apparent due to the position of the horizontal line across the mid portion of the tooth. Relocating the margin cervically removes this issue. The extension palatally may serve a different role. By creating one consistent surface for anterior guidance to transition over, the opportunity for redesigning both static and dynamic occlusal contacts arises. The practice of encasing the remaining tooth tissue may utilise the process in a positive manner. The resin will contract towards the tooth on polymerising and hence 'shrink-fitting' onto the tooth. This is likely to improve the contact between the tooth and the restoration as the composite resin tightly compacts as it polymerises. Extending the direct composite resin restoration into the pulp chamber can also be a further feature of the restoration, depending on the extracoronal tooth tissue remaining.

Where anterior teeth have near no coronal dentine or enamel, the options are expectedly more limited. In such situations, alternative options other than restoring the unit, such as phased treatment or extraction with prosthetic replacement may be considered. The former may involve electively burying the root in young patients until such time when the alveolar and soft tissue have fully developed, and alveolar growth is completed. The latter may result in the consideration for extraction and bridge or implant provision.

Where deemed favourable, the provision of an adhesive post and core restoration requires appropriate assessment and planning. Predictable post and core restorations require an appreciation of how compromised the remaining tooth tissue is when compared to the adjacent structurally intact units. The ability of the restoration to apply loading evenly to the root has now nearly diminished, and the likelihood of mechanical breakdown of the tooth is greater. The concept of the ferrule effect when providing intracanal engaging restorations has long been cited. The ferrule essentially means that there is a band of extra-coronal direct or indirect restoration encircling the remaining coronal dentine tooth structure. Without any supragingival coronal tooth tissue, the root will be directly susceptible to lever forces directed when the tooth is functionally loaded in a non-axial direction. The optimal dentine thickness for ferrule effect is considered to be between 1.5 and

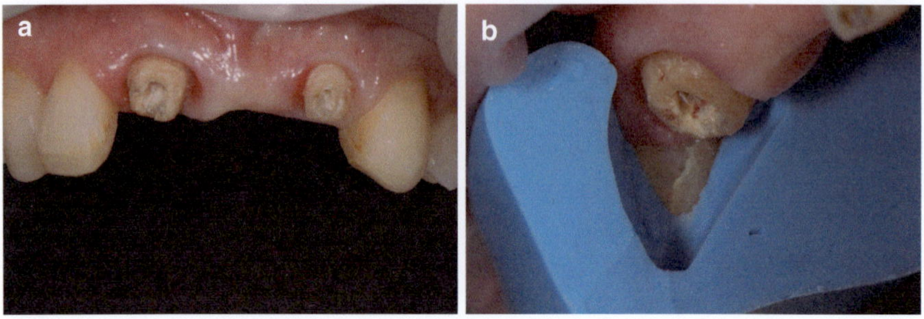

Fig. 6.5 (**a**) Teeth 11 & 22 heavily broken down with minimal coronal tooth tissue, but with adequate dentine wall height and width thickness for restoration. (**b**) Silicone matrix made from diagnostic wax-up to aid in the provision of restoration with posts

2 mm in height, the width thickness should be no less than 1 mm (Fig. 6.5). This results in the tooth and the extra-coronal restoration being loaded together when lateral forces are applied. This is then translated to the periodontal ligament more favourably.

6.5 Fibre Posts

Fibre post systems are indicated for the direct adhesive core build-up of anterior and posterior teeth that have lacking coronal supragingival tooth structure. They may be used to support and retain the coronal restoration. They have some notable advantages over traditional metal alloy post systems. The quartz fibres (approximately 60% volume) and epoxy resin (approximately 40% volume) composition of the post confers some attractive physical characteristics. Many manufacturers claim that the modulus of elasticity of the post is similar to that of human dentine (15 GPa), therefore, this theoretically confers a lower risk of fracture. The dental literature on this attractive quality when compared to metal alloy posts is evident.

The fibre posts are coloured white/opaque or are translucent in presentation, which would be aesthetically more favourable than a metal alloy post if used in conjunction with a coronal translucent restorative material. Translucency allows curing light to be transmitted throughout the length of the post surface, thus optimising photo polymerisation of the paired matched dual-cure adhesive bonding agent and resin cement in areas not readily accessible otherwise, especially in an apical direction (Fig. 6.6). Despite being translucent, the posts are identifiable radiographically as they demonstrate a degree of radio-opacity (Fig. 6.7).

Adhesive qualities of fibre posts are largely based on the surface characteristics and topography in conjunction with chemical bonding. Microporous surfaces allow for the ingress of resin to facilitate micromechanical retention (Fig. 6.6). A silanating agent is also required for the adhesion of the resin cement to the fibre

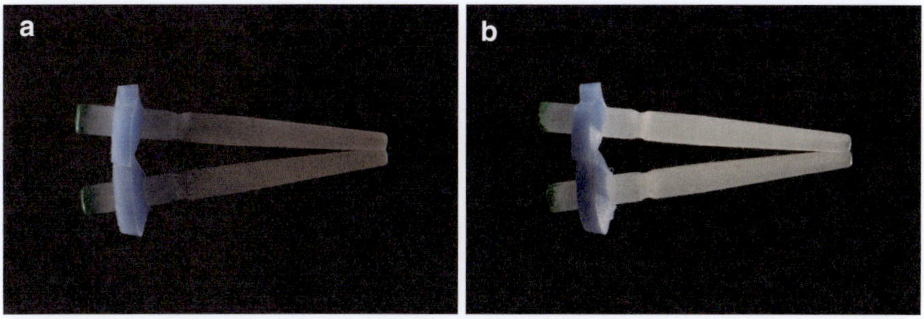

Fig. 6.6 (**a, b**) Tapered fibre post, translucent with microporous surface

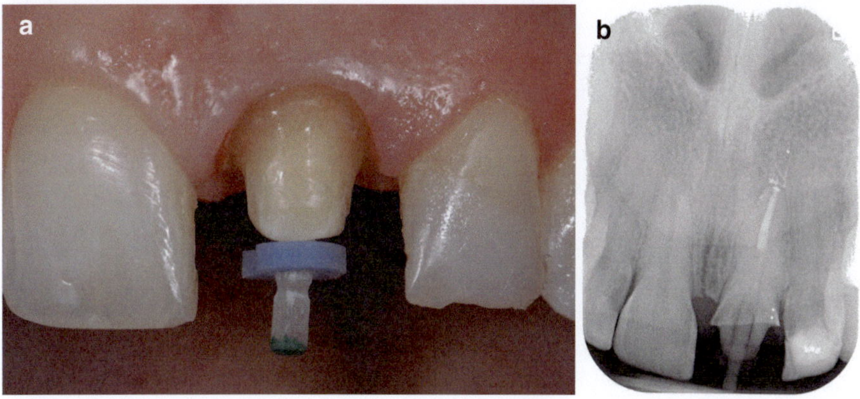

Fig. 6.7 (**a**) Tooth 21 with tapered fibre post in situ. (**b**) Diagnostic radiograph highlighting fibre post radiopacity to aid diagnostic assessment of fit of length and width, with an adequate amount of apical gutta-percha remaining

post. The micromechanical retention of the post can be improved further through sandblasting the prepared post hole in the root canal and the residual coronal tooth structure prior to the adhesive bonding procedures of post-cementation and core build-up.

Prior to deciding to provide a post, a comprehensive assessment needs to take place in addition to the relative design of the post and how the latter can optimise restoration of the former. Posts that are parallel-sided generate more stress in the residual root on cementation but provide less stress during function. The converse is true for tapered posts, where in function the wedging effect concentrated towards the apex of the tooth during function increases stress but during cementation the stresses are much less in comparison to parallel-sided. The majority of fibre post systems are tapered and hence require less preparation of the residual root due to their inherent similarity with anatomical canals, which naturally taper also (Figs. 6.6 and 6.7). A sensible post design incorporates a hybrid of both parallel and tapered features to benefit the said advantages of both shape designs (Fig. 6.8).

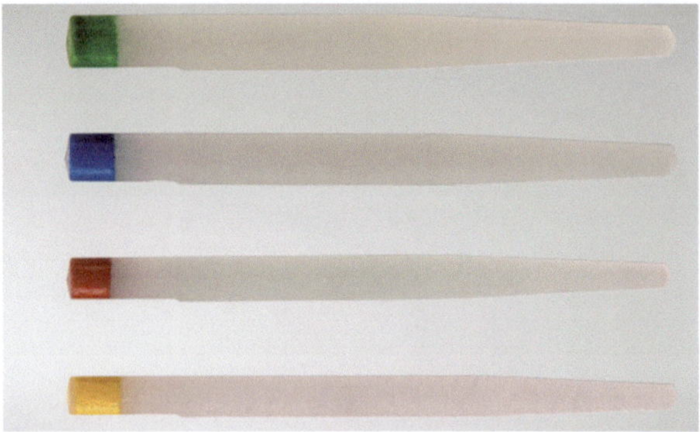

Fig. 6.8 Hybrid parallel and tapered design of fibre post. (Image courtesy of Dentsply Sirona)

The length of the post within the canal also needs to be considered. A longer post results in greater surface contact and hence improved retention. This needs to be balanced against the need to maintain the apical biological seal and the amount of gutta-percha remaining in the apical portion. The greater the amount of gutta-percha remaining at the apex, the less the likelihood that the seal would have been disturbed. A widely accepted minimum amount of gutta-percha remaining is 3–4 mm (Fig. 6.7).

The root morphology and the root diameter also need consideration. A severely curved root in either the middle or apical root third is likely to compromise the length of the post. Further, if the canal is wide, the ratio between the diameter of the post and the root and the associated resin cement becomes more unfavourable due to the greater thickness of the resin cement. The largest post diameter that remains passive within the canal is an arbitrary measure for post placement. Other arbitrary measures of post dimensions such as the post length being of a minimum length to the coronal crown are not heavily supported by evidence but are considered sensible biomechanical rules of thumb.

Once the provision of the post has been decided upon removal of the gutta-percha to accommodate the post space preparation can take place. The length of the post above the residual root should be decided upon with the final coronal restoration in mind. This may be determined by a diagnostic wax-up of the proposed external contour of the final coronal restoration. This can then be used to make a variety of silicone matrices to aid the provision of either direct composite resin or indirect ceramic restorations (Fig. 6.5).

6.6 Posterior Teeth

The internal surface area available to adhesively bond to is greater for endodontically treated posterior teeth as the pulp chamber is exposed as is the canal for the provision of the foundation restoration. The direct adhesive restoration of endodontically treated molar or premolar teeth to seal the root canal access cavity can be fairly straightforward where; the tooth may be easily isolated, matrixed and access cavity well confined with adequate thickness of dentine walls circumferentially. An IRM subseal over the gutta-percha, followed by resin-modified glass-ionomer base with a capping layer of composite resin, is more than likely to suffice in the same manner as that for anterior teeth (Fig. 6.9). In cases where there is significant loss of coronal tooth structure and volume, where the access cavity is larger, interdental marginal ridges breached, and the dentine walls thinner and undermined, the clinician may consider provision of a direct composite resin onlay cuspal coverage restoration to provide both coronal seal and mechanical protection for biomechanical assurances (Fig. 6.10). This treatment modality may also be used where the endodontic prognosis of the tooth unit is unknown and an elongated time period is required for appropriate endodontic prognostic review.

The mechanical strength and stiffness of the tooth diminish (up to 45–60%) with the breach of either or both mesial and distal marginal ridges due to the inherent increase in susceptibility of the remaining tissue to fracture propagation. In this situation, the immediate requirement for cuspal coverage increases due to the risk of flexure. The provision of a direct composite resin onlay or an indirect ceramic onlay restorations in these circumstances can achieve cusp coverage and optimally seal without unnecessary additional removal of large amounts of tooth tissue (Figs. 6.10 and 6.11).

Challenges in the provision of adhesive bonding may occur where the interproximal caries defect or existing restoration that requires removal extends deep into the subgingival area. Adequate tooth margin isolation in these deep areas may be achieved by use of a conventional matrix band and wedge in order to prevent ingress of saliva, blood and crevicular fluid contaminants into the bonding areas. A highly filled composite resin material is placed and used as a core build-up material. As such, the finish line for the definitive indirect adhesive cuspal coverage restoration may be placed on this material in a subgingival position allowing ease and improved

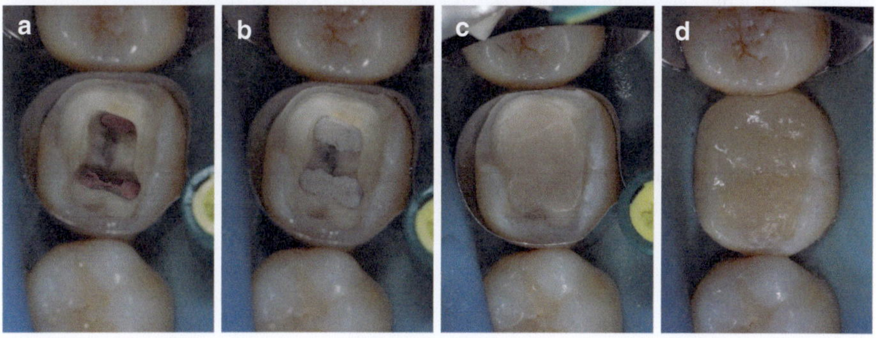

Fig. 6.9 Restoration of RCT tooth 36 with; (**a, b**) a subseal of IRM, (**c**) a glass-ionomer cement base and (**d**) a capping layer of composite resin. This tooth will require indirect cuspal coverage protection for long-term prognostic functional success

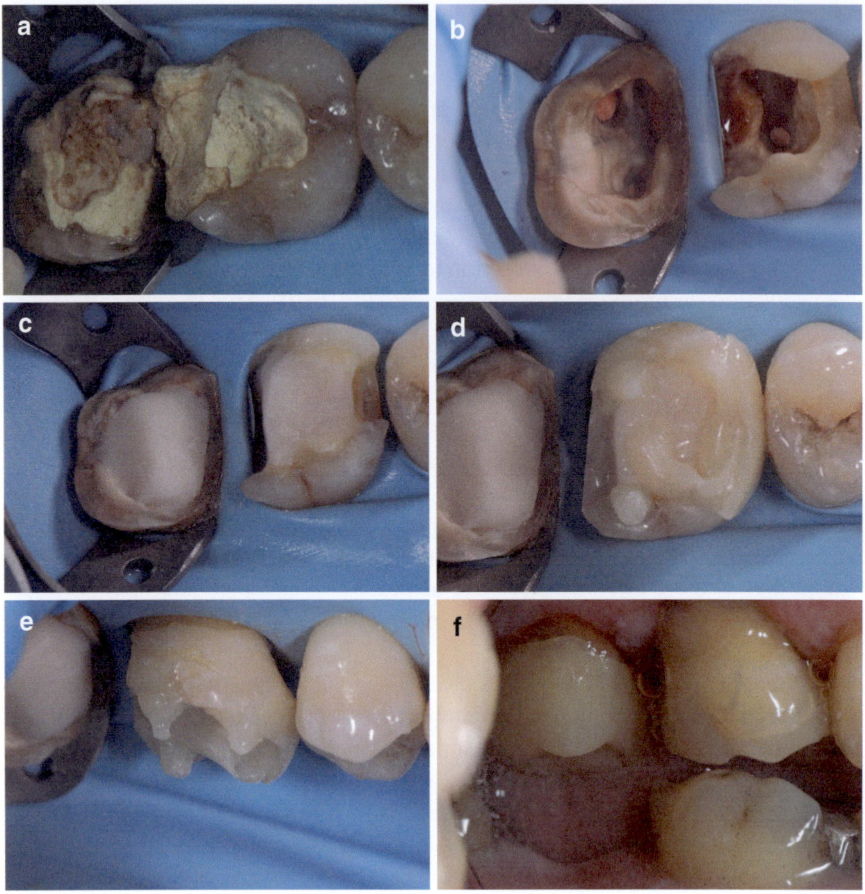

Fig. 6.10 Restoration of Re-RCT teeth 17 & 16 with direct composite resin onlay restorations; (**a, b**) isolation, temporary fillings and removal. (**c**) Sub-seal of IRM and glass-ionomer cement base. (**d, e, f**) Capping layer of composite resin incrementally anatomically built to full functional contour. These teeth will require indirect cuspal coverage protection for long-term functional success after an appropriate endodontic prognostic review

access for impression taking/digital scanning, adhesive bonding of the indirect restoration and ease of cement removal in the interproximal areas. This process is termed 'Cervical Margin Relocation (CMR)', alternatively termed 'Deep Margin Elevation (DME)' (Fig. 6.11).

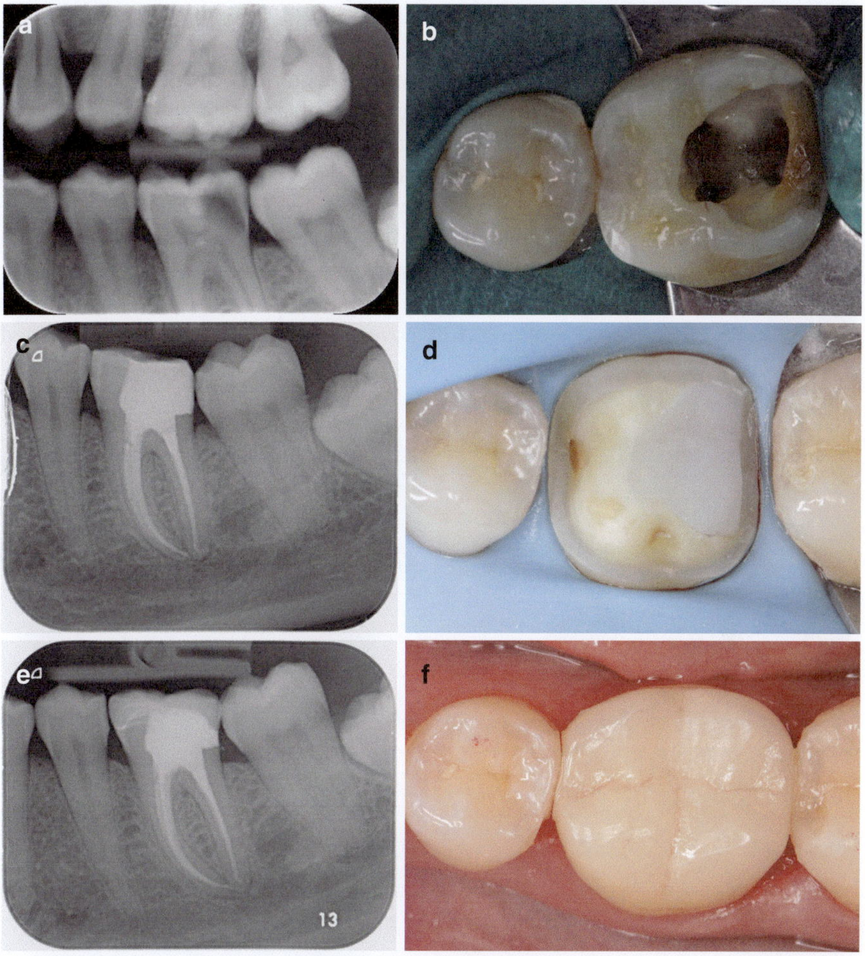

Fig. 6.11 Tooth 36 presenting with; (**a, b**) a deep distal caries lesion. (**c, d**) After root canal treatment, core build-up and onlay tooth preparation, (**e, f**) a CMR/DME technique was used to here to aid the provision and delivery of the adhesive lithium disilicate ceramic onlay restoration

6.7 Cuspal Coverage Restorations

As a cuspal coverage restoration, the onlay restoration has many advantages. The majority of the restoration margin is coronal and supragingivally placed rather than cervical near the gingival margin (defect-dependent). This makes preparation of the finish line, its capture with impression material, and its assessment post-cementation significantly easier. The restoration margin will likely predominantly have an enamel adhesive bond, hence, a superior biological seal. Due to the decreased surface area covered by the indirect restoration the hydraulic pressure generated during cementation is less and so decreased the likelihood of incomplete seating of the onlay restoration.

Onlay restorations require greater attention to detail than the standard conventional full coverage crown restorations. The onlay margin may undulate with the margin of the core restoration or in its relationship to the endodontic access cavity. The path of insertion needs careful assessment, especially if the preparation has both internal and external engaging aspects when seated on tooth tissue.

However, when there is significant coronal tooth structural damage and the engagement of tooth structure for the proposed cuspal coverage restoration is lacking for both intra-coronal and extra-coronal adhesive bonding options, a fibre post retained core can be used where a full coverage crown restoration is planned (Fig. 6.12).

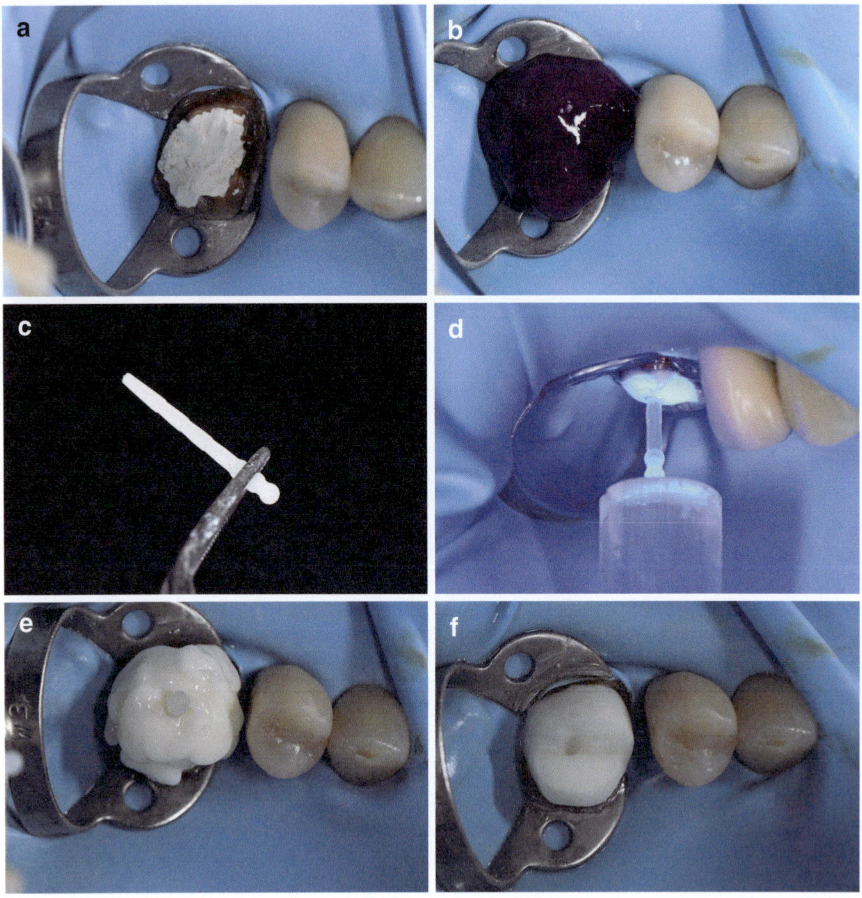

Fig. 6.12 Restoration of RCT tooth 16 with a fibre post retained core; (**a, b**) isolation, temporary filling removal and etching. (**c, d**) Tapered fibre post cementation and light curing. (**e, f**) Cured fibre post retained core, and after preparation for full coverage crown restoration

More recently, the utilisation of indirect restorations that fully engage the pulp chamber has gained popularity, otherwise known as the 'Endocrown' (Fig. 6.13). Although any material can be utilised for this technique, the overriding popular choice is the use of high-strength all-ceramic materials. As a concept, the Endocrown aims to engage the pulp chamber as a single-piece restoration without the need for a post retained core and a traditional full coverage crown restoration. This conserves tooth tissue within the root system, maximises the adhesive surface area engagement whilst providing cuspal coverage and axial loading of the restoration and tooth. It is characterised by a supra-gingival margin and is cemented with an adhesive approach. Preparation features need to incorporate occlusal reduction of at least 2 mm. Unlike more traditional preparation techniques, the internal walls of the pulp chamber require preparation to ensure no undercuts to accommodate the restoration's extension into this area. Once these stages are completed, attention can be directed to the floor of the pulp chamber. The canal orifices should have a base subseal material placed to optimise biological seal, any sharp or protruding areas can be smoothed or rounded off to reduce risk of stress concentration. Bonding under rubber dam isolation should be provided and resin cements including self-etching adhesives can be utilised (Figs. 6.13 and 6.14).

6.7.1 Immediate Dentine Sealing

Immediate dentine sealing (IDS) is a technique to treat the tooth that may be utilised in conjunction with the provision of indirect adhesive onlay restorations. It involves adhesively sealing the freshly exposed dentine surfaces immediately after they are cut during tooth preparation prior to impression taking/digital scanning and placing the definitive restoration. The etching and bonding procedures are carried out in the normal preferred manner (as described in Chap. 2), aiding in sealing the dentine substructure from dehydration, moisture and bacterial contamination; decreasing post-operative sensitivity (in the case of vital teeth) and ensuring an extended time for the dentine bond to mature for improved efficacy.

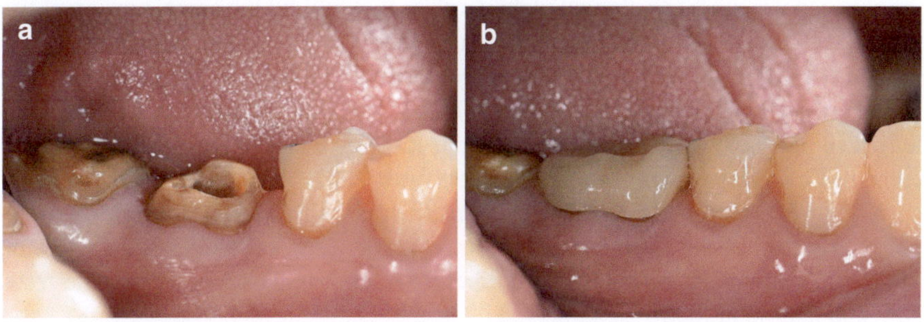

Fig. 6.13 (**a, b**) Endocrown restoration of tooth 46 before and after

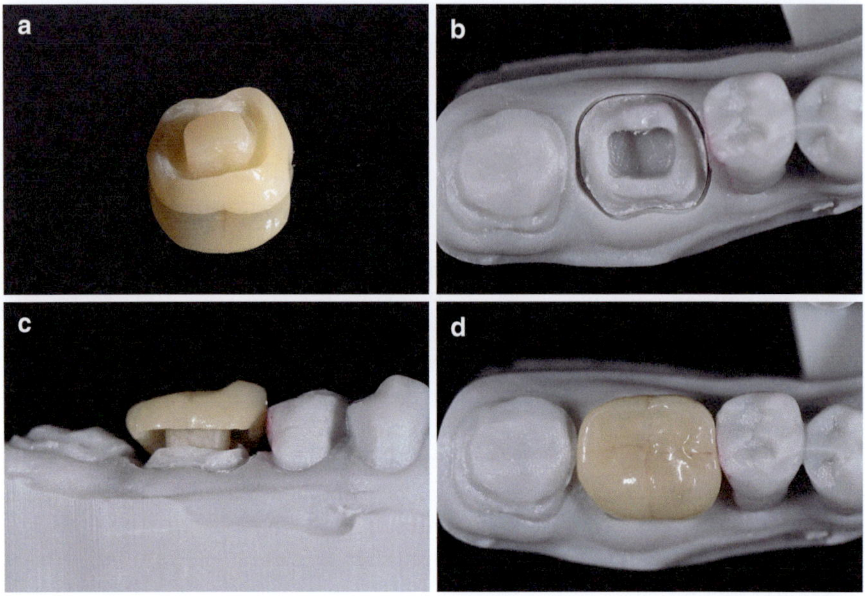

Fig. 6.14 Endocrown restoration of tooth 46 on working model. (**a**) Restoration. (**b**) Preparation. (**c**) Restoration fitting. (**d**) Restoration seated

6.8 Adhesive Technique

6.8.1 Fibre Post Cementation

Once the post diameter size, length and fit has been established and diagnostically confirmed (Fig. 6.7), the post should be disinfected and then cleaned with alcohol and air-dried. A silane primer is then applied. The root canal should be sandblasted and acid-etched. It then should be disinfected with hypochlorite and air-dried. The root canal should be coated with a dual-cure adhesive agent and air dried to allow evaporation of the solvent and prevent pooling. Application of the resin cement to the root canal requires an elongated delivery tip that will fill the apical portion of the prepared post space first. To prevent air entrapment, the tip of the applicator should remain within the cement as it is dispensed. Once filled, the post is seated with firm apical pressure within the canal. This is followed by light curing through the vertical length of the post to initiate the polymerisation of the adhesive agent and resin cement. The same cement material is then further dispensed around the post in a coronal direction to build up the core. This then is light-cured again to initiate the polymerisation of the resin cement. A time period allowing the self-cure to complete over a course of 5 min is elapsed before final shaping of the composite resin core and abutment tooth.

The summary of clinical stages for the adhesive cementation of a fibre post is listed in Table 6.1 and is shown in the presented clinical case (Figs. 6.15, 6.16, 6.17, 6.18, and 6.19).

6.8.2 Direct Composite Resin Onlay

This technique can be used for both RCT teeth and vital teeth that are cracked and require cuspal protection for structural protection.

Table 6.1 Summary of clinical stages of fibre post adhesive cementation and composite resin core build-up

Clinical stages
1. Abutment tooth and canal clean
2. Fibre post try-in & diagnostic radiograph
3. Rubber dam isolation
4. Fibre post disinfect/clean/silanate
5. Abutment tooth and root canal sand blast/etch/disinfect/dry/bond
6. Cement post & simultaneous composite resin core build-up with paired match dual-cure adhesive agent and resin cement system
7. Core and tooth preparation

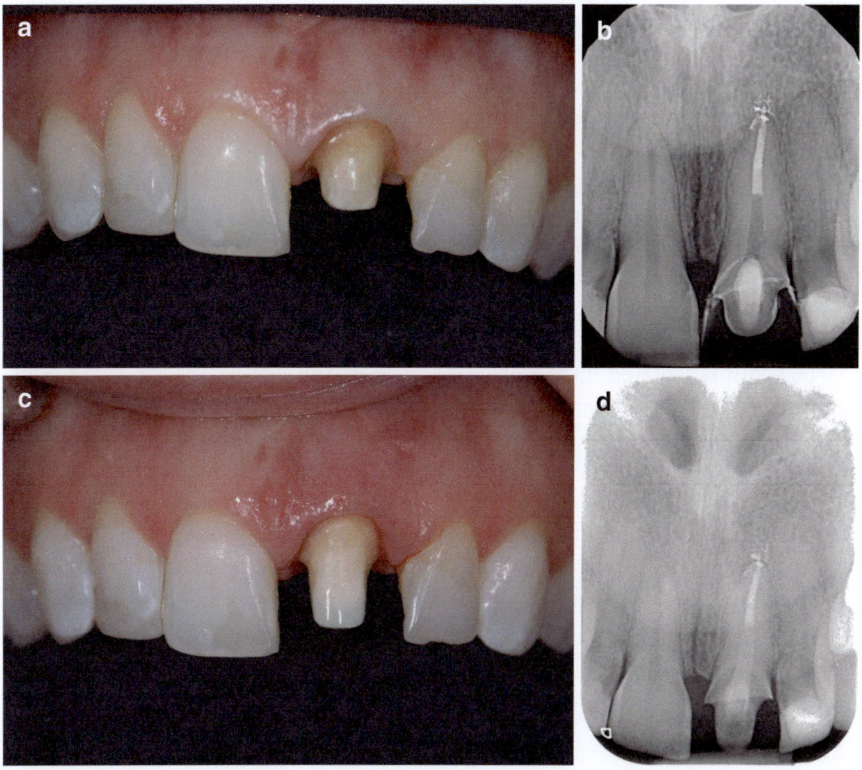

Fig. 6.15 (**a, b**) Tooth 21 before and (**c, d**) after fibre post placement and composite resin core build-up

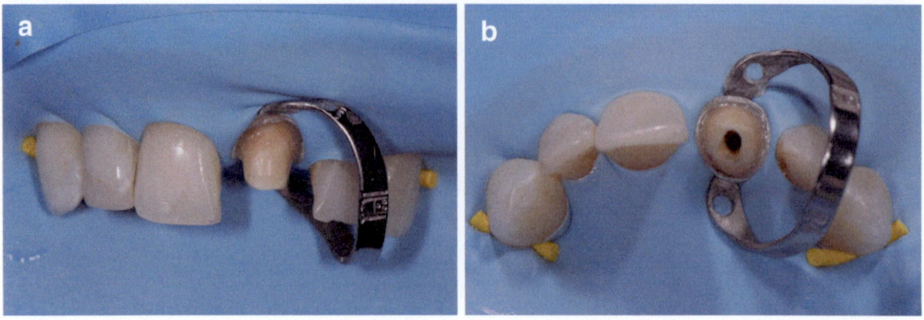

Fig. 6.16 (**a, b**) Rubber dam isolation ensuring full exposure of abutment tooth 21 and root canal bonding surfaces

A translucent and non-perforated impression tray is filled with a translucent silicone impression material, and an impression of the diagnostic wax-up or the tooth itself (depending upon what is required for the diagnostic functional and aesthetic form) is made. Alternatively, the material can be dispensed freehand without the support of an impression tray if the material's viscosity allows it. It is important that there is at least 2 mm of material thickness circumferentially.

Once removed, the inside of the matrix can be examined. Air blows, drags and void areas are likely to mean that the matrix needs to be remade. The matrix can be trimmed and tested in the mouth for fit and location. At this point, when locating the matrix intra-orally, the clinician should take note of the path of insertion of the matrix and that it seats fully on the teeth without too much flexibility. The matrix needs to be tooth supported and can be trimmed in areas where the rubber dam components may interfere with its full seating. At this stage, an injection/vent hole is required to allow for the introduction of an injectable tip to inject the composite resin material into the stent and for excess overflow material out of the matrix. The position of the injection/vent hole should correlate to the midpoint of the occlusal table. Even if venting is applied to the matrix, the composite resin overflow is likely to be spread across adjacent teeth, into the interdental embrasures and the gingiva. To reduce the likelihood of this, a separating and block out material such as PTFE tape can be utilised.

The tooth is isolated then prepared across its full occlusal surface and a circumferential finish line is made to accommodate space and engagement of the restorative material. Once the tooth is sandblasted, etched, resin bond applied and light cured, both the tooth and the matrix can be pre-loaded with composite resin material. If composite resin paste material is used, it may be heated in a composite resin warming machine to decrease its viscosity in order to allow flow of the material with limited distortion to the transparent silicone matrix carrier. The matrix needs to be loaded with the aim of limiting the amount of air bubbles

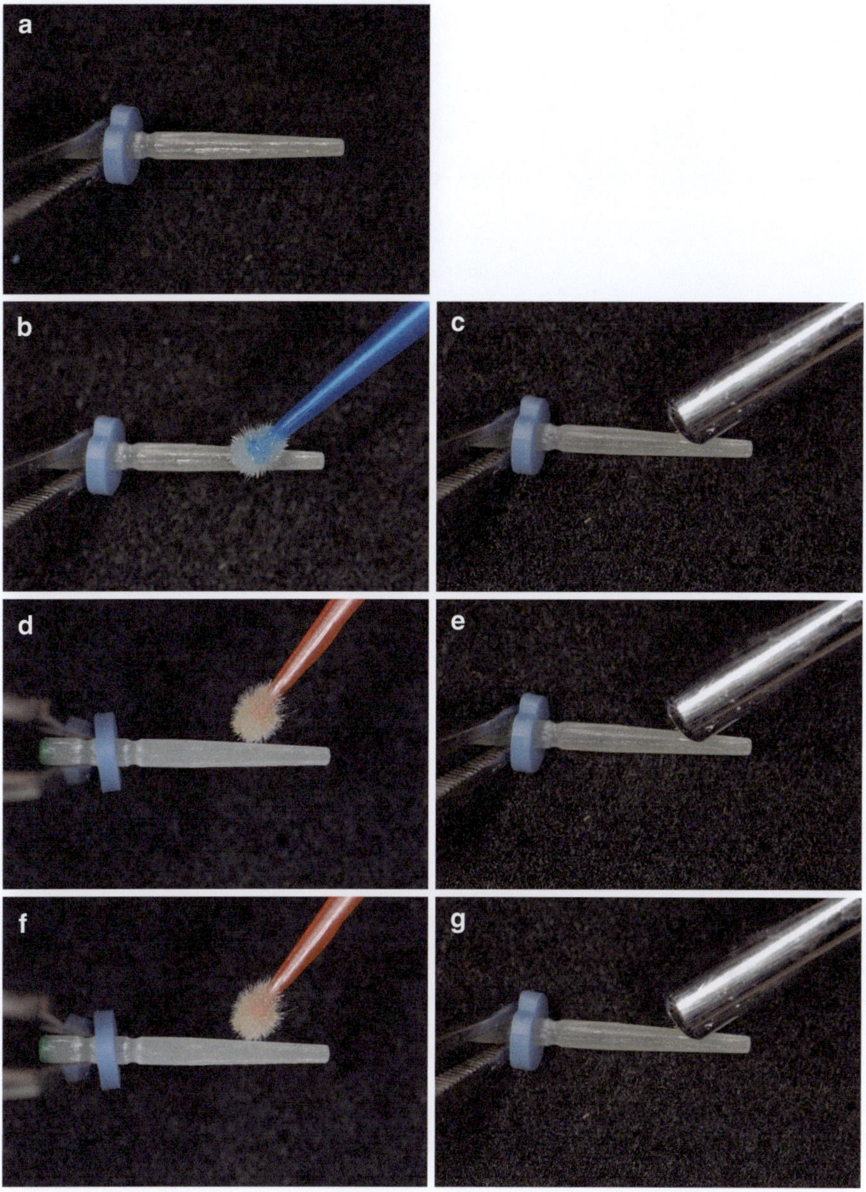

Fig. 6.17 Glass-fibre post restoration surface treatment for adhesive bonding, disinfection/clean/silanate (**a**) Steam cleaned (**b**) Alcohol clean (**c**) Air dry (**d**) Silane (60 s if post not pre-silanated) (**e**) Air dry (**f**) Adhesive (dual-cure) application (**g**) Air dry

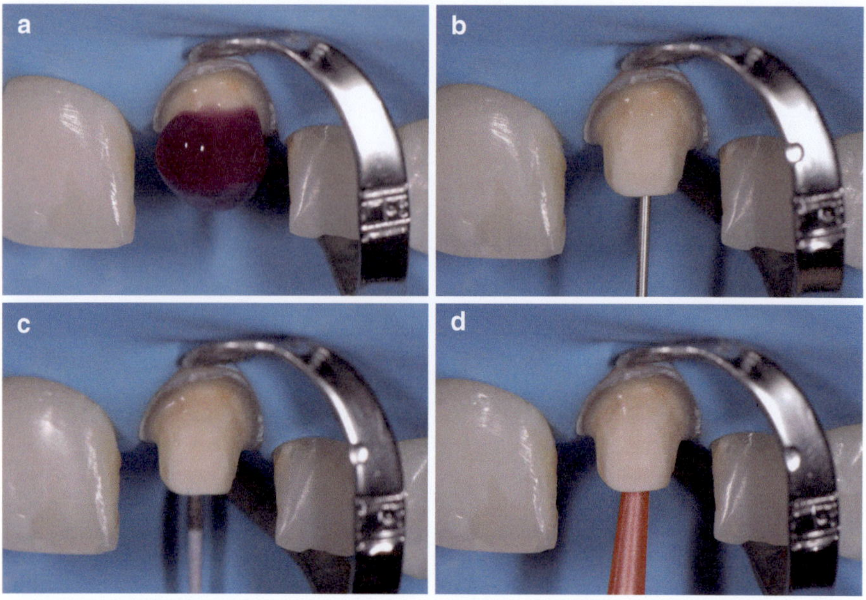

Fig. 6.18 Abutment tooth and root canal (**a**) etch, (**b**) disinfect, (**c**) dry and (**d**) dual-cure bond

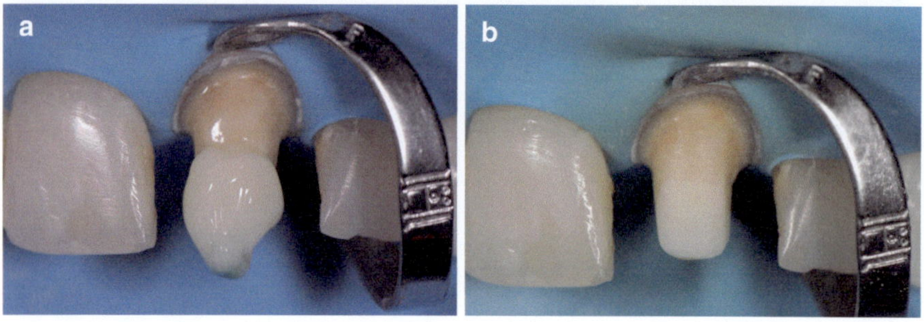

Fig. 6.19 (**a**) Cement post and simultaneous dual-cure composite resin core build-up. (**b**) Core and tooth preparation

or voids within the composite resin material. This can be minimised by loading the matrix with a monoblock mass of uncured composite resin paste from a twist delivery tube as opposed to that from an injected delivery compule. If a flowable injection material is used, care should be taken not to introduce air bubbles into the composite material by keeping the tip of the syringe buried in the expelled material.

This stage is important as suboptimal composite resin loading can result in voids or folds being introduced into the resin mass, which will also be present in the final polymerised restoration. Once loaded, the matrix is then seated onto the teeth with positive pressure. At this point, the clinician can use reference points from the previous try-in to ensure the matrix is fully located with the composite resin adapted to both the tooth and matrix. If an injection method is used, the material is injected at this point. Excess composite resin material may be removed where access allows. The composite material is then light-cured through the translucent matrix. Depending on the thickness of the matrix and the thickness of the composite resin, the curing process with the matrix in situ is likely to polymerise the outside layer only. Once the initial curing cycle is completed, the matrix is removed. This is likely to result in an outer shell of cured composite encasing an inner layer of uncured composite. The restoration is cured again through an oxygen-blocking material now that the light-cure head can be approximated onto the tooth and complete the curing of the resin, which lies deeper than the outer layer.

At the end of the light-curing phase, the composite resin is unfinished and unpolished, and there is likely excess flash over the adjacent teeth, into the interdental embrasures and over the gingiva. At this stage, the shape of the restoration is established, and the approach to completion is the removal of the gross excess material. The removal requires the use of No.11,12, 15 and 15c scalpel blades and pointed/flame fine or extra fine grit (red or yellow band) diamond burs, to gently trim the excess material to reveal the PTFE tape. After the rubber dam has been removed, an occlusal check is performed and required occlusal adjustments made to allow for final restoration, marginal finishing and surface polishing utilising appropriate polishing burs.

Where multiple teeth require modification, a variation of the technique to reduce composite overspill onto adjacent teeth involves the use of PTFE tape, or any removable inert material, to occupy the void between the teeth and the matrix for the teeth on either side of the tooth to be bonded to.

The summary of clinical stages for the provision of a direct composite resin onlay is listed in Table 6.2 and is shown in the presented clinical case (Figs. 6.19, 6.20, 6.21, 6.22, 6.23, 6.24, 6.25, 6.26, and 6.27).

Table 6.2 Summary of clinical stages of direct composite resin onlay restoration

Clinical stages
1. Production of a clear silicone stent at least 2 mm thick
2. Rubber dam isolation
3. Abutment tooth preparation occlusal surface and circumferential finish line
4. Abutment tooth sandblast/etch/bond
5. Composite resin loading of tooth and matrix
6. Matrix seating and composite resin material excess removal
7. Light curing
8. Composite resin material excess removal
9. Occlusal check
10. Restoration finishing and polishing

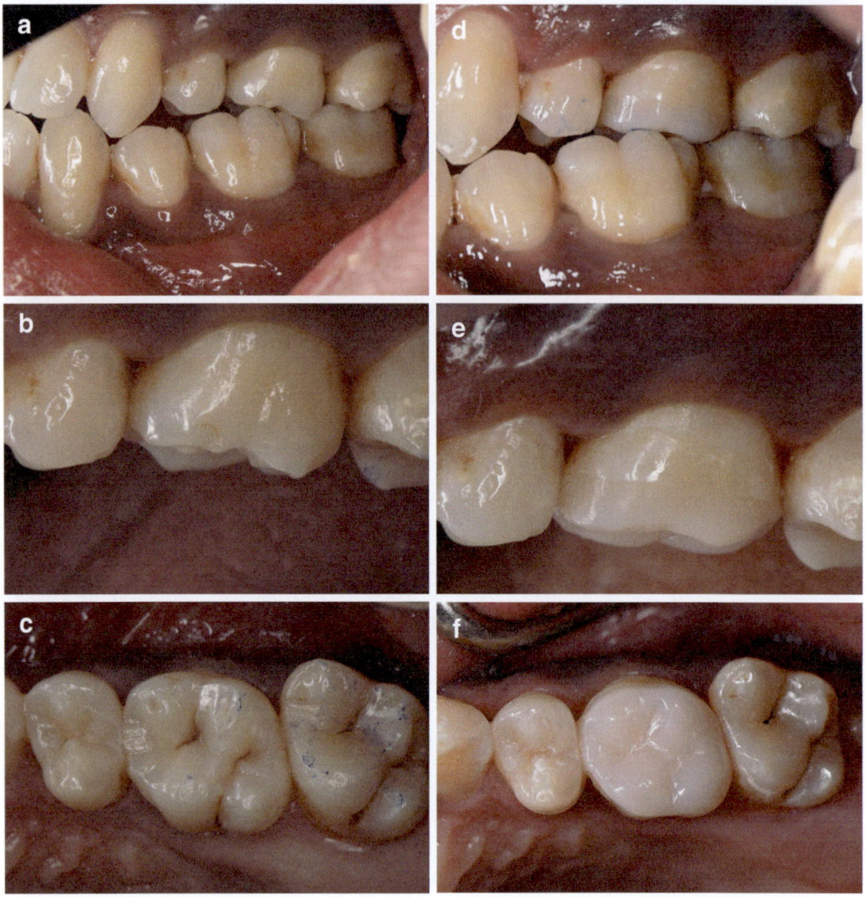

Fig. 6.20 Tooth 26 (**a–c**) before and (**d–f**) after direct composite resin onlay restoration

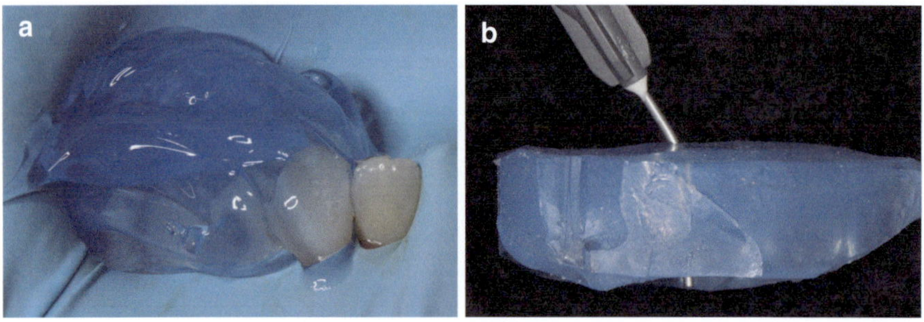

Fig. 6.21 (**a**) Production of a clear silicone stent at least 2 mm thick, (**b**) with an injection tip/vent hole

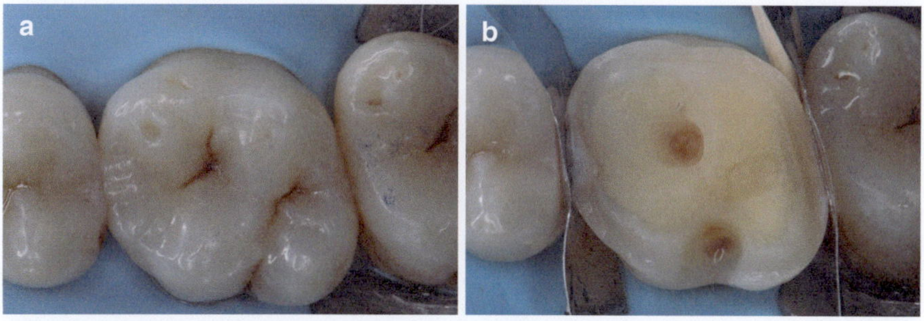

Fig. 6.22 (**a, b**) Abutment tooth 26 preparation occlusal surface and circumferential finish line (with caries removal cavity defects)

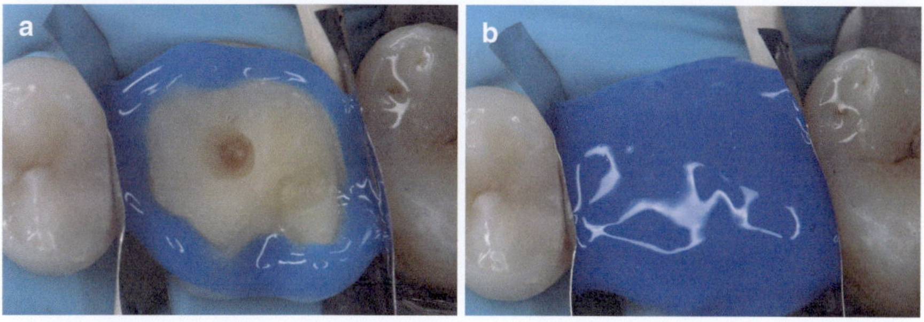

Fig. 6.23 (**a, b**) Abutment tooth etch, total etch technique

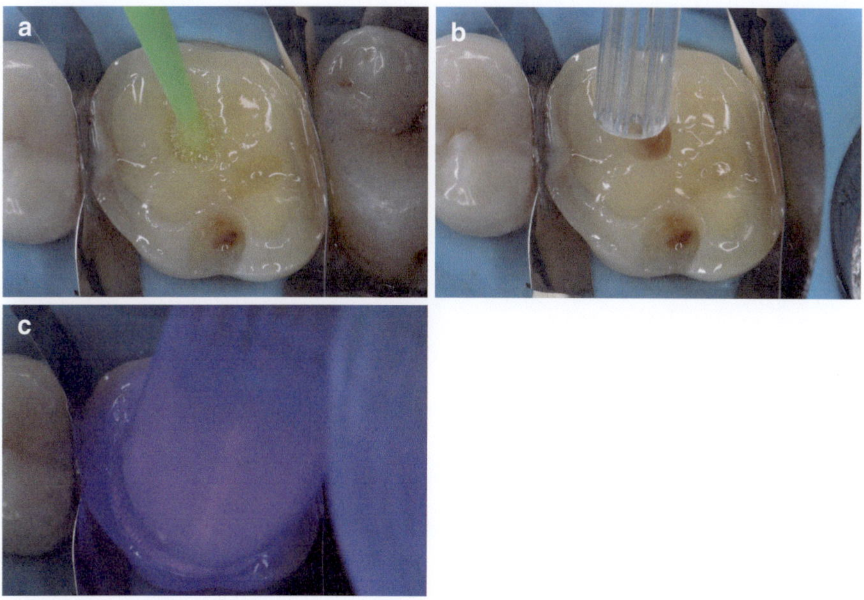

Fig. 6.24 Abutment tooth (**a**) bond application, (**b**) air dry for solvent evaporation and (**c**) light curing

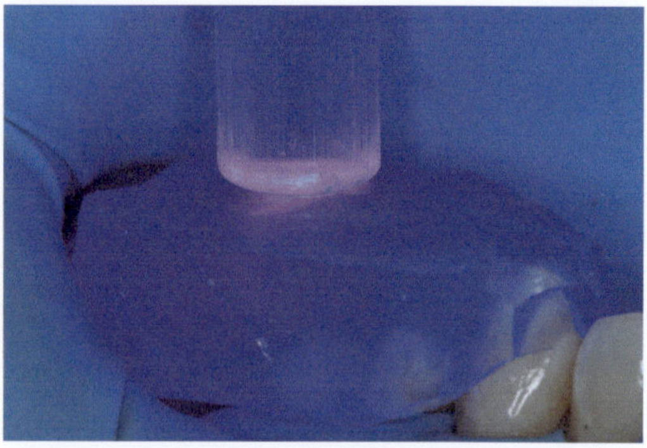

Fig. 6.25 Matrix seating, injection of composite resin material and light curing

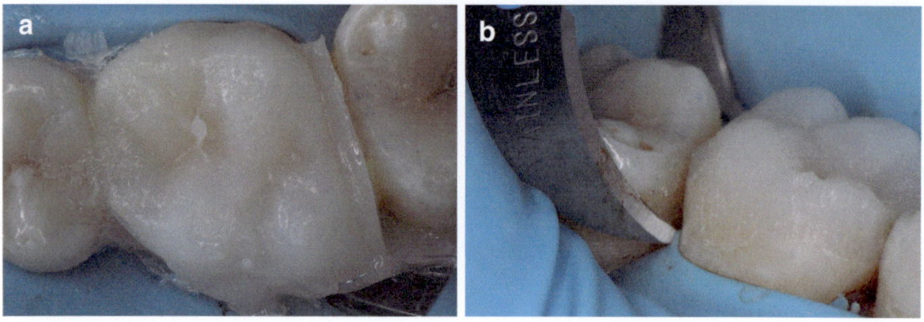

Fig. 6.26 (**a**) Composite resin material excess and (**b**) removal with scalpel no. 12 blade

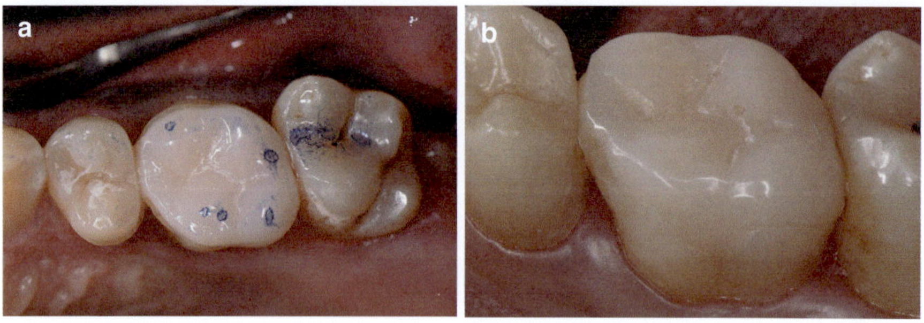

Fig. 6.27 (**a**) Occlusal check and (**b**) onlay restoration finished and polished

Further Reading

1. Cagidiaco MC, Goracci C, Garcia-Godoy F, Ferrari M. Clinical studies of fibre posts: a literature review. Int J Prosthodont. 2008;21:328–36.
2. Dawood A, Patel S. The dental practicality index—assessing the restorability of teeth. Br Dent J. 2017;222:755–8.
3. Dietschi D, Spreafico R. Current clinical concepts for adhesive cementation of tooth-colored posterior restorations. Prac Periodont Aesthet Dent. 1998;10:47–54.
4. Dietschi D, Spreafico R. Evidence-based concepts and procedures for bonded inlays and onlays. Part I. Historical perspectives and clinical rationale for a biosubstitutive approach. Int J Esthet Dent. 2015;10:210–27.
5. Grubbs TD, Vargas M, Kolker J, Teixeira EC. Efficacy of direct restorative materials in proximal box elevation on the margin quality and fracture resistance of molars restored with CAD/CAM onlays. Oper Dent. 2020;45:52–61.
6. Juloski J, Köken S, Ferrari M. Cervical margin relocation in indirect adhesive restorations: a literature review. J Prosthodont Res. 2018;62:273–80.
7. Magne P. Immediate dentin sealing: a fundamental procedure for indirect bonded restorations. J Esthet Restor Dent. 2005;17:144–55.
8. Magne P, Spreafico R. Deep margin elevation: a paradigm shift. Am J Esthet Dent. 2012;2:86–96.
9. Magne P. IDS: Immediate Dentin Sealing (IDS) for tooth preparations. J Adhes Dent. 2014;16(6):594.
10. Magne P, Kim TH, Cascione D, Donovan TE. Immediate dentin sealing improves bond strength of indirect restorations. J Prosthet Dent. 2005;94:511–9.
11. Mannocci F, Bertelli E, Sherriff M, Watson TF, Ford TR. Three-year clinical comparison of survival of endodontically treated teeth restored with either full cast coverage or with direct composite restoration. J Prosthet Dent. 2002;88:297–301.
12. McDonald AV, Setchell DJ. Developing a tooth restorability index. Dent Update. 2005;32:343–8.
13. Reeh ES, Messer HH, Douglas WH. Reduction in tooth stiffness as a result of endodontic and restorative procedures. J Endodont. 1989;15:512–6.
14. Sorensen JA, Engelman MJ. Ferrule design and fracture resistance of endodontically treated teeth. J Prosthet Dent. 1990;63:529–36.

Further Reading

Treating Anterior Tooth Surface Loss

7

Contents

Learning Outcomes

- Appreciate the difference in functional loading that restorations on anterior teeth have to manage when compared to posterior teeth.
- Understand that anterior restoration material choice can accommodate functional and aesthetic needs.
- Recognise that direct adhesive restorations on anterior teeth are best provided with a pre-determined diagnostic wax-up of the desired final result.
- Appreciate that adhesive restorations on anterior teeth may require no tooth preparation.

A. Alani, M. Patel, *Adhesive Techniques in Restorative Dentistry*, BDJ Clinician's Guides, https://doi.org/10.1007/978-3-032-07346-4_7

7.1 Introduction

Tooth surface loss (TSL) is a multifactorial process resulting in the loss of enamel and dentine through a number of different modes that do not involve a bacterial component. This process, much in the same as carious tissue loss, threatens the survival of the tooth and results in a number of identifiable symptoms that patients report and signs that are readily clinically identifiable. For example, patients may readily complain about the increasing sensitivity of their teeth due to the progressive exposure of underlying dentinal tubules or the continual diminishing coronal height of their teeth as an aesthetic concern. Younger patients are presenting with more severe aspects of the disease and, as such, threaten the longevity of tooth retention during their lifetime. This needs to be balanced against the awareness that our patients are living for longer, and for such a process to be severe so early will undeniably result in a greater chance of tooth loss even in the short term.

TSL differs in its pattern of enamel and dentine destruction and as such the approach in its treatment will also differ from that for teeth requiring regular restoration or those needing crowns subsequent to plaque-associated disease. One overriding principle in managing TSL is the focus on maintenance of tooth tissue to retain pulp vitality and make the ability to replace restorations in the future a lot more achievable. In essence, as has been previously described, the enamel and dentine should not be considered perishable in the process of TSL management. On the contrary, maintenance of tooth tissue is the main focus.

7.2 Aetiology and Pattern of TSL

7.2.1 Erosion

Erosive tooth surface loss is the chemical dissolution of tooth tissue by way of non-bacterial related exposure to acid from extrinsic or intrinsic sources. Extrinsic sources include the consumption of acidic fizzy drinks as well as alcoholic beverages to levels that create erosive lesions. Intrinsic sources can be potentially more challenging to identify and manage. Patients can present with emotive issues such as alcohol dependence or bulimia, resulting in acid insult due to the continual contact between regurgitated acidic contents of the stomach. The amount, duration and episodes of contact the teeth are exposed to the acid directly correlate, up to a degree, with the amount of tooth tissue that is lost. Erosive features of enamel include the presence of a smooth, shiny and reflective tooth surface with the loss of tertiary anatomical features such as perikymata, mamelons and the shape of the cingulum. As the erosion progresses, the tooth surface becomes progressively flatter and darker as the darker subsurface dentine shines through the now thinner enamel. One milestone in this process is the change in pattern and urgency for the need for treatment once the dentine has been breached. Once the harder enamel is removed, the softer dentine will dissolve at a greater rate, resulting in the characteristic 'cupping' defect. At this point, the patient's symptoms may increase due to the closer proximity to the pulp chamber and the presence of the open dentinal tubules. In fast progressing lesions, the pulp may blush through the dentine. This is a further sign of the aggressiveness of the erosion. Slow-progressing lesions allow the pulp to defend itself through the laying down of reactionary dentine to insulate the pulp. Where constant repeated acid insults occur over a short period, the opportunity for dentine deposition may not be possible. Another prominent feature of erosion is the palatal cervical area. A band of enamel is maintained in the cervical area despite the destruction towards the central portion of the palatal area (Fig. 7.1). This observation has been theorised to signify neutralisation of the acid by the gingival crevicular fluid. This aspect of the pathological process is important as it provides an avenue for a bonded restoration to seal the periphery of the margin with an enamel bond rather than the weaker and less robust dentine bond.

A key aspect of erosive tooth surface loss progression is the nature of the acid exposure and its duration. Extrinsic sources, such as the consumption of fizzy drinks, have a characteristic halo shape centred on the mesial portion of the central incisors. This clearly correlates to the shape and manner in which the fizzy drink is consumed. Patients who may "swirl" or "swish" acidic liquids may present with an additional sign where there may be a more generalised pattern of tooth surface loss. This, of course, increases the relative exposure of the teeth to the acid and is likely to result in more severe tissue loss. Another factor to consider is the relative number of exposures to acidic liquids. Where patients tend to sip contents continually throughout the day, this cumulative insult is more damaging than consuming the beverage over a shorter period of time. One salient feature that can be confused with an attritive aetiology is patients reporting the "fracturing" of teeth. This may represent the presence of progressive erosion, which results in the hollowing out of the palatal surface of the tooth, resulting in the labial surface becoming progressively thinner and weaker, culminating in the fracturing of the remaining incisal portion (Fig. 7.2). This may result in the first indication to the patient that advice or treatment is needed for their condition.

Intrinsic acid erosion can present in a similar manner to extrinsic sources, where the brunt of erosion occurs on the maxillary central incisors, reducing progressively

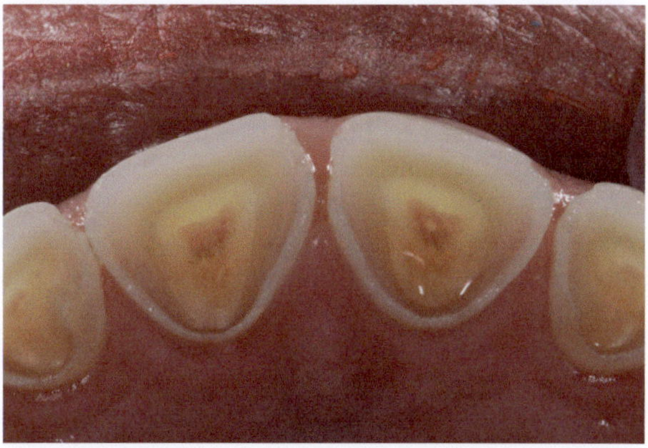

Fig. 7.1 Acid erosion tooth surface loss highlighting band of cervical enamel

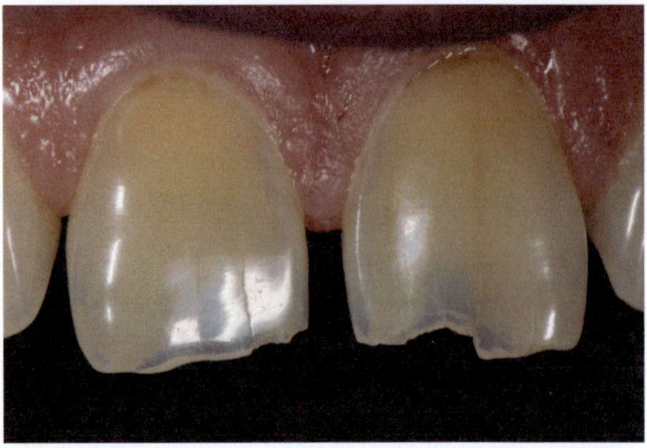

Fig. 7.2 Acid erosion affecting the thickness of incisal edges

to the lateral incisors and the canine teeth as the intensity of acid flow diminishes. The majority of the initial erosion in these situations occurs on palatal surfaces due to the protection extended by the tongue when gastric contents are expelled. If the erosion continues and progresses, the protective mechanism diminishes, and it may be inevitable that other teeth are affected with erosive lesions progressing further posterior in the maxillary arch to the molar teeth, whilst also involving the mandibular molar teeth (Fig. 7.3).

7.2.2 Attrition

Attrition is tooth surface loss caused by frictional tooth-to-tooth contact and is largely localised to the incisal and occlusal surfaces of teeth and is common amongst patients who present with parafunction or bruxism. The pattern of tooth surface loss contrasts with that of erosion, as the manner in which the teeth are obliterated differs. Unlike erosive lesions, there is a definite demarcation between the area that is being worn and those areas of the tooth that are being spared. For example, there is a greater tendency, but not exclusively, for the enamel and dentine to wear at the same rate. Such is the relative definition of the lesion that teeth can be sharp at the worn and unworn surfaces. The nature of the lesions is flat and rough, having been essentially worn by the opposing unit (Fig. 7.4).

When examining the dentition, the teeth that are being worn tend to lose their natural tooth contacts. In anterior segments, the natural anatomy of the maxillary cingulum and mandibular incisal edge is gradually diminished, resulting in both surfaces becoming flat and the contact becoming as wide and broad as the attritive lesion. This will change the pattern of anterior guidance, which may the over the longer period of time may culminate in its loss. The maxillary and mandibular teeth mirror each other in the shape of the occlusal plane. In a similar manner to erosive lesions, the pulp lays down tertiary dentine if provided the opportunity. In its most severe and progressed form, there is a complete loss of occlusal anatomy resulting in widespread flat surfaces both anterior and posterior segments (Fig. 7.5).

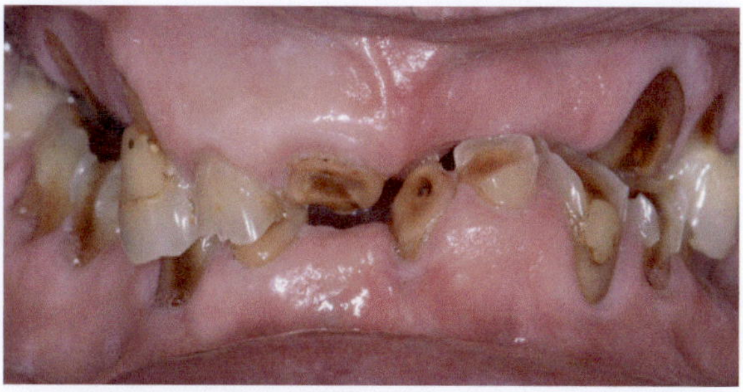

Fig. 7.3 Maxillary and mandibular dentition severely affected by acid erosion. Note the teeth contact due to dentoalveolar compensation, leading to severe disruption in the occlusal planes

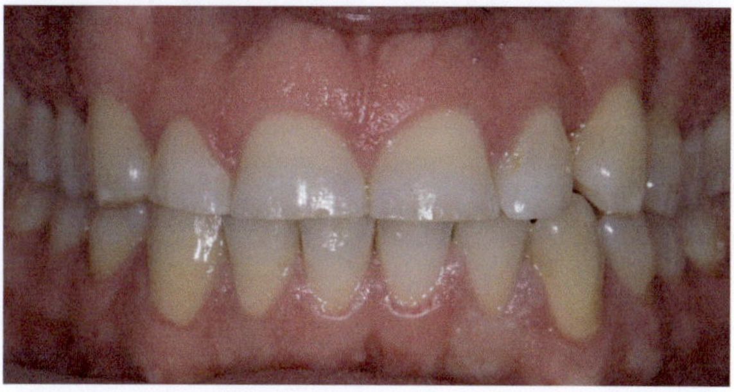

Fig. 7.4 Attrition tooth surface loss highlighting flat incisal surfaces

7.2.3 Abrasion

This mechanism of tooth surface loss involves mechanical wearing of tooth tissue other than that caused by the opposing natural tooth tissue. This, in its most common form, may present as a cervical lesion due to abrasion from tooth brushing (Fig. 7.6). Other rarer manifestations include sand chewing habits and the presence of tongue piercings that may sit between anterior teeth. One emerging aetiological factor in abrasion cases is the iatrogenic development of tooth surface loss through previous treatment. Patients with historical treatment for localised tooth surface loss may have been provided with metal ceramic restorations that are inherently rougher than natural tooth tissue. This classically presents where the maxillary anterior teeth are restored with crowns and the mandibular anterior teeth are unrestored. Over time, the mandibular anterior teeth are chronically exposed to the rougher ceramic surfaces opposing them, resulting in abrasion.

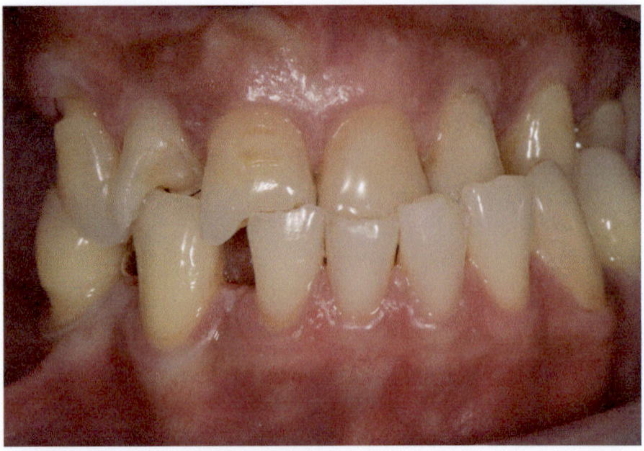

Fig. 7.5 Maxillary and mandibular dentition severely affected by attrition. Note the teeth contact due to dentoalveolar compensation, leading to severe disruption in the occlusal planes

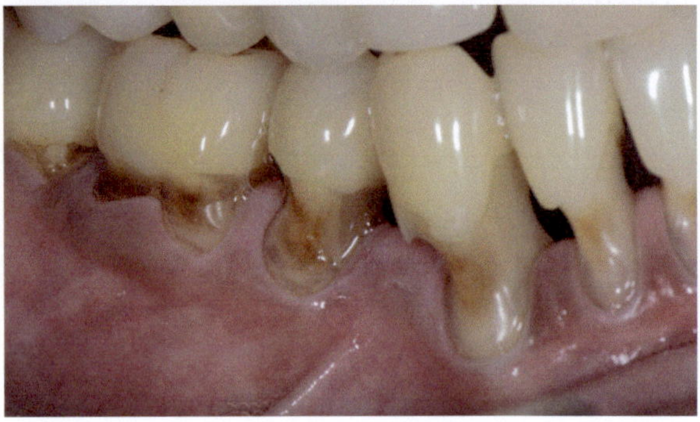

Fig. 7.6 Abrasion tooth surface loss affecting cervical surfaces of teeth 46, 45, 43, 42

7.2.4 Abfraction

Abfraction is a form of tooth surface loss that occurs around the cervical portion of teeth on the buccal surface. Abfraction is thought to take place when excessive cyclic, non-axial tooth loading leads to cusp flexure and stress concentration in the vulnerable cervical region of teeth. Such stress is then believed to directly or indirectly contribute to the loss of cervical tooth substance. This, in its most common form, may present as a cervical lesion without the presence of associated gingival recession, as may be seen with abrasion lesions (Fig. 7.7).

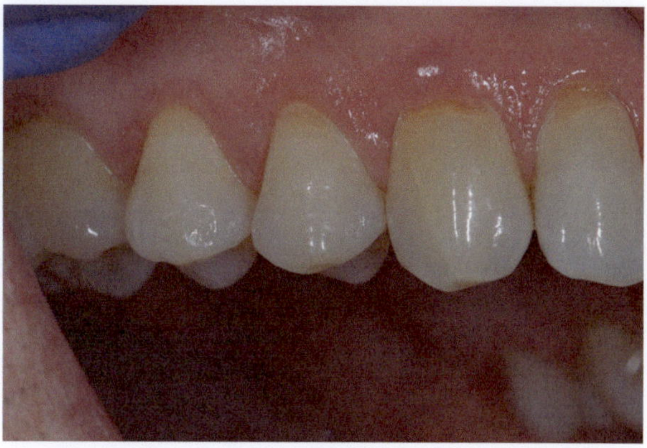

Fig. 7.7 Abfraction tooth surface loss affecting cervical surfaces of teeth 22, 23, 24 & 25

7.3 Management and Treatment Strategies

The most precious commodity in oral health is the presence of healthy, natural tooth tissue. The less tooth tissue is lost, the less extensive the restoration, and so the greater the longevity of the latter and the improved survival of the former. The second most precious commodity in oral health, especially when considering the need for tooth replacement or restoring individual teeth, is 'restorative space'. This need can take the form of occlusal space or space between a restoration and the pulp canal system, in an effort to avoid the need for root canal treatment. The additive provision of adhesive restorations in supra-occlusion is a minimally invasive technique that protects and preserves underlying tooth tissue whilst simultaneously creating restorative space.

7.3.1 Prevention

This aspect of management is of paramount importance in the management of tooth surface loss and is linked to a successful diagnostic process. The eradication of the tooth surface loss process is most ideal before the instigation of treatment. It is common to require the input of medical colleagues in instigating a preventive regime.

A patient suffering from gastro-oesophageal reflux disease (GORD) may benefit from a consultation with their general medical practitioner for the prevention of further regurgitation. This may take the form of prescribed medicines such as proton pump inhibitors or further investigation by a gastroenterologist. Where clinicians suspect an eating disorder such as bulimia or anorexia nervosa, the situation can become more difficult to manage if the patient does not readily admit to their condition. Psychology and psychiatric management are invaluable in trying to achieve the optimal outcome for this cohort of patients. Invariably, if patients are aware that empowering their dentist with information on the aetiology of the tooth surface loss could potentially aid their treatment they may be more likely, despite the stigma and embarrassment, to admit to their problem.

In terms of the consumption of acidic drinks and other less conspicuous sources of acid intake, this may distil down to the ability of the dentist to communicate how important the diet control and reduction of consumption is to the future of their dentition.

The use of a high fluoride-containing toothpaste and mouthrinse to be used daily for topical application is important to help strengthen biologically weakened areas of teeth by remineralisation. The use of occlusal splints also will be of benefit for those patients (where the oral acid has been controlled) requiring mechanical protection of the teeth in the interim period whilst diagnostic and treatment planning measures are being undertaken.

7.3.2 Restorative Challenges

The physiological process of dentoalveolar compensation brought about by pathologic tooth surface loss creates a dilemma for the clinician. One option may be to conform to the current occlusal scheme without changes in the vertical dimension. This may be intuitive, but unfortunately, it may expose the patient and the dentist to risk. When lacking, conformative approaches require restorative space obtained by tooth tissue removal. This is more specifically problematic for the tooth surface loss patient because of the already reduced tooth volume and height. An option may be to consider surgical crown lengthening to increase the supra-gingival tissue volume. This results in a reduction in periodontal support and a crown restoration shape that has root dentine as a significant portion. Due to the inherent difference between the root shape and circumference, and the need for a tapered full crown preparation, this is also likely to result in weakening of the tooth and further pulp insult. Such a tapering preparation may be unavoidably aggressive due to the existing tooth form shape and produce reduced proximity to the root canal system. Not only does this also result in reduced periodontal ligament support but it also increases the crown-to-root ratio.

An alternative treatment option to create restorative space is the use of orthodontic treatment to allow localised or generalised bodily tooth movements. This is likely to prolong treatment time and increase treatment financial expense. It may also be challenging achieve due to the limited coronal tooth tissue to bond orthodontic brackets to, and the high anchorage requirement needs. Communication between restorative and orthodontic colleagues and patients for this management strategy is key to its success.

Outside of conforming to the current occlusal scheme and orthodontic treatment to create restorative space is to increase the occlusal vertical dimension (OVD). Due to the challenges discussed, additive adhesive strategies could be considered more conservative. Depending on the manner in which this is delivered, this can navigate around these issues. The traditional approach is likely to involve the provision of a combination of direct and indirect restorations as a comprehensive full-mouth rehabilitation. This may reduce some risk by the avoidance of conforming but can expose the patient to other forms of risk. This approach, by definition, aims to restore all teeth regardless, if they require restoration or not (i.e. the restorative status of the tooth). For example, in localised erosive cases, only a succinct number of teeth may be affected and require treatment. This approach may not only remove sound tooth tissue and potentially damage the pulp but also commit the patient to increased lifelong restoration maintenance by entering a repeated cycle of restoration replacement, otherwise known as the "restorative failure spiral".

7.3.3 Dahl Concept

What may be fairly daunting from the outset in the treatment of tooth surface loss is the multiple teeth it is affecting and the need to manage these units collectively. It is rare for a solitary tooth unit to be affected, and it is not possible to treat one tooth in isolation when other teeth have lesions. Further treatment challenges exist where the shape of the lesion itself inherently does not provide an avenue for retention and resistance form for the restoration of the tooth. The cupping and flat nature of erosive and attrition defects requires a wholly adhesive approach if the tooth is not to be prepared for a more destructive crown restoration. Reliance on the adhesion of resin cements to restorative materials requires an attention to detail of how best they are applied and an awareness of the advantages and limitations of such techniques.

One notable challenge in tooth surface loss treatment is the management of the occlusion and more crucially dentoalveolar compensation. This is a physiological compensatory process through which teeth maintain occlusal contact with the opposing teeth units. The OVD and the freeway space are unaltered as the occlusal contacts are maintained by alveolar bone remodelling, resulting in axial elongation of the alveolar process. As teeth gradually wear, a space is created inter-occlusally, which allows the tooth-periodontal ligament-alveolar process complex to erupt and maintain occlusal contact. The process of erosion, attrition or abrasion reduces the enamel and dentine thickness overlying the pulp, whilst axial tooth movement during the gradual process of dentoalveolar compensation diminishes the interocclusal space. The pulp recognises this process as a threat and lays down reactionary dentine depending on the severity. If the rate of tooth surface loss is greater than the eruptive potential of the teeth, an open bite will develop. As the tooth surface loss progresses, there is a net reduction in supragingival tooth tissue, a reduction in the interocclusal space due to the dentoalveolar compensation and disruption of the occlusal planes (Figs. 7.3 and 7.5). This lack of coronal tooth tissue and absence of any interocclusal space to tore to amongst a number of teeth units may appear daunting if more conventional approaches to treatment are considered. An approach that conforms to the current vertical dimension would involve a fairly invasive approach with significant tooth morbidity. Also, surgical crown lengthening followed by conventional crown preparations exposes patients to a variety of risks and potential complications. The alternative approach to conforming to the presenting vertical dimension is to reorganise the occlusal scheme to provide the requisite restorative space for the provision of restorations. Increasing the OVD in this manner may still commit teeth to extra-coronal restorations, depending on the approach. In essence, the most amicable approach in managing this situation is the 'reversal' of the dentoalveolar compensation by way of manipulating occlusal contacts to induce a favourable change in tooth movements to create space for restorations. This is largely achieved through a process of axial tooth movements by a combination of intrusion and extrusion of teeth.

The Dahl concept is a method of purposefully inducing physiological tooth movement that serves to create restorative space in worn dentitions in the presence of a lack of interocclusal space where dentoalveolar compensation has maintained functional teeth contact (Fig. 7.8). This is achieved through imposed changes to isolated arch occlusal contacts on anterior teeth with the provision of fixed restorations with the absence of restorations and occlusal contacts on posterior teeth. Therefore, the OVD is solely increased by the restoration of the anterior teeth. Axial tooth movements will be induced, and the posterior tooth occlusal contact is later re-established by the compensatory dentoalveolar mechanism over a period of time. The time for re-establishment to occur is dependent upon the amount of OVD increase. Occlusal contact re-establishment is a combination of the eruption of posterior teeth and the intrusion of anterior teeth that are in contact. The split between the processes is 60:40, respectively. For example, if the OVD is increased by 2 mm, re-establishment of occlusal contact would involve 1.2 mm of over-eruption and 0.8 mm of intrusion. This fairly crude calculation is not entirely accurate as 2 mm of change in occlusion anteriorly equates to approximately 1/3 of the amount posteriorly due to distance from the hinge action of the mandible.

The concept was first investigated by Dahl and colleagues in 1975 and developed further by clinicians in the United Kingdom from 1997 onwards to managing localised anterior TSL with a lack of interocclusal restorative space. This resulted in a series of clinical reviews and subsequent cohort studies that examined the utilisation of fixed 'Dahl' appliances provided through the restoration of worn teeth with adhesive composite resin restorations. During this period, clinicians were beginning to appreciate improvements in the predictability of adhesive bonding to tooth tissue.

7.3.4 Restoration Design

To achieve axial intrusion of anterior teeth, the palatal portions of maxillary teeth restorations need to consider the vector of the forces applied and the angle of the long axis of the teeth. In general, the coronal portion of the maxillary anterior teeth are inclined buccally with the apical portion angled further palatally, this is in contrast to mandibular anterior teeth which are more perpendicular in their axis. To compensate for both of these aspects the palatal portion of the maxillary teeth restorations need to be designed with these factors in mind.

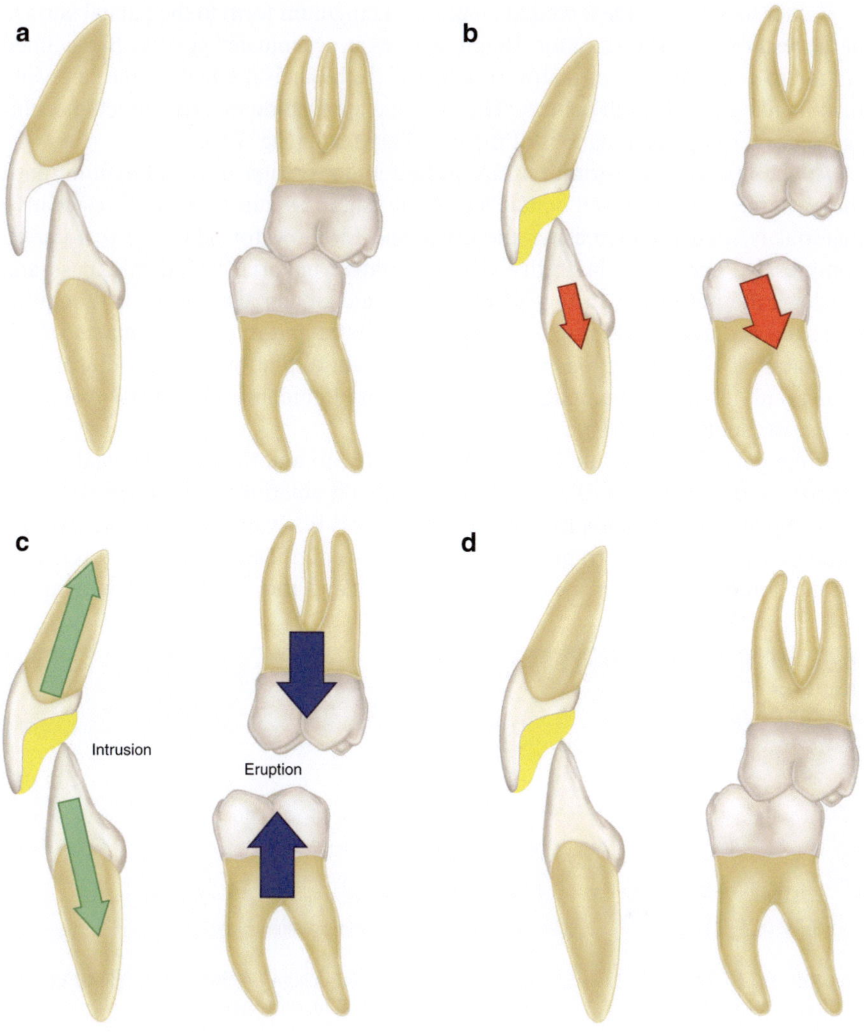

Fig. 7.8 (**a**) Localised anterior erosive tooth wear on the upper anterior units results in a lack of space to restore the palatal surfaces due to dentoalveolar compensation. (**b**) Provision of a resin-bonded palatal platform to restore the anterior units, loading the teeth axially, results in an increase in the occlusal vertical dimension and creation of an open bite posteriorly. (**c**) Through a combination of intrusion of the maxillary and mandibular anterior units and eruption of the posterior units, the process results in the re-establishment of occlusal contacts posteriorly. (**d**) Establishment of contact posteriorly

Rather than to provide a natural anatomical cingulum form to the palatal surface of the restoration, the restoration design requires an accentuated positive flat inclined cingulum occlusal contact platform onto which the incisal edges of the opposing mandibular anterior teeth contact. This aids the application of axial directed occlusal forces through the long axis of the maxillary teeth (Fig. 7.9).

As the restorative restorations are placed under greater occlusal loading until the posterior teeth occlusal contacts re-establish, a 2+ mm volume of restorative material is used for increasing the OVD and to allow for adequate restoration compressive and wear durability. The restorative material added thickness and insulates the pulp from further insult. The clinician can also more easily equilibrate the occlusal markings to achieve ideal static and dynamic contacts of the restorations. The restorations create a stable occlusal platform with occlusal contacts evenly distributed amongst teeth with shared guidance in protrusive and lateral movements (Fig. 7.10).

If the palatal surface and cingulum are created to a normal dimensional shape, the palatal incline may still contact the mandibular anterior teeth but the vector of force applied is more likely to be angled and so less likely to apply the force axially through the central root trunk of the tooth. A steep guidance plane may result in greater forces applied in a non-axial direction and thus be more damaging. If

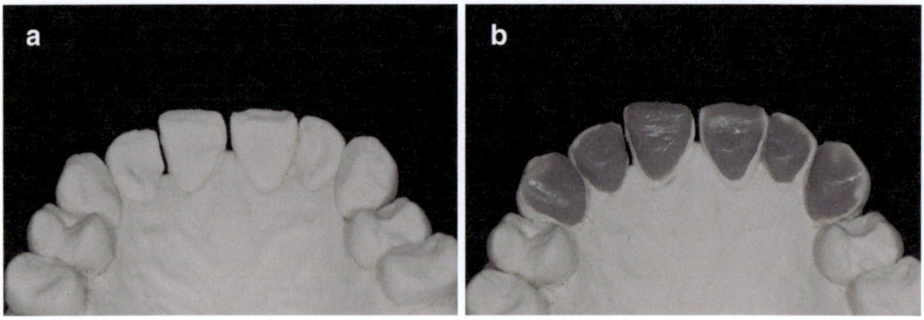

Fig. 7.9 (**a, b**) Teeth 13–23 palatal diagnostic restoration design of cingulum occlusal contact platforms. Wax extension is 0.5 mm away from the gingival margins

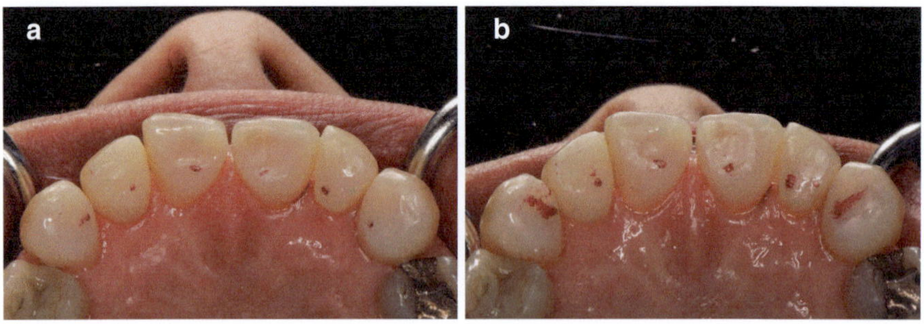

Fig. 7.10 Direct hybrid composite resin restorations highlighting a stable occlusal platform with occlusal contacts evenly distributed amongst teeth in (**a**) static and (**b**) dynamic movements

shallow guidance is created, the vector of force will be predominantly exerted down the central trunk of the tooth. Loading exerted in this manner results in the force being dissipated more evenly to the periodontal ligament with intrusion more likely and reducing the chance of debonding restorations, fremitus or tipping movement resulting in an unwanted increased overjet and splaying of the anterior teeth. The clinician needs to be mindful of the importance of these anterior occlusal contacts as the patient will be contacting on these restorations in isolation without posterior support until the process is completed (Fig. 7.11).

7.3.5 Restoration Material Choice

The most efficient method of applying this technique is through the provision of adhesive restorations, where the volume of tooth structure allows. This largely involves the bonding of composite resin to the palatal aspects of affected maxillary anterior teeth, thus increasing the OVD. The worn incisal surfaces of the mandibular anterior teeth may also be treated in this manner. However, material choice is variable for the provision of the bite platform as further consideration is given to the nature of the tooth surface loss, where an attritive aetiology requires a more durable, harder occlusal surface to contact against in situations where bruxing or parafunction may be ongoing. For these clinical presentations, indirect restorative materials may be used, such as indirect composite resin, CAD–CAM resin-nano ceramic and metal alloy restorations.

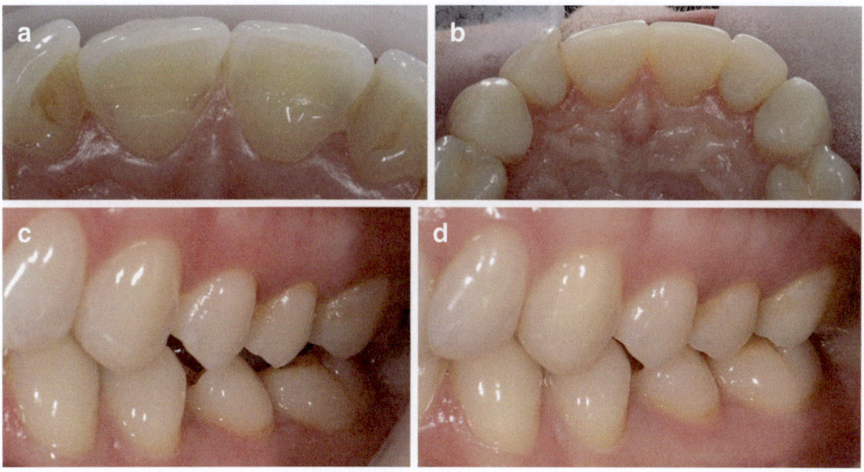

Fig. 7.11 (**a**) Localised anterior tooth surface loss (**b**) Direct composite platforms placed at an increased occlusal vertical dimension on 13–23, resulting in posterior open bite (**c**). Over a period of 8 months, the posterior units begin to re-establish contact (**d**)

7.4 Direct Restorations

Where the TSL is minimal to moderate, such as incisal edge wear and Class V defects, direct composite resin restorations can be provided for the recreation of tooth morphology. A choice of a hybrid composite resin may be more favourable to provide greater resistance to further restoration wear and for an acceptable aesthetic result. Class V restorations can be restored with glass-ionomer cement as an alternative material.

Where more extensive restorations are planned, the advantages of the direct approach include efficiency of time and reduced financial cost as well as the serviceability of the restoration and any future subsequent revisions (Fig. 7.10).

The direct adhesive restoration of teeth requires a template to work towards to provide an optimal final functional restoration contour. This, in the main, is achieved through a diagnostic wax-up prescribed through diagnostic study casts, a facebow record and an appropriate interocclusal record. The diagnostic wax-up prescription is key to a successful definitive restoration as it forms the blueprint. Focus on details such as the incisal edge position, proportion ratio of the teeth, interdental embrasure spaces, design of the palatal occlusal platform, the nature of the contact points occlusal, and interdental and the marginal interface are immensely important (Fig. 7.9). The diagnostic wax-up constructed can provide patients with a preview of the proposed future treatment via mock-up with a temporary Bis-acryl material or can also be used to give the technician a guide for the construction of indirect restorations (Fig. 7.12).

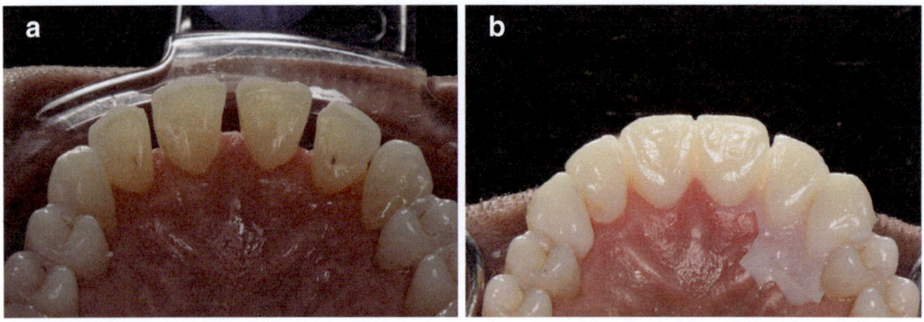

Fig. 7.12 (**a**) Before and (**b**) after mock-up with a temporary Bis-acryl material to preview the proposed future treatment

7.5 Indirect Restorations

The provision of indirect restorations for anterior teeth may allow improved functional and aesthetic control in comparison to the labour burden that multiple extensive restorations may provide, utilising direct techniques. Laboratory-fabricated indirect restorations are likely to result in a more resilient restoration with superior physical properties and potentially better shape control with regard to the restoration contour design of the palatal occlusal platform for static and functional contacts points (Fig. 7.13). However, if diagnostic and working occlusal records are not accurately obtained, it can result in the need for gross restoration adjustment post-cementation.

Choosing indirect over direct restoration provision is clinician-dependent based upon their individual knowledge of material selection, clinical skill set and

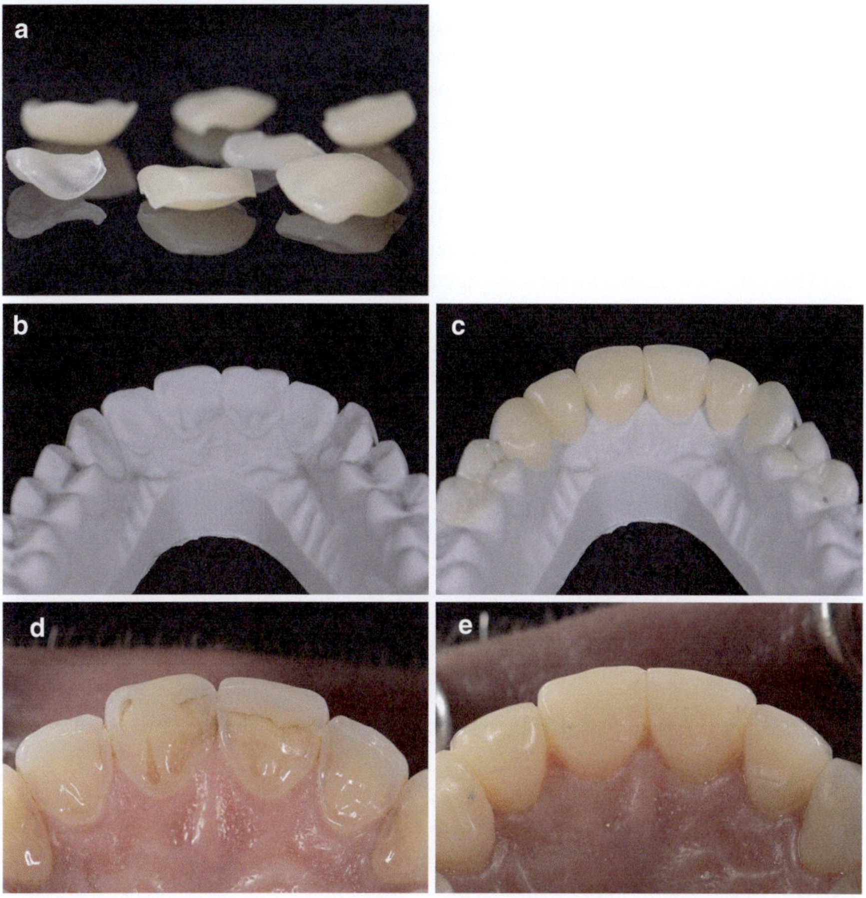

Fig. 7.13 (**a**) Indirect CAD–CAM resin palatal veneer restorations (**b, c**) in vitro and (**d, e**) in vivo

experience. The choice may also be governed and influenced by patient finances. Clinicians can consider a variety of adhesively retained indirect materials, which vary with the benefits of differing aesthetic and physical properties. The planning, choice and execution of the adhesive restoration depend heavily on the individual nature of the presenting clinical case.

If the teeth are already crowned or lend themselves to be provided with a full extra-coronal adhesive or conventional restoration, then the palatal occlusal platform can be applied to the full crown design. Where teeth are otherwise unrestored, there are numerous options. A palatal veneer can be constructed, which creates the occlusal platform and is bonded to the palatal tissues. This can be constructed from resin-based materials or metal alloys (Figs. 7.13 and 7.14).

The design of the adhesive indirect restoration needs to consider two aspects. The first is the ability to successfully locate the abutment tooth and secondly to utilise maximise bonding surface area. The basis of restoration location relies on the tooth's incisal edge and the anatomy and defect features on the palatal surface upon which the restoration can engage. A restoration lip over the junction between the palatal tissue and the incisal edge surface can make positive location easier. To reduce bonding or composite resin ingress into the gingival sulcus, 0.5 mm clearance will allow the clinician to visualise the restoration margin in this area and ensure the absence of overhangs and chronic gingival irritation (Fig. 7.9).

In situations where there is severe TSL, these features will not be defined enough to ensure adequate location, a restoration location jig may be used to ensure adequate and consistent seating at the cementation stage. A restoration wholly fabricated in composite resin can then engage all available surfaces in a positive manner.

7.5.1 Tooth Coloured Palatal Veneers

The indirect restoration tooth coloured material choice includes composite resin or resin nano-ceramic materials. These can be produced by either analogue or digital CAD–CAM processes or a combination of both processes (Figs. 7.13 and 7.15).

In cases where the indirect palatal restoration will increase the incisal length of the tooth, a composite resin material directly added to the buccal surface may be employed for improved aesthetics (Fig. 7.16). However, this incisal area can also be incorporated into the final indirect restoration if required (Fig. 7.17).

7.5.2 Metal Alloy Palatal Veneers

Where it is envisaged that restorations are to be put under greater occlusal loads or the patient requests a restoration that may be more durable than composite resin, metal alloy restorations can be considered. This decision needs to be balanced with the risks and benefits borne in mind and communicated to the patient. One clear disadvantage is that metal is not tooth coloured and patients may be more likely to reject this as an option because of this.

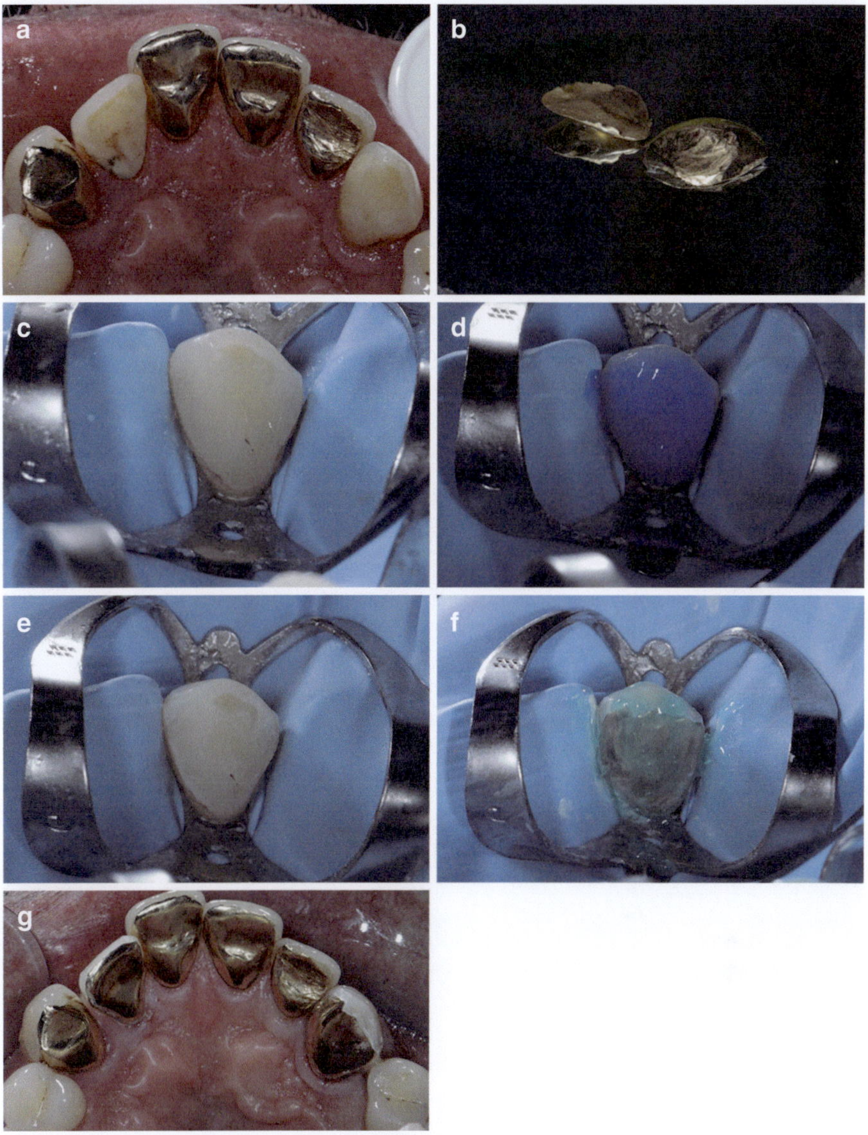

Fig. 7.14 (**a**) Indirect Type III gold alloy palatal veneers retained on the 13, 11, 21 and 22. Veneers on the 12 and 23 had failed but were kept by the patient. The original treatment was provided at the Eastman Dental Institute, London, in 1996 (**b**) The debonded gold palatal veneers, which were retrieved from the patient and recycled through a process of recasting and recementation as depicted in the following figures. (**c**) 23 isolated (**d**) 23 with etchant in place (**e**) 23 post etch (**f**) New veneer located and cemented in place on the 23 with oxygen-inhibiting gel. (**g**) The new 'recycled' restorations in place on the 12 & 23

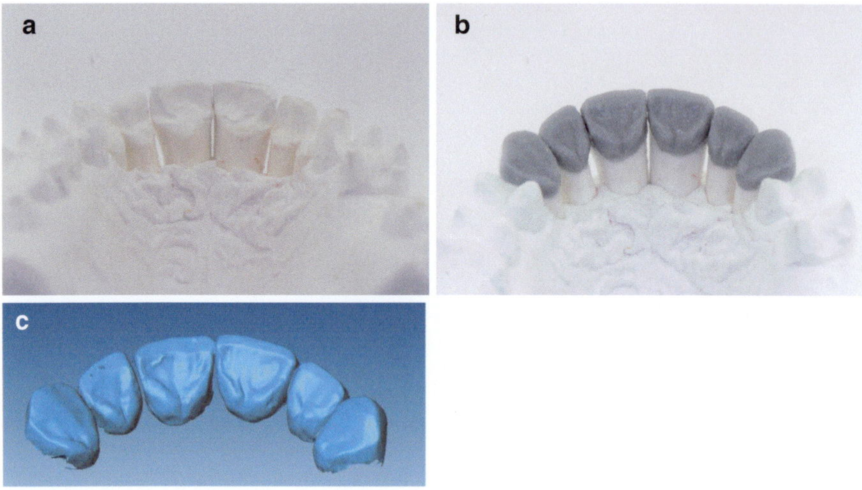

Fig. 7.15 Laboratory production of palatal veneers utilising a combination of (**a, b**) analogue and (**c**) digital CAD–CAM processes. (Images courtesy of Lab 39 United Kingdom)

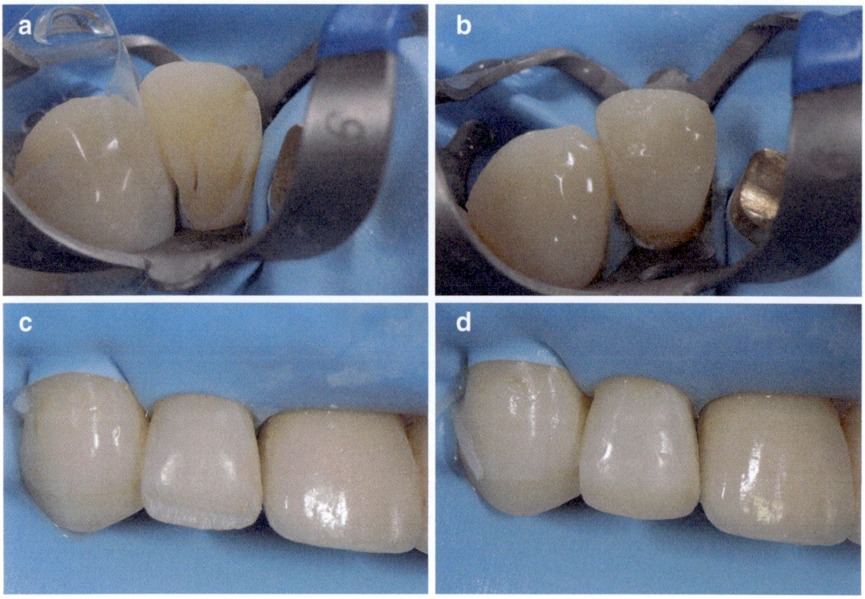

Fig. 7.16 (**a–c**) Tooth 22 indirect composite resin palatal veneer restoration to increase the incisal length, and (**d**) composite resin material directly added to the buccal surface to improve aesthetic integration

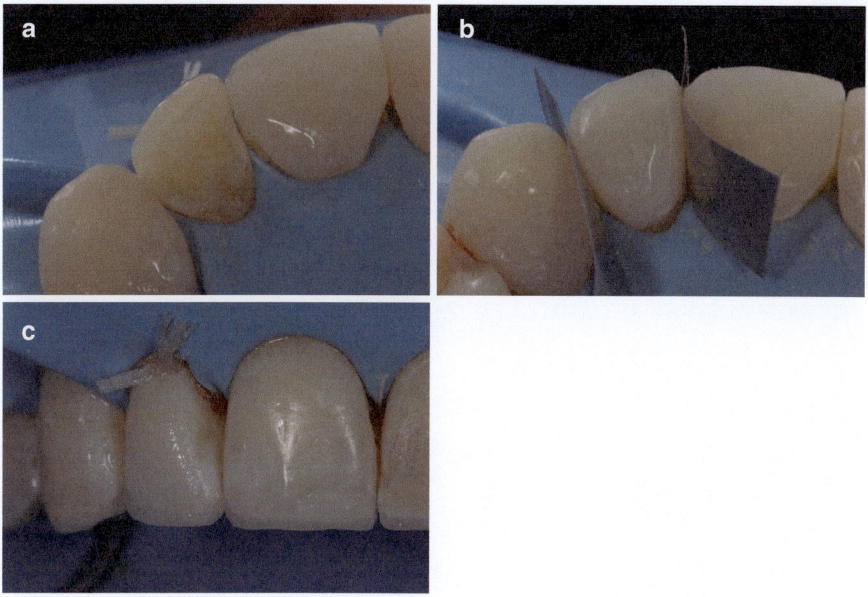

Fig. 7.17 (**a**) Tooth 22 restored with (**b, c**) indirect CAD–CAM resin nano-ceramic palatal veneer restoration to restore palatal surface and increase the incisal length, where the incisal area is incorporated into the final indirect restoration

Metal alloy palatal restorations will be more robust and harder wearing than resin-based materials. The indirect restoration metal alloy material choice includes nickel or cobalt chromium and Type III gold alloy (60% gold content) materials (Fig. 7.14). When compared to nickel or cobalt chromium, gold alloy is kinder to opposing teeth from an abrasive aspect. When used in these situations, it can be cast into sections of 1+ mm occlusal thickness with nickel or cobalt chromium, potentially less than this thickness due to their greater rigidity. This said, the advantages of producing thicker restorations have been previously specified.

Metal alloy restorations, due to their largely superior physical characteristics, are still relevant to the management of anterior TSL, where patients recognise a compromise in aesthetics that needs to be considered for teeth in different positions of the anterior sextant. A good example of customising material choice to tooth type can be illustrated with the provision of metal alloy palatal veneers to only canine teeth in order to provide durable functional surfaces to aid a canine guided occlusion to serve the patient in the long term. This results in a more resilient canine-guided occlusal scheme where the restored contacting canine teeth maintain the established change in occlusal vertical dimension.

Again, where the palatal restoration will also increase the incisal length of the tooth, a composite resin material directly added to the buccal surface may be employed for improved aesthetics to block out the darkness of the matt metal area. In this respect, yellow gold is likely to be more harmonious aesthetically than nickel or cobalt chromium, for example. To mitigate against the underlying colour issue, an opaquer can be used on the fit surface of the veneer prior to the addition of the composite resin material (Fig. 7.18).

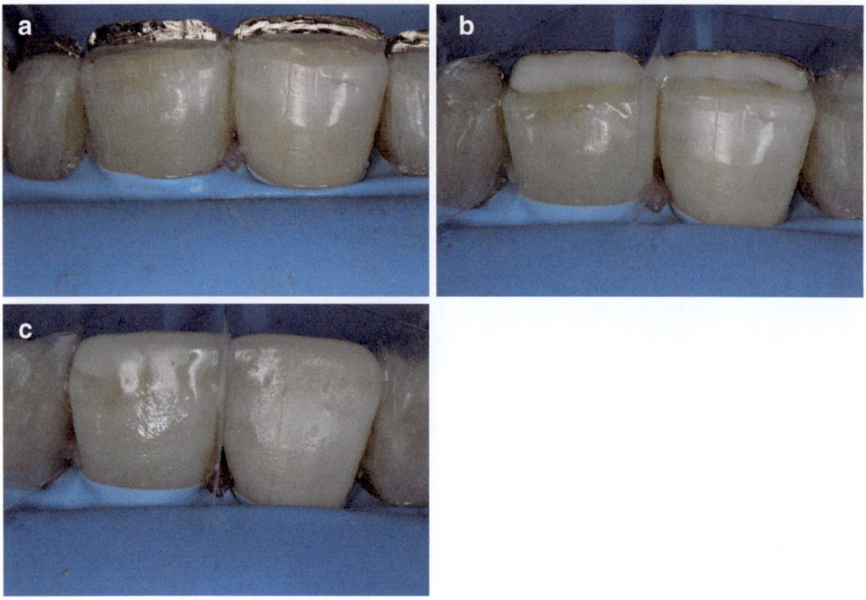

Fig. 7.18 Teeth 11 & 21 indirect palatal veneer restorations made of Type III gold alloy (**a**) to increase the incisal length and (**b**) opaquer and (**c**) composite resin material directly added to the buccal surface to improve aesthetic integration

7.6 Adhesive Technique

7.6.1 Direct Composite Resin

The following techniques utilise the diagnostic wax-up and transfer the proposed restoration shape directly to the mouth using a variety of silicone matrices. For the purposes of cleansability and ease of delivery, the technician needs to ensure that the interproximal areas are clearly defined and that the contact points between teeth are not too wide from a bucco-palatal aspect. The wider the wax-up is in this dimension, the bigger the contact point, the more difficult it will be to ensure a cleansable restoration and marginal integrity interproximally. Some clearance of the gingival margin area from the wax-up is also beneficial.

Once the teeth are isolated, they should be cleaned with prophy paste to ensure the absence of any plaque that can compromise etching and bonding. Bevelling the tooth margin can reduce the visibility of the restoration margin. A further stage of intra-oral sandblasting can improve the bonding potential of the tooth substrate.

7.6.1.1 Palatal/Lingual Silicone Matrix Technique

The major advantage of the palatal/lingual silicone matrix technique is the ability to chromatically layer and characterise the direct resin restoration. The palatal/lingual matrix involves the layered incremental build-up of teeth using a variety of different types of resin, if desired. The technique allows the clinician to utilise different materials for different roles within the restoration, functional and optical. This technique is the same as what has been previously described to treat an isolated Class IV restoration on a single unit. The exception is that it is at the discretion of the clinician to determine the number of teeth to be built-up per curing cycle. This may be easier to achieve as the clinician can build up the multiple units in unison, free from the need to match to adjacent units. Alternate teeth build-up is advised for the aid of restoration separation, finishing and polishing procedures.

The summary of clinical stages for the provision of a direct layered composite resin restoration is listed in Table 7.1 and is shown in the presented clinical case (Figs. 7.19, 7.20, 7.21, 7.22, 7.23, 7.24, 7.25, 7.26, 7.27, 7.28 and 7.29).

7.6.1.2 Translucent Matrix Technique

This technique allows direct build-up of teeth with monoshade composite resin utilising compression or injectable techniques.

The technique for the utilisation of a translucent matrix technique for the build-up of incisor teeth along their palatal/lingual/incisal/buccal surfaces is exactly the same as previously described for the provision of direct composite resin onlay restorations.

The summary of clinical stages for the provision of a direct monoshade composite resin restoration is listed in Table 7.2 and is shown in the presented clinical case (Figs. 7.30, 7.31 and 7.32).

Table 7.1 Summary of clinical stages of direct layered composite resin restorations

Clinical stages
1. Production of a palatal/lingual silicone matrix at least 2 mm thick
2. Rubber dam isolation
3. Teeth cleaning/preparation, finish lines/sandblasting
4. Teeth separation/etch/bond (alternate teeth)
5. Composite resin translucent shade loading of matrix for palatal/lingual shell
6. Matrix seating and composite resin material transfer to teeth
7. Light curing
8. Composite resin dentine body shade application
9. Composite resin enamel shade application
10. Composite resin material excess removal
11. Repeat steps 4–10 for alternate teeth
12. Restoration finishing and polishing
13. Occlusal check

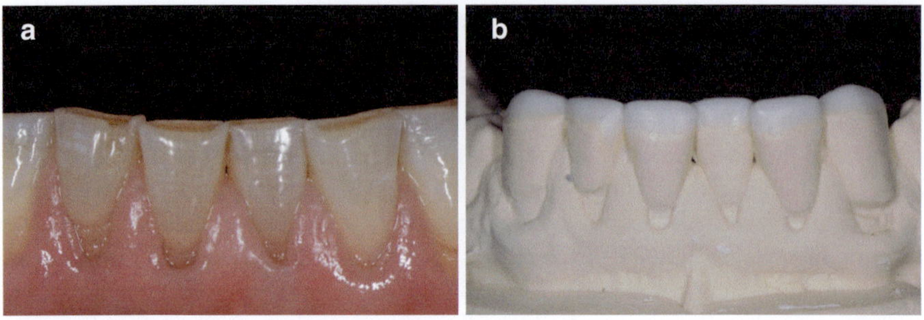

Fig. 7.19 (**a**) Teeth 33–43 with attrition and abrasion. (**b**) Diagnostic wax-up of aesthetic and functional contours of proposed restorations

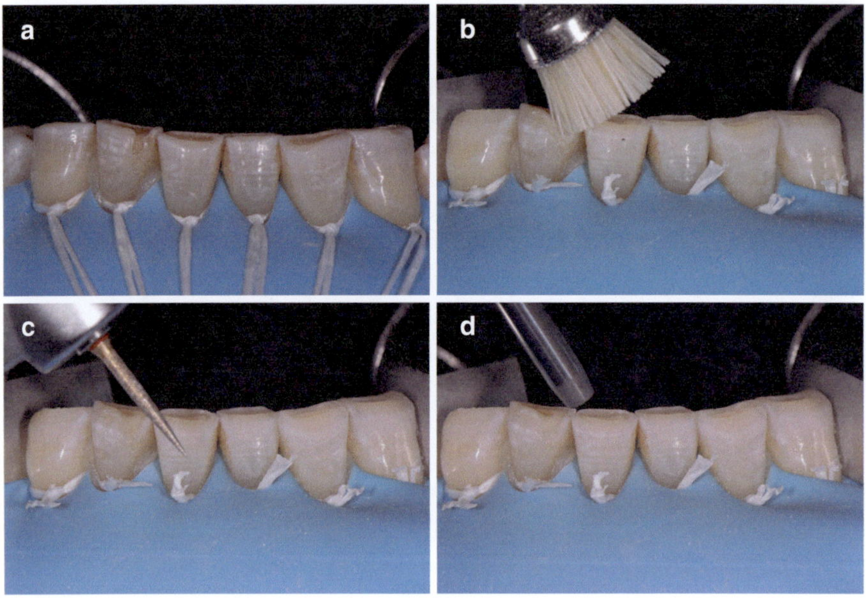

Fig. 7.20 (**a**)Teeth 33–43 rubber dam isolation; (**b**) prophylactic clean, (**c**) bevel finish line placement and (**d**) sand blasting

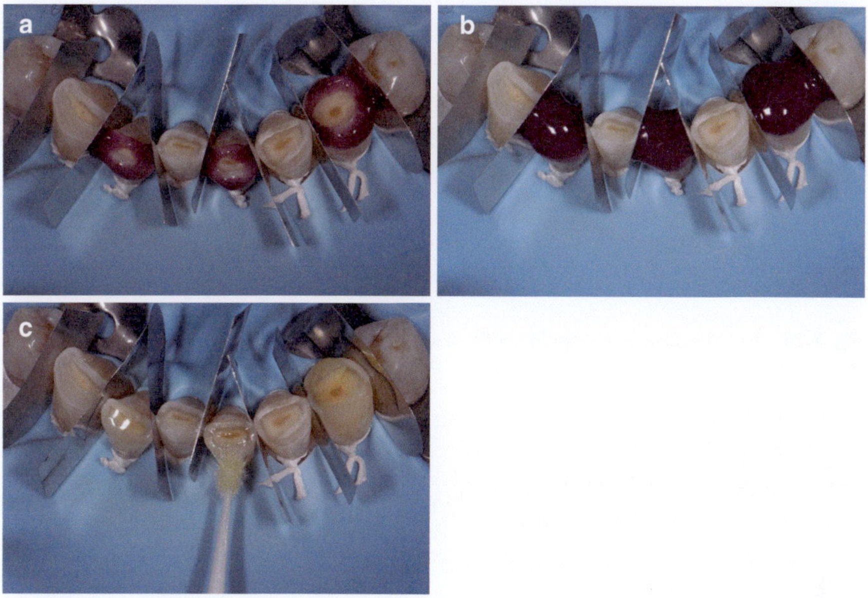

Fig. 7.21 (**a**, **b**) Teeth separation and total etching of alternate teeth with (**c**) application of bonding agent

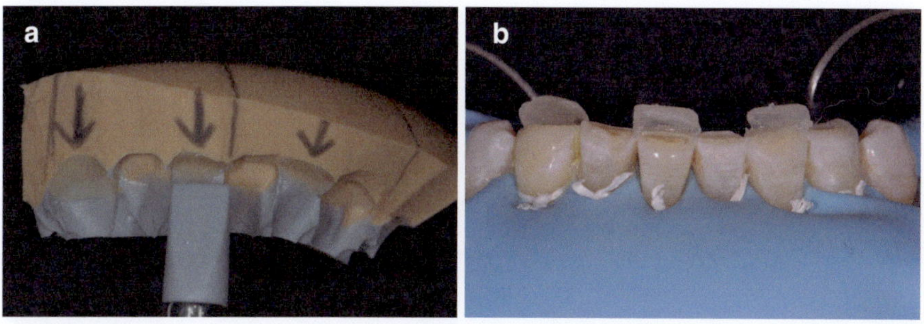

Fig. 7.22 (**a**) Composite resin translucent shade loading of matrix for palatal/lingual shell; (**b**) matrix seating and composite resin material transfer to teeth

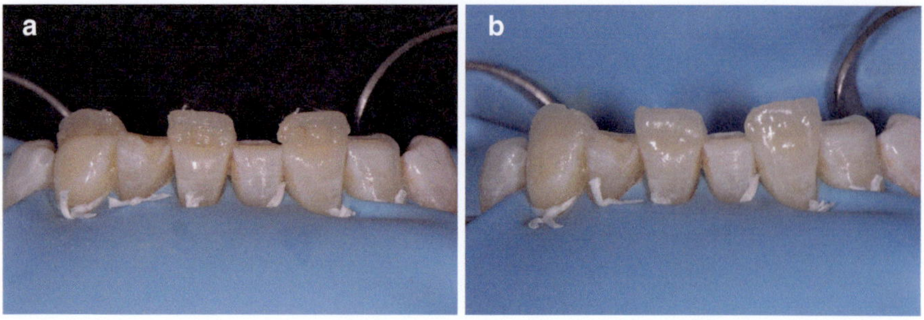

Fig. 7.23 (**a**) Composite resin dentine body shade and (**b**) enamel shade applications

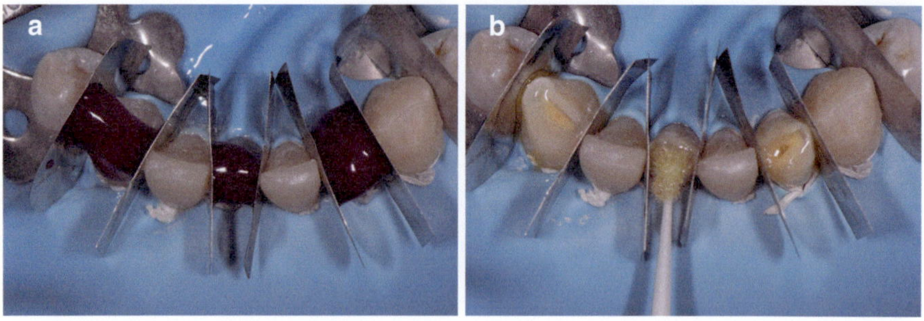

Fig. 7.24 (**a**) Teeth separation and total etching of alternate teeth with (**b**) application of bonding agent

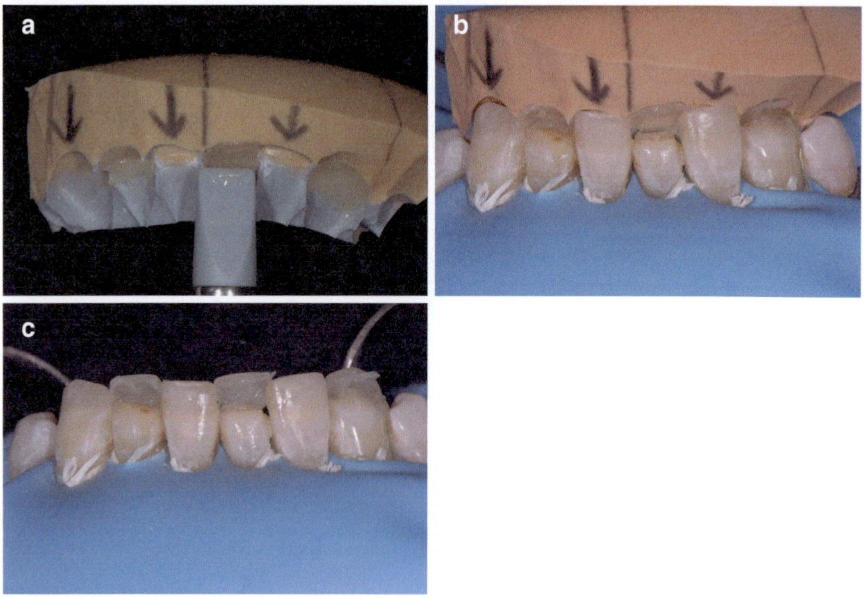

Fig. 7.25 (**a**) Composite resin translucent shade loading of matrix for palatal/lingual shell; (**b**) matrix seating and (**c**) composite resin material transfer to alternate teeth

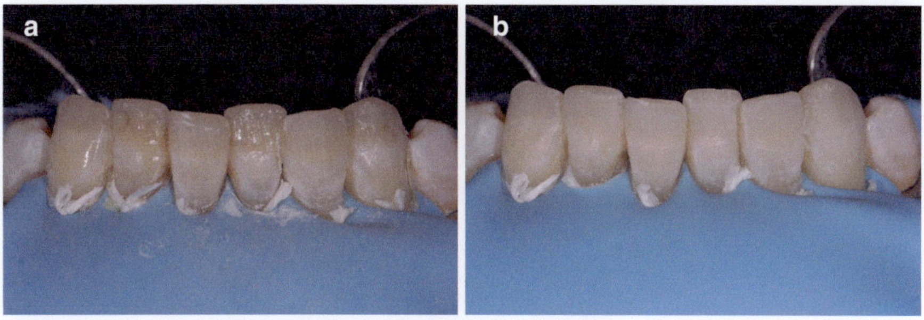

Fig. 7.26 (**a**) Composite resin dentine body shade and (**b**) enamel shade applications

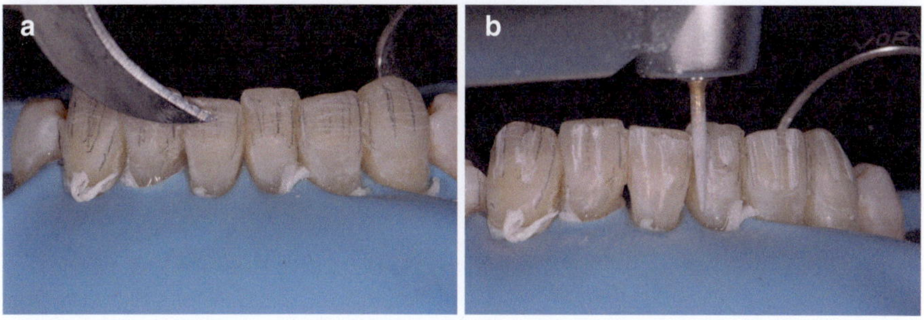

Fig. 7.27 Composite resin material (**a**) excess removal and texture placement with scalpel blade no. 12 and (**b**) restoration finishing with fine-grit diamond bur

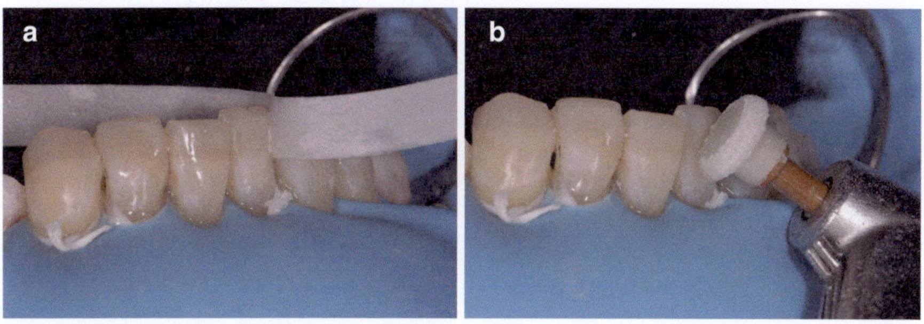

Fig. 7.28 Restoration (**a**) interdental finishing and (**b**) polishing

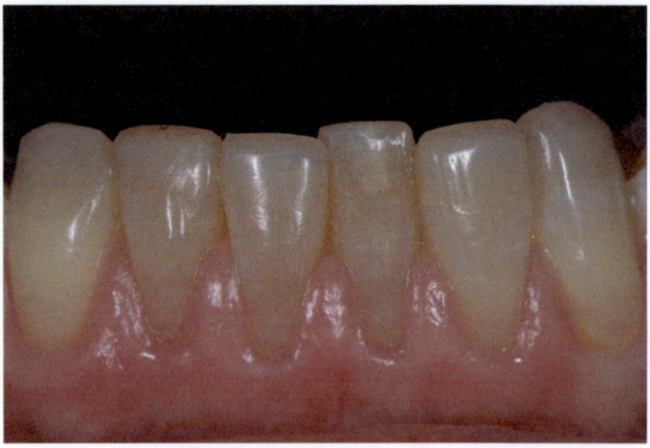

Fig. 7.29 Completed case showing teeth 33–43 with provision of Class IV layered & Class V composite resin restorations

Table 7.2 Summary of clinical stages of direct monoshade composite resin restorations

Clinical stages
1. Production of a clear silicone stent at least 2 mm thick
2. Rubber dam isolation
3. Teeth cleaning/preparation, finish lines/ sandblasting
4. Teeth separation/etch/bond (alternate teeth)
5. Composite resin loading of the tooth and matrix
6. Matrix seating and composite resin material excess removal
7. Light curing
8. Composite resin material excess removal
9. Repeat steps 4–8 for alternate teeth
10. Restoration finishing and polishing
11. Occlusal check

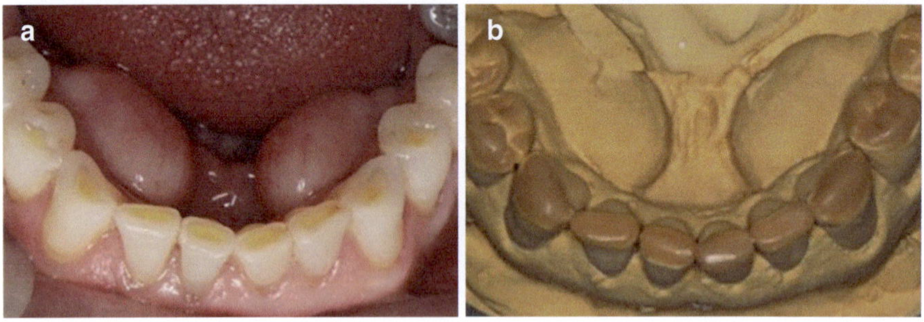

Fig. 7.30 (**a**) Teeth 34–44 with attrition. (**b**) Diagnostic wax-up of aesthetic and functional contours of proposed restorations

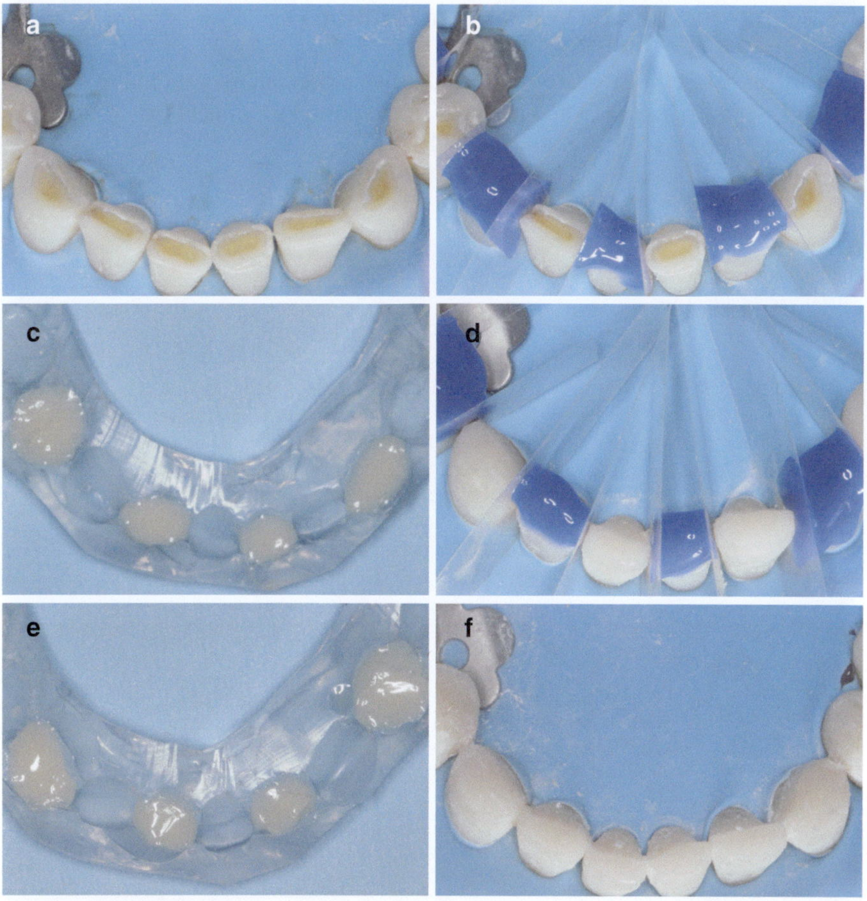

Fig. 7.31 Restoration of teeth 34–44 showing; (**a**) rubber dam isolation, (**b, d**) teeth separation with alternate teeth etching. (**c, e**) Loading of translucent matrix and (**d, f**) subsequent delivery of monoshade composite resin restorations

Fig. 7.32 Completed case showing teeth 34–44 with provision of Class IV monoshade composite resin restorations

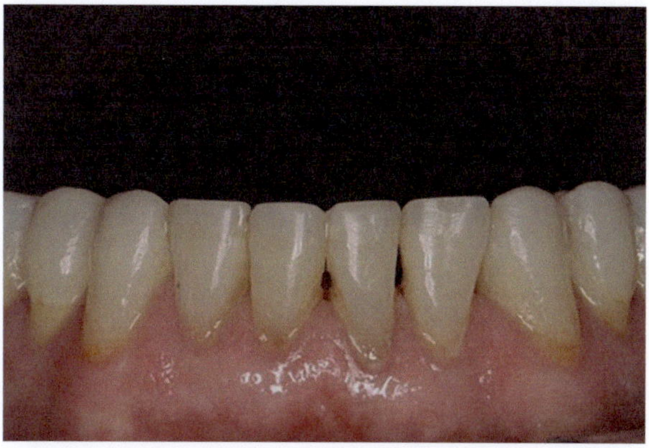

7.6.2 Indirect Palatal Veneer Cementation

The summary of clinical stages for the adhesive cementation of an Indirect palatal veneer is listed in Table 7.3 and is shown in the presented clinical case (Figs. 7.33, 7.34, 7.35, 7.36, 7.37, 7.38, 7.39 and 7.40).

Table 7.3 Summary of clinical stages of indirect palatal veneer adhesive cementation

Clinical stages
1. Abutment tooth clean
2. Veneer try-in
3. Rubber dam isolation
4. Restoration re-try
5. Abutment tooth sandblast/etch/bond
6. Veneer intaglio surface sandblast/clean/silanate/ cement loading
7. Cement veneer
8. Light cure (with oxygen block barrier)
9. Clean excess cement
10. Polish restoration margins

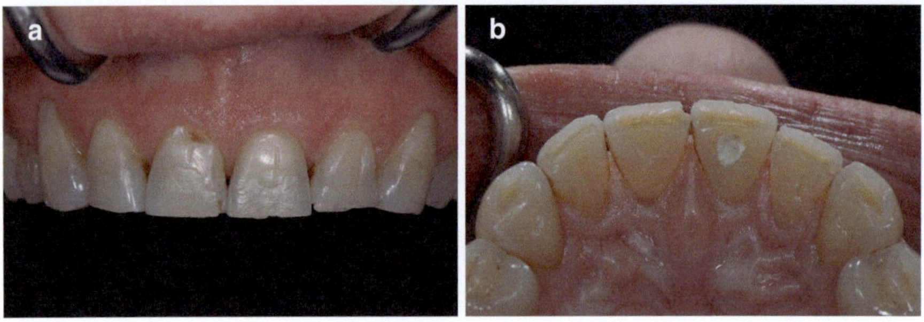

Fig. 7.33 (**a, b**) Teeth 13–23 with attrition to be restored with indirect palatal veneers

Fig. 7.34 Teeth 13–23 rubber dam isolation

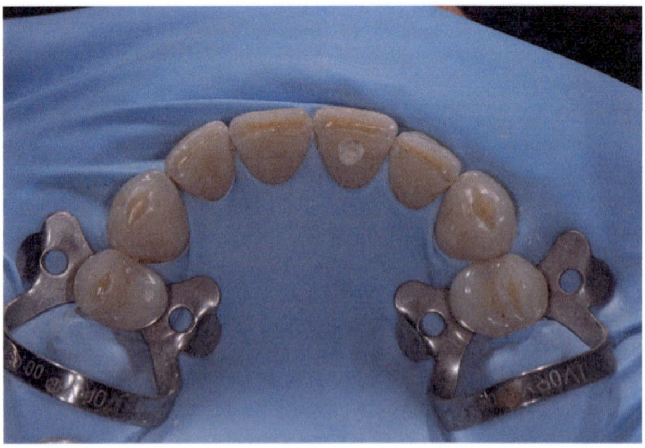

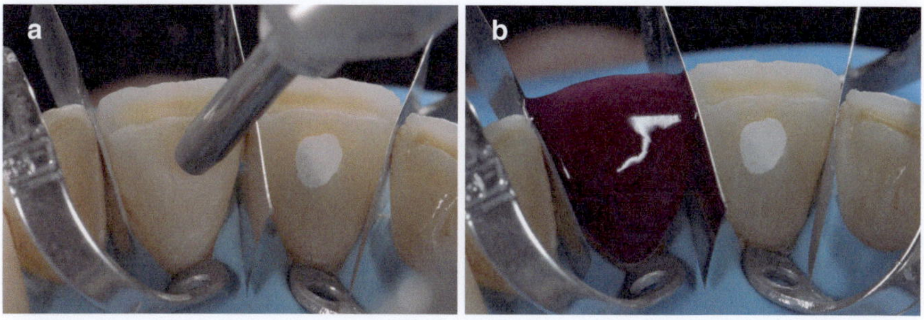

Fig. 7.35 Abutment tooth 11; (**a**) sand blast and (**b**) etch

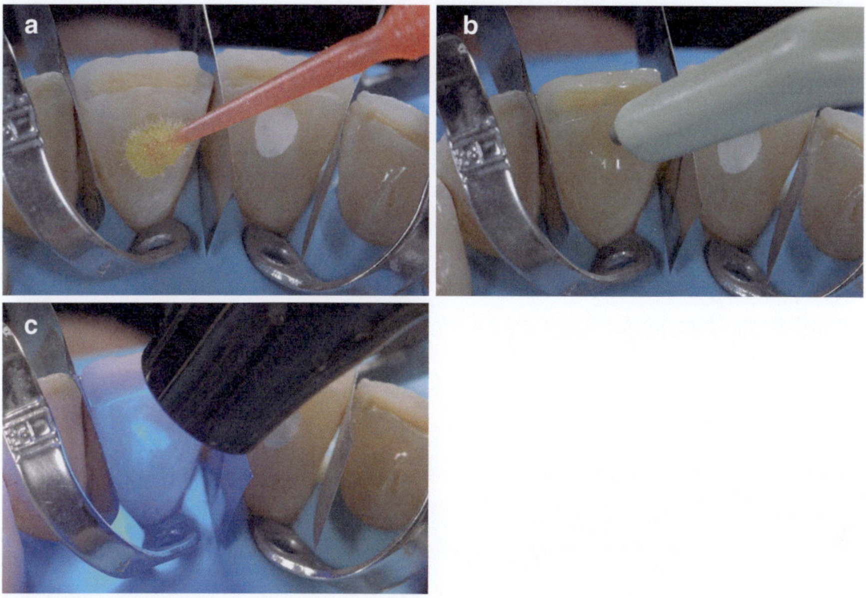

Fig. 7.36 Abutment tooth 11; (**a**) bond application, (**b**) air dry and (**c**) light cure

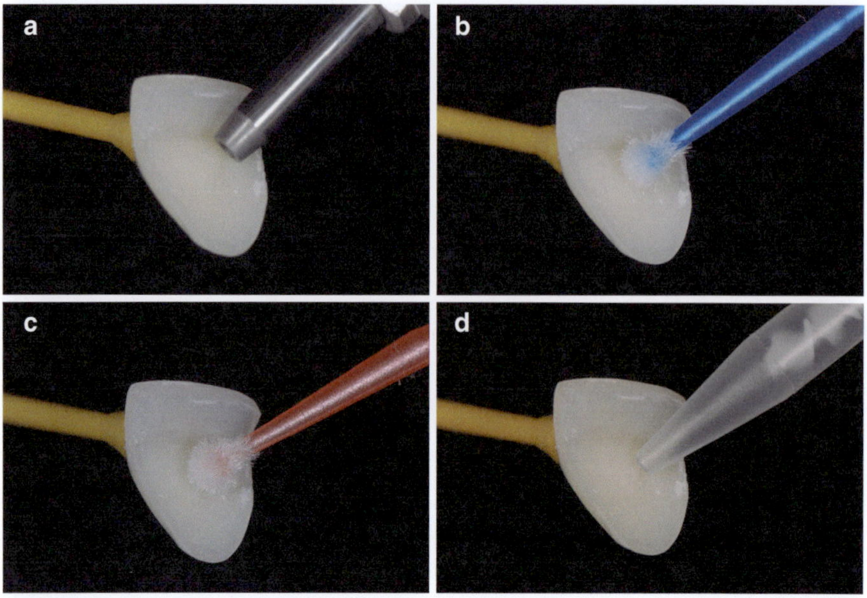

Fig. 7.37 Veneer (indirect composite resin) intaglio surface; (**a**) sandblast, (**b**) clean, (**c**) silanate and (**d**) cement loading

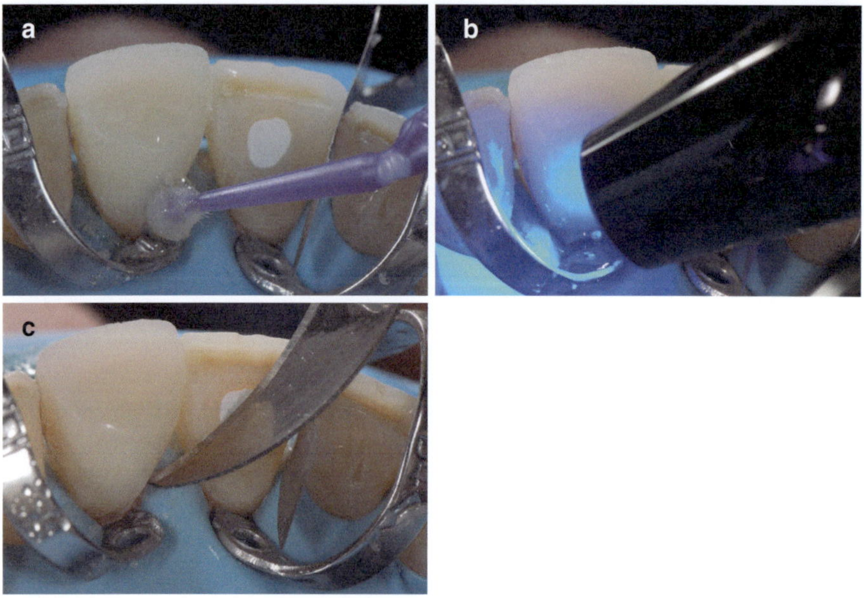

Fig. 7.38 (**a**) Abutment tooth 11 palatal veneer cemented and oxygen block barrier application. (**b**) Light cure and (**c**) excess cement removal with scalpel blade no. 12

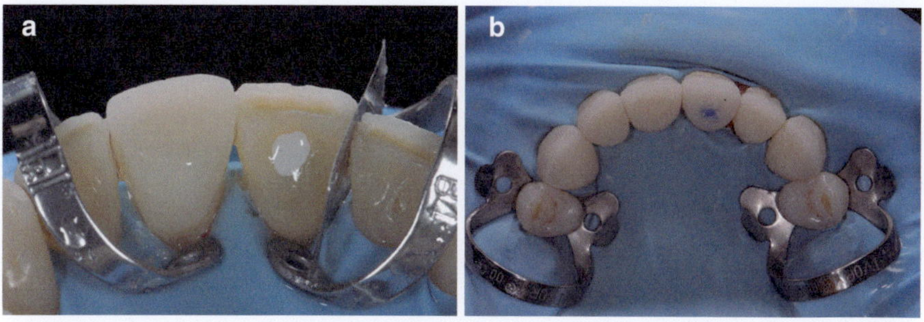

Fig. 7.39 (**a**) Tooth 11 palatal veneer cemented and (**b**) completion of individual fitting of teeth 13–23 unit palatal veneer restorations

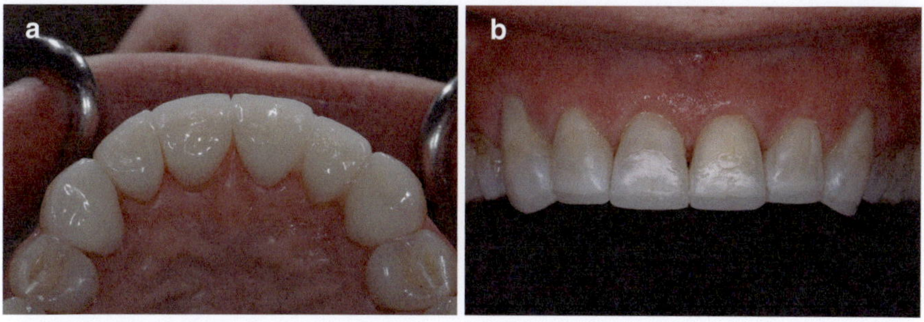

Fig. 7.40 (**a, b**) Teeth 13–23 restored with indirect palatal veneers, completed case

Further Reading

1. Alani A, Patel M. Clinical issues in occlusion - part I. Singap Dent J. 2014;35:31–8.
2. Alani A, Mehta S, Koning I, Loomans B, Pereira-Cenci T. Restorative options for moderate and severe tooth wear: a systematic review. J Dent. 2025;156:105711.
3. Dahl BL, Krogstad O, Karlsen K. An alternative treatment in cases with advanced localised attrition. J Oral Rehabil. 1975;2:209–14.
4. Gulamali A, Hemmings K, Tredwin C, Petrie A. Survival analysis of composite Dahl restorations provided to manage localised anterior tooth wear (ten year follow-up). Br Dent J. 2011;211:E9.
5. Patel M. Treating tooth surface loss: adhesive restoration of the worn anterior dentition. Prim Dent J. 2016;5(3):43–57.
6. Patel M, Alani A. Clinical issues in occlusion—part II. Singap Dent J. 2015;36:2–11.
7. Vailati F, Belser UC. Palatal and facial veneers to treat severe dental erosion: a case report following the three-step technique and the Sandwich approach. Eur J Esthet Dentist. 2011;6(3):268–78.

Treating Posterior Tooth Surface Loss

8

Contents

Learning Outcomes

- Appreciate the difference in functional loading that restorations on posterior teeth have to manage when compared to anterior teeth.
- Understand that posterior restoration material choice can accommodate functional and aesthetic needs.
- Recognise that direct adhesive restorations on posterior teeth are best provided with a pre-determined diagnostic wax-up of the desired final result.
- Appreciate that adhesive restorations on posterior teeth may require less tooth preparation.

8.1 Introduction

The management of tooth surface loss (TSL) on posterior teeth, much in the same with anterior teeth, is heavily dependent on the aetiology of the tooth surface loss, whether it is ongoing and on the amount/volume of coronal dental hard tissue remaining. Intact posterior teeth manage loads by crushing food on a relatively flat

A. Alani, M. Patel, *Adhesive Techniques in Restorative Dentistry*, BDJ Clinician's Guides, https://doi.org/10.1007/978-3-032-07346-4_8

occlusal table. This, unlike anterior teeth, lends themselves to an adhesive approach. Anterior teeth tend to shear food in function; this shear force can translate to the restoration tooth junction, resulting in adhesive bond failure. Molar and premolar teeth, in comparison, restored with an adhesively bonded cuspal coverage restoration will load the tooth-restoration complex in compression, which is tolerated much better than shear forces at the adhesive bond junction. As a result of this difference in loading, adhesive restorations may be more amenable in the posterior than the anterior dentition. This greater likelihood of compressive loading of the tooth lends itself to the greater expected loading due to the closer proximity to the masseter muscle and temporomandibular joint.

8.2 Aetiology and Pattern of TSL

Tooth topography subsequent to erosive TSL can vary from patient to patient and is directly related to the nature and source of the erosion and its severity. A bulimic patient is likely to confer protection on the mandibular teeth through the tongue, which will result in the majority of stomach contents contacting the maxillary teeth. This manifests clinically as asymmetric tooth volume, where the palatal surfaces are almost non-existent in severe cases and the buccal surfaces are entirely intact. Such an asymmetric shape may daunt the clinician due to the non-existent palatal aspect, which has limited potential to create resistance and retention form for indirect conventional cemented restorations. This lack of palatal tooth structure volume will result in a wholly short preparation if the tooth is going to be prepared for a conventional crown.

In contrast, patients with parafunction attritive tendencies essentially plane the tooth flat resulting in loss of all morphology and, in severe cases, revealing the underlying dentine. The topography of tissue in these cases may require greater thought, if not due to the non-axial forces that may or may not continue post-restoration.

Both TSL presentations can not only result in compromised tooth height for indirect conventional restoration but also compromised adhesive bonding potential due to the exposure of the underlying dentine, or more severely, tertiary dentine where the pulp previously resided, in the central portion of the tooth. Both conditions can also prospectively have an enamel margin for the restoration, but the bonding technique needs to be as optimal as possible due to the reduced amount of enamel substrate present. Dentine bonding, in severe cases, will be more likely and greater in volume than the enamel bond.

One aspect that may not be entirely apparent but needs appreciation is the positional change of posterior teeth in relation to neighbouring teeth in the same arch and those that they oppose. As teeth wear across their occlusal surfaces, they are likely to maintain occlusal contact through dentoalveolar compensation. This results in the need to plan the increase in occlusal vertical dimension due to the reduced volume of dentine mass between the opposing teeth pulps. As the worn occlusal surfaces diminish the cusp anatomy, the teeth develop an end-to-end

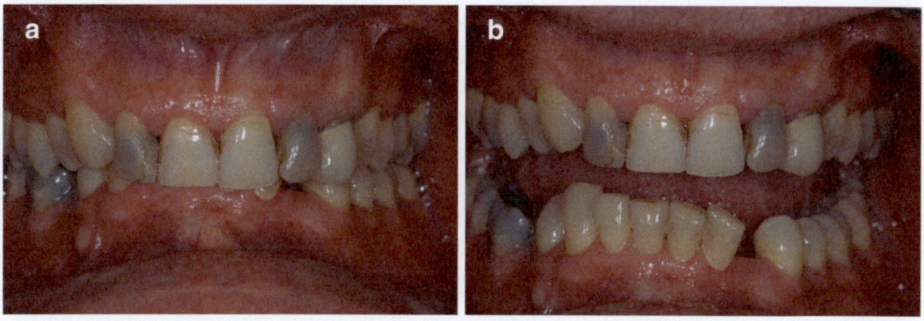

Fig. 8.1 (**a**, **b**) Malocclusion and unfavourable tooth positions make restorative correction challenging without orthodontic management

relationship with both flat surfaces abutting each other. In severe cases, this develops further into a pseudo Angle's Class III relationship with no easily referenced points of contact in the intercuspal position. With progressive occlusal wear and loss of a stable intercuspal position, teeth can migrate into very unfavourable positions, resulting in cross-bites or unfavourable vertical migration, either resulting in a locked-in occlusal relationship or tooth malposition that cannot accommodate a stable contact post-rehabilitation. In these instances, orthodontic treatment may be considered; however, a compromise may need to be considered if this is not possible (Fig. 8.1). Such changes may preclude the ability of the clinician to recreate a traditional cusp fossa relationship where mesial drift or rotations have occurred. Other aspects of posterior wear include changes in the interproximal contact which progressively becomes wider and flatter. This makes designing restorations more difficult as the contact becomes tighter and more difficult to create a cleansable interface. The pattern of wear in the posterior dentition is inextricably linked to the wear of anterior teeth. If anterior guidance is lost through wear, lack of posterior teeth disclusion on lateral and protrusive excursions will inevitably result in further wear on posterior teeth resulting in a progressive and rapid cycle of tooth surface loss.

8.3 Direct Restorations

Where the TSL is minimal, such as cupping on the occlusal surface, direct restoration can be achieved relatively easily. The cupped area is bounded by enamel, and the recreation of tooth morphology is likely to be straightforward with direct composite resin. These relatively early lesions within molar teeth need to be recognised early. Lesions wholly in enamel can be restored predictably prior to the lesion breaching into dentine. Once dentine is exposed, the rate of TSL progresses at a faster rate due to the inherent porosity and softness of dentine when compared to enamel. The lesions then broaden and widen as a result. Where more extensive restorations are planned, these cupping lesions can be incorporated into the restoration, providing a locating feature in the intaglio surface of the restoration. Due to posterior teeth likely to undergo greater functional occlusal loading, the choice of a more heavily filled composite resin, however more viscous, may be more favourable to provide greater resistance to further occlusal restoration wear.

In situations where the TSL is more extensive, the direct adhesive restoration of teeth requires a template to work towards to provide an optimal final functional restoration contour. This, in the main, is achieved through a diagnostic wax-up prescribed through diagnostic study casts, a facebow record and an appropriate interocclusal record. The diagnostic wax-up prescription is key to a successful definitive restoration as it forms the blueprint. Focus on details such as the design of the occlusal table, the nature of the contact points occlusal and interdental, and the marginal interface is immensely important. Diagnostic wax-ups are constructed to either provide patients with a preview of future treatment or to give the technician a guide for indirect restorations, also these can be utilised to transfer the restoration shape directly to the mouth from the chairside.

A direct restoration in composite resin does not rely on the need for a path of insertion. Direct provision can also mitigate against areas of undercut within the residual tooth tissue. The advantages of the direct approach include efficiency of time and cost, as well as the serviceability of the restoration and any subsequent revisions.

It should be noted that direct composite onlay restorations may be provided for both vital and non-vital teeth. These restorations can act as provisional or definitive restorations for single or multiple teeth, depending upon the planning of the case (Figs. 8.2 and 8.3).

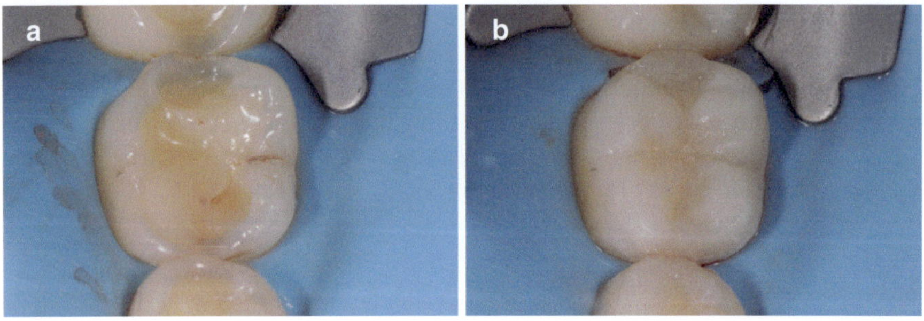

Fig. 8.2 (**a**) Tooth 46 erosive and attritional tooth surface loss and (**b**) after definitive restoration utilising a direct composite resin onlay restoration

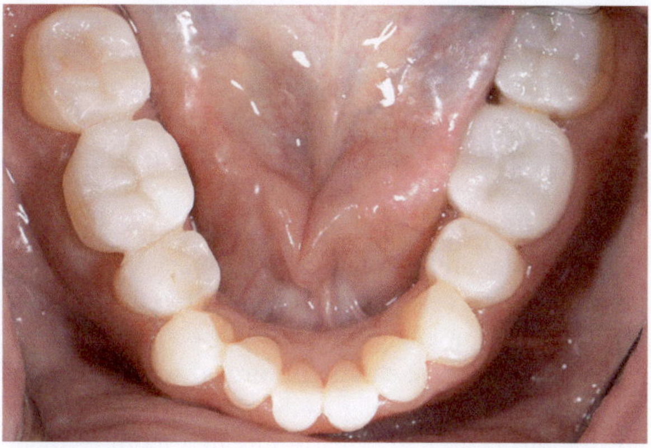

Fig. 8.3 Adhesive reconstruction of mandibular attritive Tooth Surface Loss utilising direct composite resin restorations on all teeth. These restorations can act as provisional or definitive restorations depending upon the planning and management of the case

8.4 Indirect Restorations

The indirect restoration of posterior teeth has historically been the accepted mode of treatment due to a lack of awareness of the ability or progression in the mode of direct restoration provision as previously described. Essentially, indirect restorations are more likely to be easier to deliver, especially in terms of management of the interproximal areas and labour burden that multiple extensive restorations may provide utilising direct techniques. Indirect restorations fabricated in a laboratory are likely to result in a more resilient restoration with superior physical properties and potentially better shape control with regard to the restoration design of the occlusal table for static and functional contact and interdental surfaces for contact points.

Choosing indirect over direct restoration provision is clinician-dependent based upon their individual knowledge of material selection, clinical skill set and experience. The choice may also be governed and influenced by patient finances. Clinicians can consider a variety of adhesively retained indirect materials, which vary with the benefits of differing aesthetic and physical properties. The planning, choice and execution of the adhesive restoration depend heavily on the individual nature of the presenting clinical case.

8.4.1 Metal Alloy Onlays

The indirect restoration metal alloy material choice is confined to either nickel or cobalt chromium and type III gold alloy (60% gold content). When compared to nickel or cobalt chromium, gold alloy is kinder to opposing teeth from an abrasive aspect. When used in these situations, it can be cast into sections of 1–1.5 mm occlusal thickness, with nickel or cobalt chromium potentially less than this thickness due to their greater rigidity. However, with any material, the thicker the restoration, the stronger it will be.

Type III gold alloy onlay restorations that are to be adhesively bonded may be heat treated to improve their adhesive efficacy. The heat treatment process is carried out in a furnace after fabrication of the final restoration and creates a copper oxide layer that allows improved bonding. The dark appearance of the layer can then be polished off the exterior surface of the restoration, or if left will dissipate over time through exposure in the oral cavity (Fig. 8.4).

Metal alloy restorations on posterior teeth due to their largely superior physical characteristics are still relevant to the management of TSL, where patients recognise compromises in aesthetics that need to be considered for teeth in different positions of the mouth, utilising different roles. A good example of customising material choice to tooth type can be illustrated with the provision of gold alloy onlays to molar teeth, and premolar teeth are provided with more aesthetic 'tooth coloured' restorations (Fig. 8.5). This results in a more resilient occlusal scheme where the restored contacting molar teeth maintain the established change in occlusal vertical dimension. As these opposing contacting occlusal units have the same restorative material across their occlusal surfaces, this should minimise wear progression.

The design of the preparations for these restorations needs to consider two aspects.

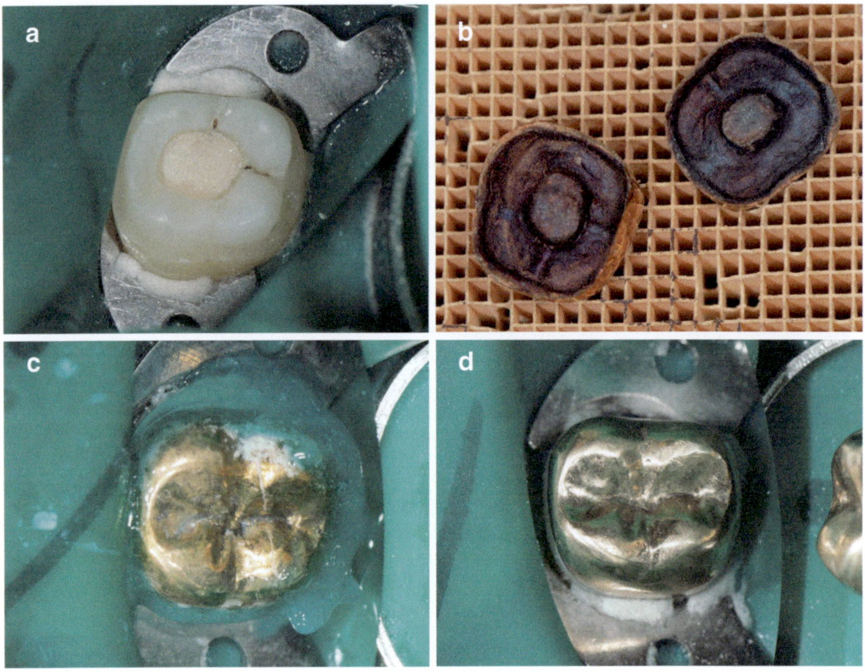

Fig. 8.4 (**a**) Molar tooth preparation and isolation. (**b**) Appearance of Type III gold alloy adhesive onlay restorations intaglio surfaces with oxide layer immediately after heat treatment. (**c**) Onlay restoration adhesively bonded and (**d**) after removal of oxide layer by restoration polishing. (Images courtesy of Dr Guy Stephens)

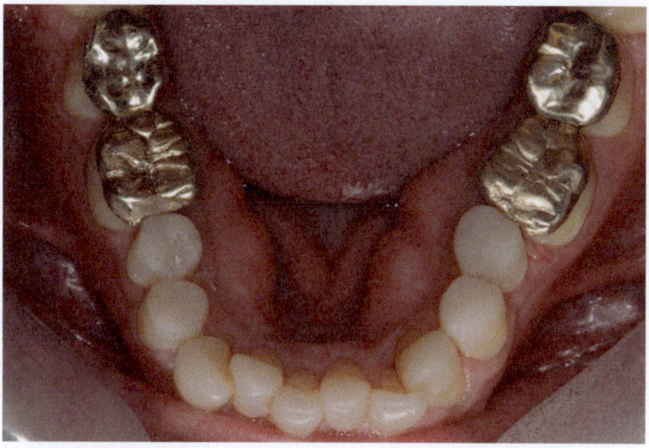

Fig. 8.5 Adhesive reconstruction of mandibular erosive tooth surface loss utilising type III gold alloy restorations on molar teeth and direct composite resin restorations on premolar, canine and incisor teeth

The ability to successfully locate the restorations with ease and maximise bonding surface area. The basis of location relies on creating a single path of insertion, the clinician may consider some form of anti-rotation feature within the preparation merely to allow for ease of restoration location intra-orally and less so for the path of insertion. Depending on what stage the tooth presents with, there may be natural morphological features which the restoration can engage for purposes of location. Residual cupping or the presence of fissure patterns can aide this. In situations where there is severe TSL then, these features will not be present. Creation of defined grooves or slots on axial wall areas or in the occlusal surface will limit the path of insertion and ensure adequate and consistent seating at the cementation stage.

8.4.2 Tooth Coloured Onlays

The indirect restoration tooth coloured material choice are composite resin, resin nano-ceramic or all-ceramic materials. High-strength lithium disilicate glass-matrix ceramic materials are the preferred choice of the all-ceramic material selection.

Resin-based materials can be made into sections of 1.5–2 mm occlusal thickness with lithium disilicate potentially made less than this thickness due to its greater strength.

The designs of the preparations for these restorations take into account the same two aspects as required for the metal alloy restorations, location and maximising bonding surface area. However, the creation of defined grooves or slots on axial wall areas is not advised for these materials.

8.5 Adhesive Technique

8.5.1 Direct Composite Resin Onlay

This technique has been described previously in Chap. 6.

The summary of clinical stages for the provision of direct composite resin onlays is listed in Table 8.1 and is shown in the presented clinical case (Fig. 8.6).

Table 8.1 Summary of clinical stages of direct composite resin onlay restorations

Clinical stages
1. Production of a clear silicone stent at least 2 mm thick
2. Rubber dam isolation
3. Teeth cleaning/preparation, finish lines/ sandblasting
4. Teeth separation/etch/bond (alternate teeth)
5. Composite resin loading of the tooth and matrix
6. Matrix seating and composite resin material excess removal
7. Light curing
8. Composite resin material excess removal
9. Repeat steps 4–8 for alternate teeth
10. Restoration finishing and polishing
11. Occlusal check

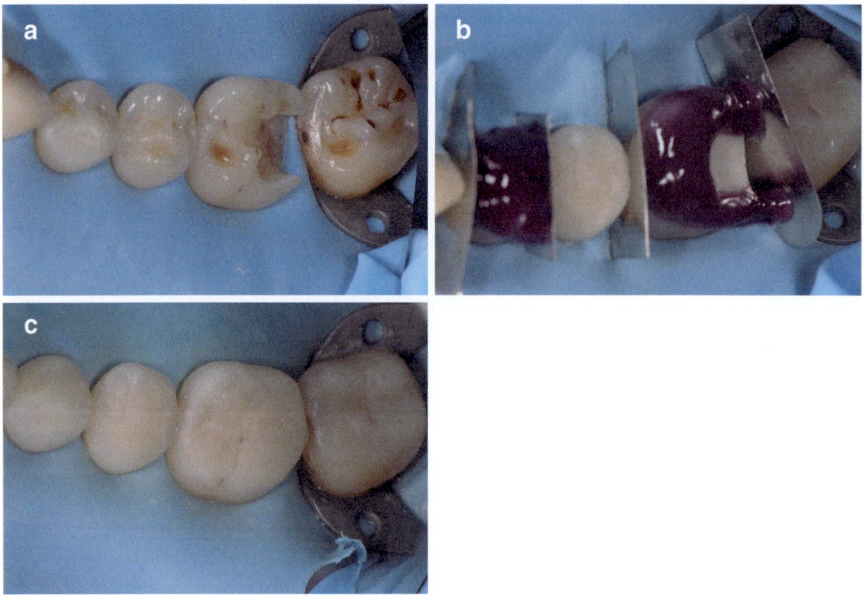

Fig. 8.6 Provision of direct composite resin onlays for teeth 37–34; (**a**) rubber dam isolation; (**b**) teeth separation/etch (alternate teeth) and (**c**) completed restorations after finishing and polishing

8.5.2 Indirect Onlay Cementation

This technique has been described previously in Chap. 7, where the summary of clinical stages for the adhesive cementation of an indirect palatal veneer is listed.

The summary of clinical stages for the adhesive cementation of an indirect onlay is listed in Table 8.2 and is shown in the presented clinical cases (Figs. 8.7, 8.8, 8.9, 8.10, 8.11, 8.12, 8.13, 8.14, 8.15 and 8.16).

Table 8.2 Summary of clinical stages of indirect onlay adhesive cementation

Clinical stages
1. Abutment tooth clean
2. Onlay try-in
3. Rubber dam isolation
4. Restoration re-try
5. Abutment tooth sandblast/etch/bond
6. Onlay intaglio surface sandblast/clean/silanate or prime/cement loading
7. Cement onlay
8. Light cure (with oxygen block barrier)
9. Clean excess cement
10. Polish restoration margins

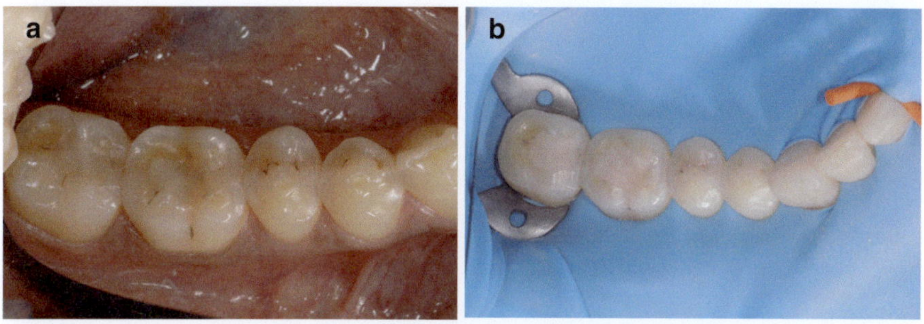

Fig. 8.7 (**a**) Teeth 44–47 with erosion and attrition to be restored with indirect onlays. (**b**) Rubber dam isolation of lower right side quadrant

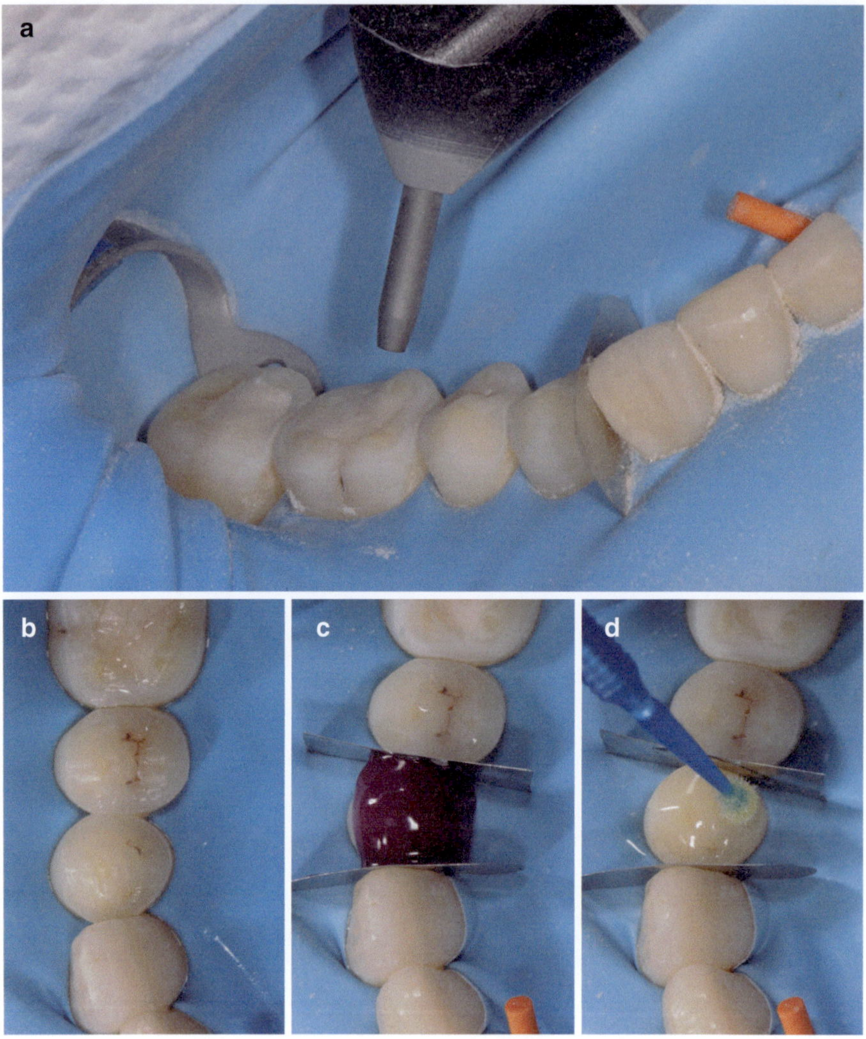

Fig. 8.8 (**a**) Lower right quadrant abutment teeth sand blasting. (**b**) Abutment tooth 44; (**c**) total etch and (**d**) bonding agent application

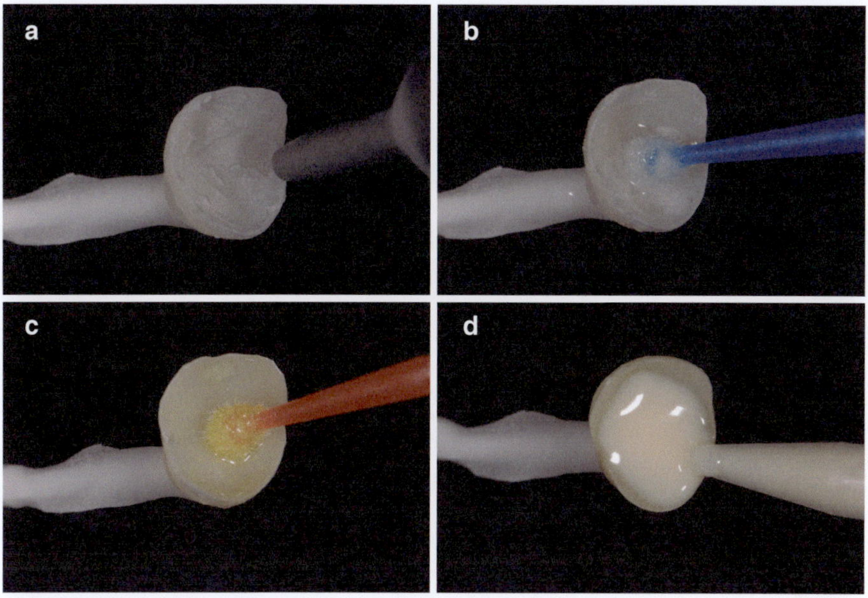

Fig. 8.9 Onlay (indirect resin nano ceramic) intaglio surface; (**a**) sandblast, (**b**) clean, (**c**) silanate and (**d**) cement loading

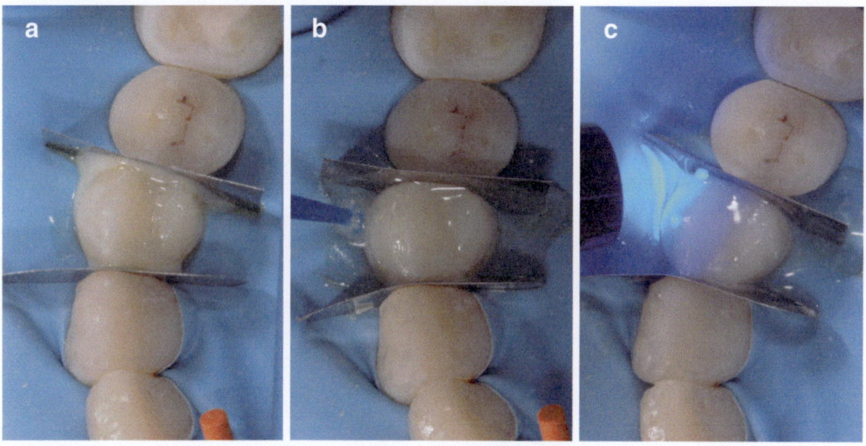

Fig. 8.10 (**a**) Onlay cemented, (**b**) oxygen block barrier application and (**c**) light cure

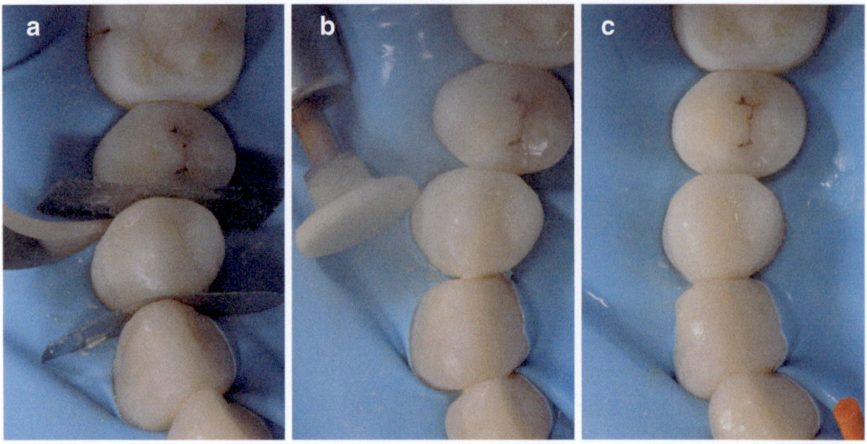

Fig. 8.11 (**a**) Onlay excess cement removal with scalpel blade no. 12, (**b**) restoration margins polish and (**c**) restoration in-situ

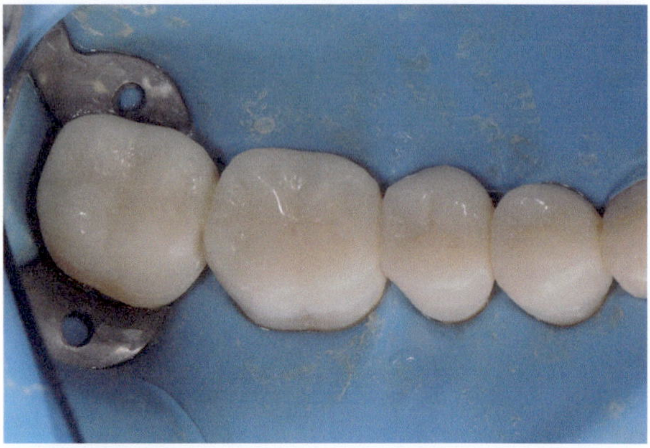

Fig. 8.12 Completion of individual fitting of teeth 44–47 unit onlay restorations

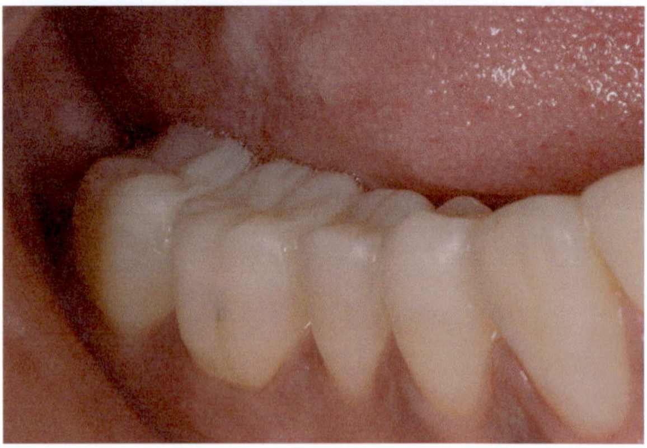

Fig. 8.13 Teeth 44–47 restored with indirect onlays, completed case

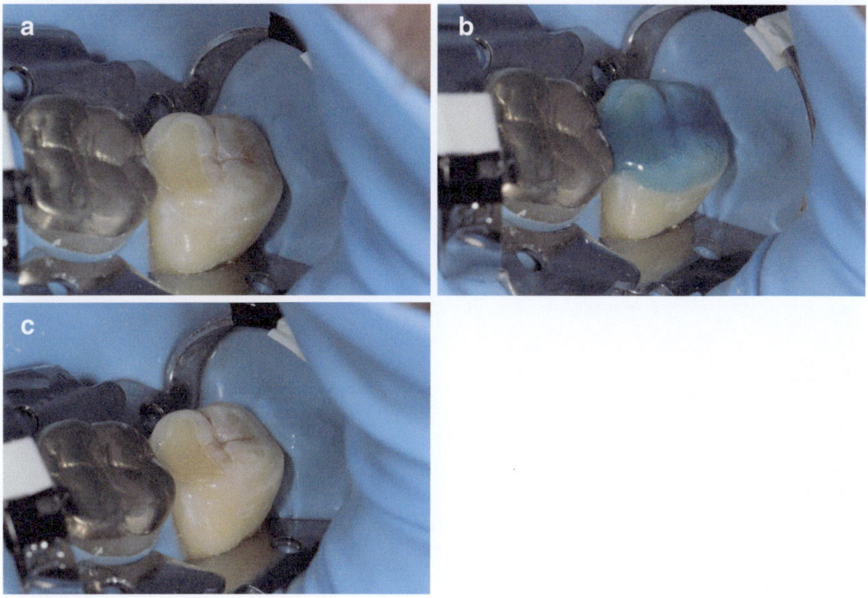

Fig. 8.14 (**a**) Abutment tooth 37 rubber dam islolation, (**b**) total etch and (**c**) bonding agent application

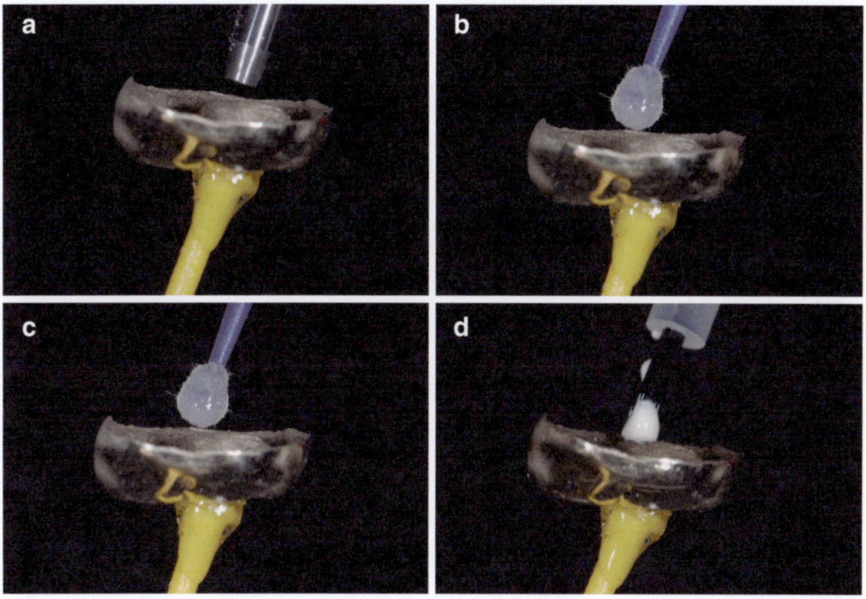

Fig. 8.15 Onlay (Type III gold alloy) intaglio surface; (**a**) sandblast, (**b**) clean, (**c**) prime and (**d**) cement loading

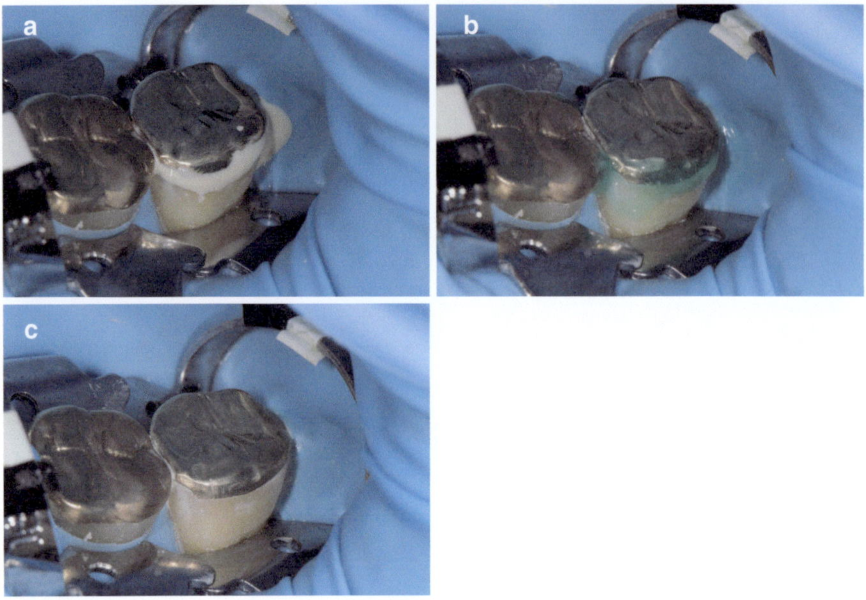

Fig. 8.16 (**a**) Onlay cemented, (**b**) oxygen block barrier application and (**c**) restoration in-situ

Further Reading

1. Alani A, Patel M. Clinical issues in occlusion - part I. Singap Dent J. 2014;35:31–8.
2. Alani A, Mehta S, Koning I, Loomans B, Pereira-Cenci T. Restorative options for moderate and severe tooth wear: a systematic review. J Dent. 2025;22(156):105711.
3. Chana H, Kelleher M, Briggs P, Hooper R. Clinical evaluation of resin-bonded gold alloy veneers. J Prosthet Dent. 2000;83(3):294–300.
4. Eder A, Wickens J. Surface treatment of gold alloys for resin adhesion. Quintessence Int. 1996;27(1):35–40.
5. Patel M. Treating tooth surface loss: adhesive restoration of the worn anterior dentition. Prim Dent J. 2016;5(3):43–57.
6. Patel M, Alani A. Clinical issues in occlusion—part II. Singap Dent J. 2015;36:2–11.

Managing Tooth Replacement

9

Contents

Learning Outcomes

- Identify current materials used for resin-bonded bridge restorations, how they may be applied and their limitations.
- Understand the principles governing design parameters of resin-bonded bridge restorations and their components.
- Identify parameters that will influence the predictability of resin-bonded bridge restoration success.

9.1 Introduction

Resin-bonded bridge (RBB) restorations are an efficient and predictable method of restoring edentulous spaces. Since their inception in the 1970s as a method for splinting periodontally involved teeth, the technique has gradually evolved due to improvements in adhesive resin technology and knowledge on failure mechanisms. In the 1980s to early 1990s, the technique came under scrutiny due to a number of studies documenting poor survival rates. The initial popularity was stunted as failure rates were less than acceptable, and as such, the technique fell out of favour. In

A. Alani, M. Patel, *Adhesive Techniques in Restorative Dentistry*, BDJ Clinician's Guides, https://doi.org/10.1007/978-3-032-07346-4_9

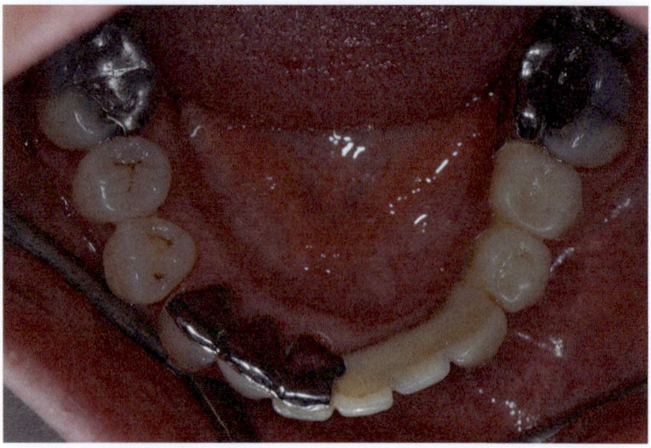

Fig. 9.1 Overengineered RBB restoration utilising multiple abutment units

hindsight, this period was likely attributed to poor bonding technique, as well as suboptimal retainer wing design and inadequate attention to occlusal factors. In addition, and in keeping with certain prosthodontics ethos' from this era, the RBB may also have suffered from over-engineering where multiple abutments were engaged (Fig. 9.1) when a more simple design would later be revealed as more successful. Fortunately, a cohort of further studies maintained the excellent promise shown during this period. This culminated in the publication of a long-term follow-up of 832 resin-bonded bridges by Djemal et al. in 1999. This study outlined specific requirements relating to the design of the bridgework whilst also emphasising the need for an optimal bonding technique. Single pontic single abutment bridges provided the greatest survival time, with bridges on anterior teeth, and this was greater than on posterior units. A sound enamel substrate surface was shown to be another significant variable. This was subsequently followed by a study by King et al. in 2015, illustrating excellent survival over 15 years, especially with single-unit single cantilever designs. Some important proven points from this landmark study were that a lack of abutment preparation resulted in greater longevity than prepared abutments and that operators with greater experience generally exhibited longer restoration survival. History shows that a lack of understanding or apathy towards 'good adhesive bonding' has resulted in less than expected outcomes. These results could be considered timely when considering the emerging complication rates of both single-unit implants and implant-supported bridgework.

9.2 Planning Tooth Replacement

Tooth replacement provision requires some basic baseline information in order to establish which prosthesis is suitable and how this will be achieved. From the information obtained, the method and mode through which the treatment can be delivered can be decided. Information gathering can vary from the clinical and radiographic examination up to and including full records with clinical photographs and casts mounted on a semi-adjustable articulator with a diagnostic wax-up of the

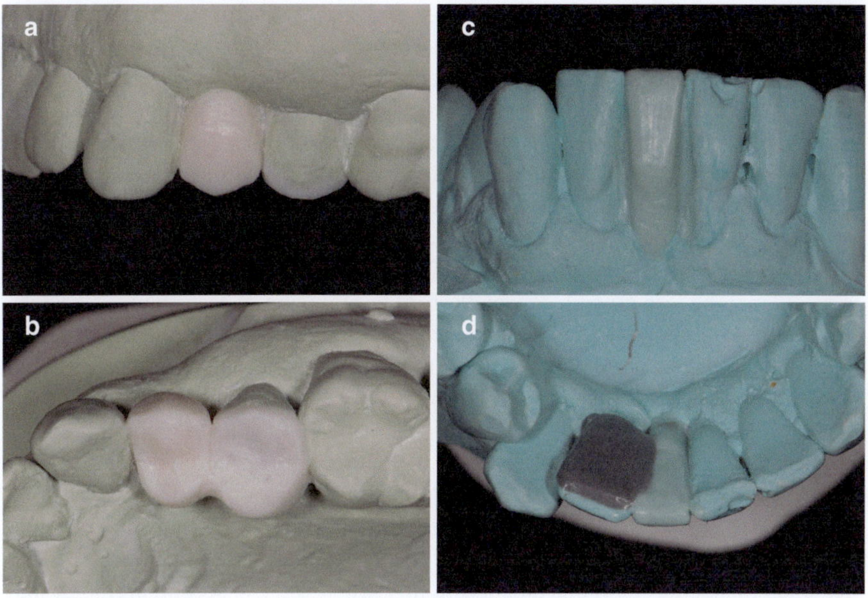

Fig. 9.2 Diagnostic wax-up of two proposed RBB treatment cases; including the retainer and abutment replacing (**a, b**) tooth 24 and (**c, d**) tooth 41

proposed treatment (Fig. 9.2). The amount of information required varies with the complexity of the case and the potential invasive nature of the prosthesis. For example, where interocclusal space is reduced, bone volume and quality are unknown, and abutment teeth have a questionable prognosis, the full plethora of investigative techniques will be required. In contrast in a healthy minimally restored mouth where proposed abutment teeth are unrestored and the potential pontic space is adequate, the ability to plan prosthetic replacement is easier.

9.3 Abutment Tooth Selection

Examination of the proposed abutment teeth is vital as the mode of restoration retention is adhesive. The restorative status of the tooth is important as this will be directly related to the amount of enamel available for bonding (i.e. unrestored vs heavily restored teeth). Sound enamel for adhesion is a key factor to consider when choosing potential abutments. Where a proposed abutment tooth requires restoration, the tendency may be to choose alternative unrestored abutment teeth in favour of larger tooth units with a compromised quantity of enamel tissue. However, if proposed abutment teeth have existing restorations, replacement of these with a composite resin material is likely to optimise adhesive bonding with an adhesive resin cement. A fresh resin surface void of long-term exposure to the oral environment will reduce water absorption into the composite resin and improve the adhesive bond of the retainer wing. Where the available clinical crown height is short, assessment of the periodontal status can provide information on the feasibility of gingivectomy or crown lengthening procedures to increase the availability of the enamel surface (Fig. 9.3). Soft tissue assessment extends to the pontic site also. Where the gingiva in the missing tooth span overlying the alveolus is thick and well keratinised, there is more potential for tissue augmentation to improve the emergence profile of the pontic. This may be achieved via the gingival manipulation process' (Figs. 9.4, 9.5 and 9.6).

With the advent of adhesion, those traditional bridge design and bridge abutment concepts may be less crucial, especially for the provision of resin-bonded bridges. Outside of patients with parafunction, teeth occlude approximately 15 minutes a day. As such, the emphasis on structural robustness of the abutment may diminish in favour of the enamel available for bonding. Where restorations are present that are confined to the occlusal, palatal or lingual surface of the teeth without breaking the marginal ridges, the restoration void can either be incorporated into the wing design or restored with composite resin to maximise further bonding with resin if the underlying restoration is amalgam, for example (Fig. 9.7). The nature and type of tooth has repercussions on the mode of loading of the abutment wing. For example, when managing the replacement of a first premolar. The second premolar may naturally provide a flat platform once restored with a wing. In contrast, without designing a horizontal platform into the wing, the canine will produce a sloped surface, which will naturally load the tooth differently and potentially non-axially.

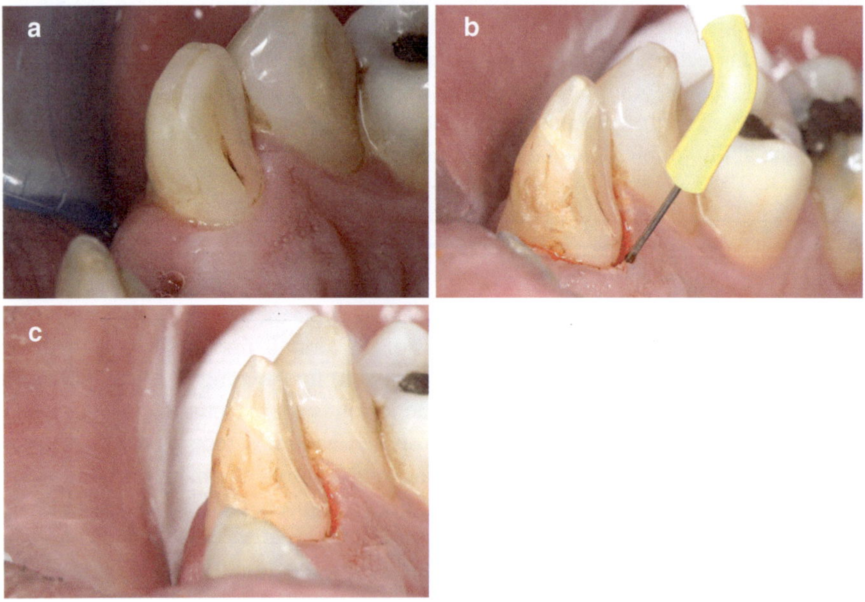

Fig. 9.3 (a–c) Tooth 22 palatal gingival tissue removal on tooth 22 with an electrosurgery unit to increase bonding surface area and expose palatal cingulum for RBB wing retainer provision

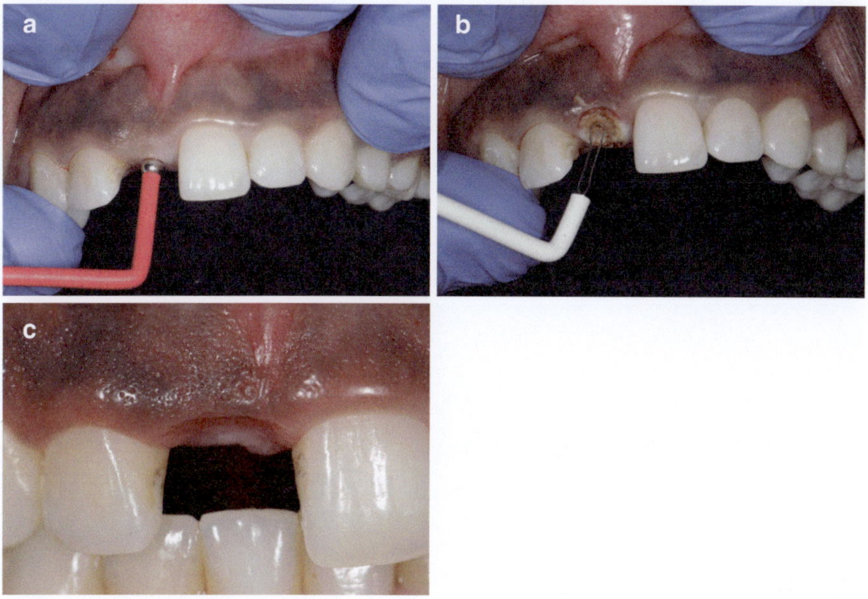

Fig. 9.4 (**a, b**) Pontic site gingival tissue sculpting to allow improvement of the emergence profile of the bridge pontic and (**c**) healed site

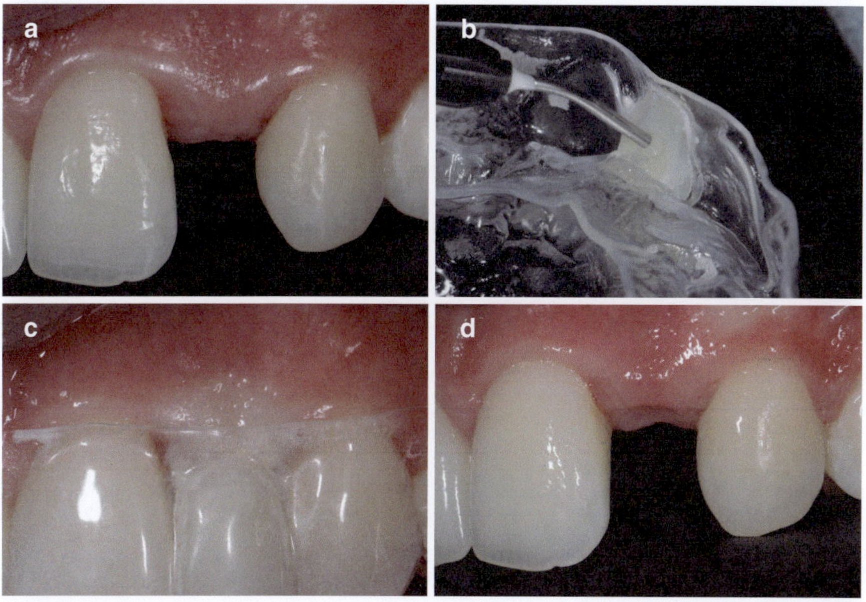

Fig. 9.5 (**a**) Tooth 22 pontic site modified through controlled pressure necrosis (**b**) by adding flowable composite resin within an Essix retainer. (**c**) Note the gingival blanching on the fit of the retainer, which later subsided. (**d**) The modification to the gingival architecture now allows for an ovate pontic to be fitted

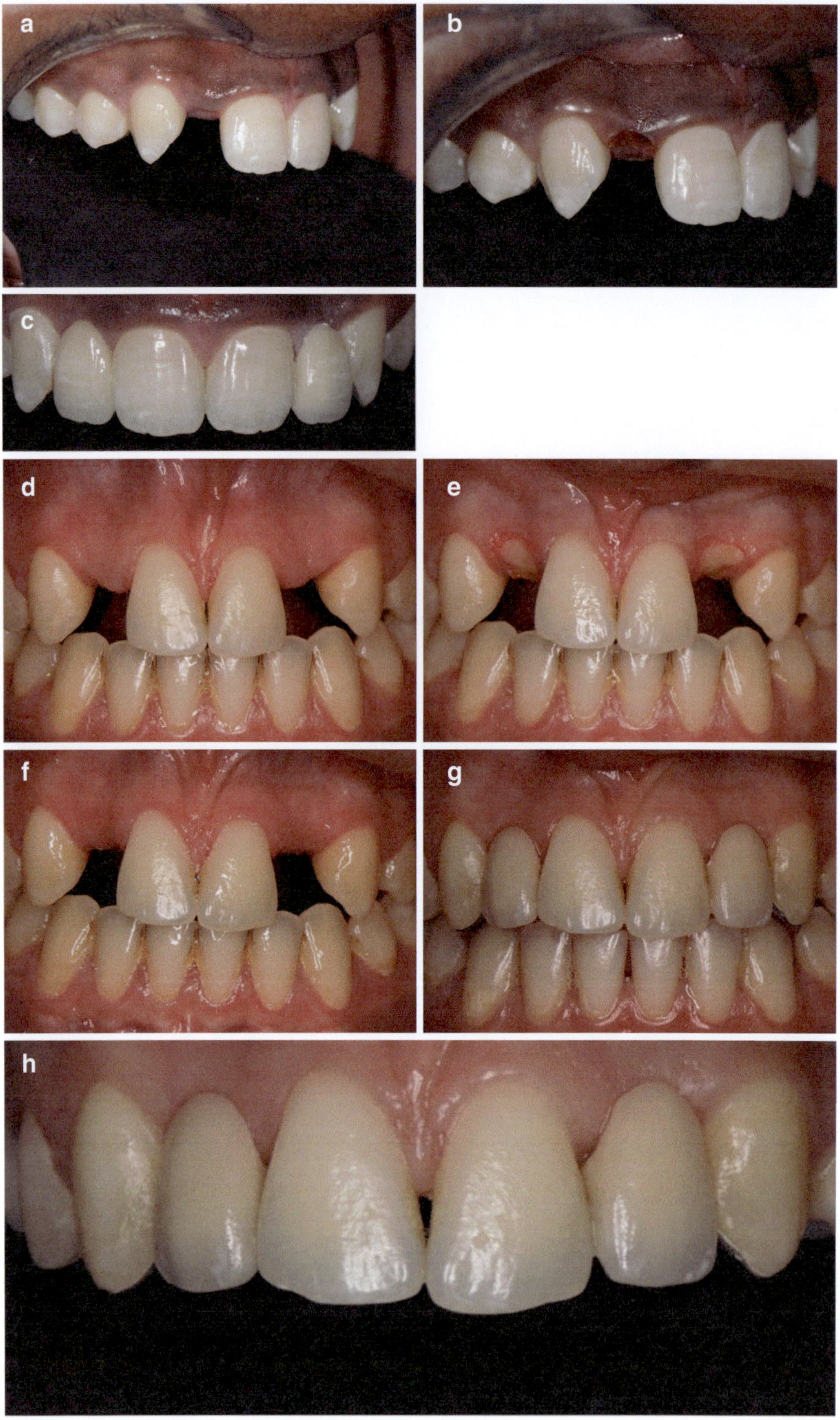

Fig. 9.6 (**a–h**) Two clinical cases showing the use of gingival tissue manipulation and healing to allow aesthetic integration of the RBB pontics in lateral incisor sites

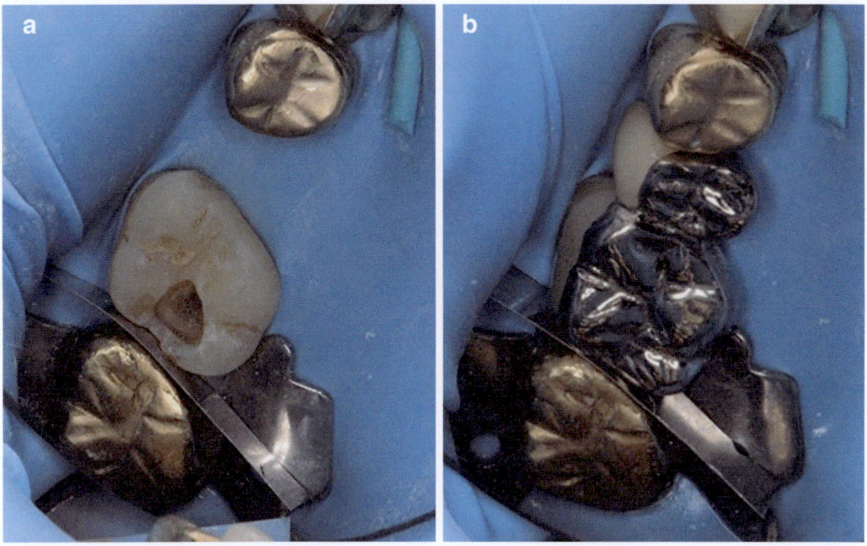

Fig. 9.7 Tooth 16; (**a**) occlusal amalgam removal void and cavity defect preparation to allow (**b**) engagement of RBB retainer wing to improve bonding surface area and the path of insertion of the restoration

Other factors to consider include the angulation and position of the potential abutment teeth. Grossly tilted or rotated teeth impact the connector height and the shape of the pontic. In certain cases, orthodontic treatment to optimise tooth position may be required to improve prosthodontic provision for these reasons.

9.4 No Tooth Preparation

As a concept, a 'no tooth preparation' bridge design may initially be counterintuitive to most. With a lack of any abutment preparation, there is an absence of restorative space to accommodate the thickness of the bridge retainer and a lack of resistance and retention form with a total reliance on micromechanical and chemical adhesion of the retainer, cement lute and hard dental tissue substrate. The evidence for such an approach is established largely through two British studies based in secondary care specialist units. Djemal and King and colleagues in 1999 and 2015, respectively, demonstrated predictable success rates with this approach. This may be explained as the abutment surface is unblemished, resulting in a totally enamel substrate adhesive bond which is significantly superior and more predictable in comparison to a dentine substrate adhesive bond.

The evidence also points towards the single retainer pontic cantilever design being the most successful in most anterior and posterior situations (Fig. 9.8). The clinician may also consider abutments on either side of multiple pontics (fixed–fixed) to provide greater bonding surface area as well as support from two separate teeth (Fig. 9.9). However, these 'rules' may not necessarily apply where the method

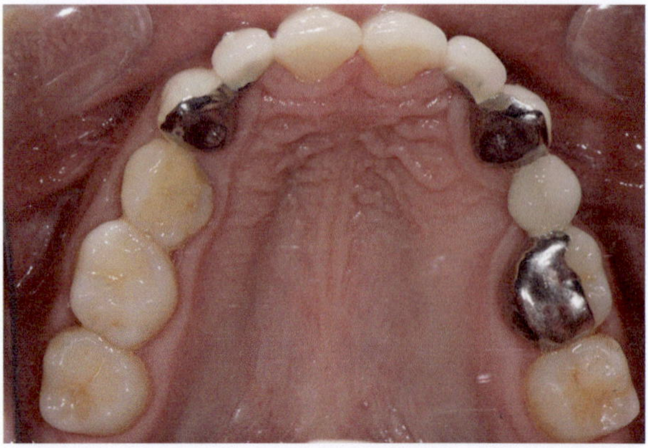

Fig. 9.8 Single retainer pontic cantilever design for three RBBs replacing teeth 12, 22 & 25

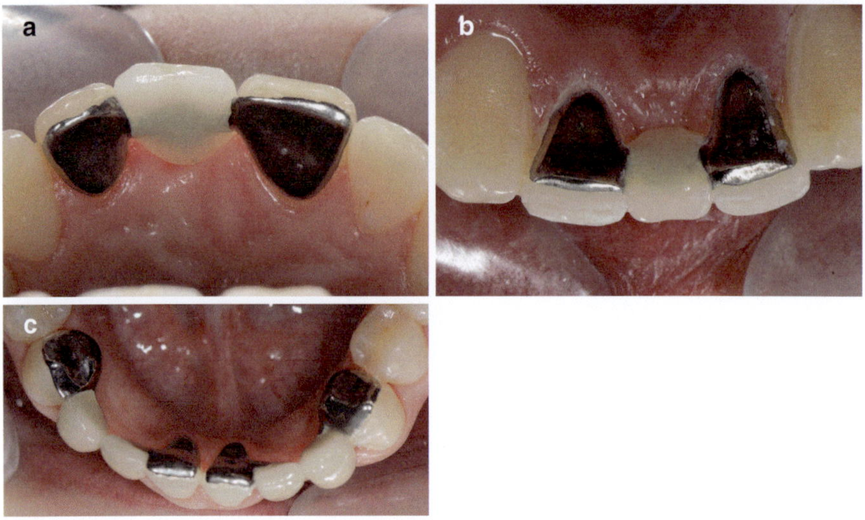

Fig. 9.9 Fixed–fixed RBBs showing replacement of (**a, b**) single and (**c**) multiple tooth units

of retention is largely based on adhesion. Where there is no abutment teeth preparation, tooth bulbosity on either side of a pontic limits the amount of hard tissue covered by the retainer wings. This is due to the limitations on coverage by the path of insertion of the prosthesis. A further consideration is the differential movement of the two abutment units that can also result in failure of the adhesive bond at the minor retainer and therefore debond of the bridge prosthesis. It may seem counter-intuitive to consider a single abutment over the seemingly advantageous fixed–fixed design, but there are notable biological and mechanical advantages.

The cantilever design has an inherent fail-safe mechanism when compared to multiple retainer designs. If microleakage, resin cement breakdown and caries develop under the retainer wing in either design, the outcomes of each can be very different. With the single retainer design, partial or complete debond is likely to result in the bridge losing retention and the patient subsequently presenting to the clinician requesting recementation or the need for revised bridge provision. Where multiple abutments are present, debond on one wing is likely to go undetected by the patient and can be difficult to diagnose for the clinician. This debonded retainer can harbour plaque and debris, providing a niche for bacteria within which can develop and could result in catastrophic failure. This debond may be due to differential movements between the two abutments, and in most cases, it is the 'weaker' abutment, which has less surface area and less root size, that is likely to suffer the failure (Fig. 9.10).

Further to this, tooth preparation incorporating finish lines, guide planes, grooves or slots can also achieve a more defined path of insertion and creation of occlusal space, but it is more difficult to achieve passivity of fit and could be more difficult for the technician to construct. Nonetheless, these designs can be very successful when delivered optimally (Figs. 9.7 and 9.11).

A key component in any restoration, and more acutely where teeth are being replaced, is the manner in which abutment teeth are loaded statically and dynamically. The outcome may become more dependent on the nature of the interocclusal space and whether the occlusal vertical dimension is planned to change post-cementation. Where there is sufficient interocclusal space, the design of the functional surface of the bridge is much less crucial other than the potential for a thicker palatal portion causing annoyance to the patient (Fig. 9.12). Where the interocclusal retainer thickness cannot be accommodated both statically and dynamically, the

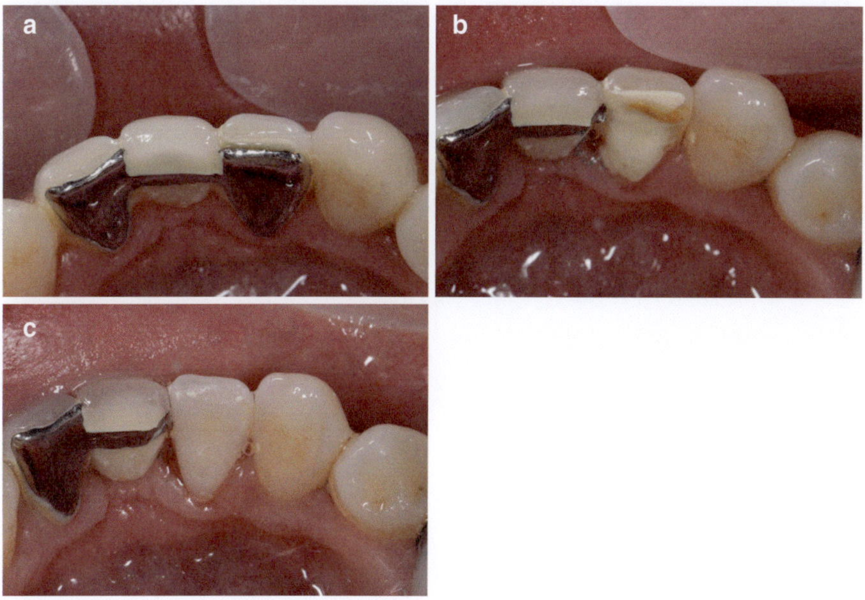

Fig. 9.10 (**a**) Fixed–fixed RBB showing debond of retainer wing at abutment tooth 42, (**b**) sectioning and removal of the debonded retainer and (**c**) cleaned of abutment tooth surface

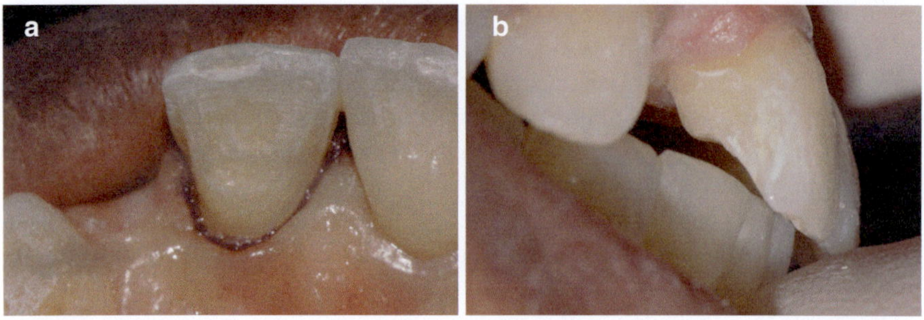

Fig. 9.11 (**a, b**) Tooth preparation incorporating finish lines, guide planes, achieving a defined path of insertion and creation of occlusal space

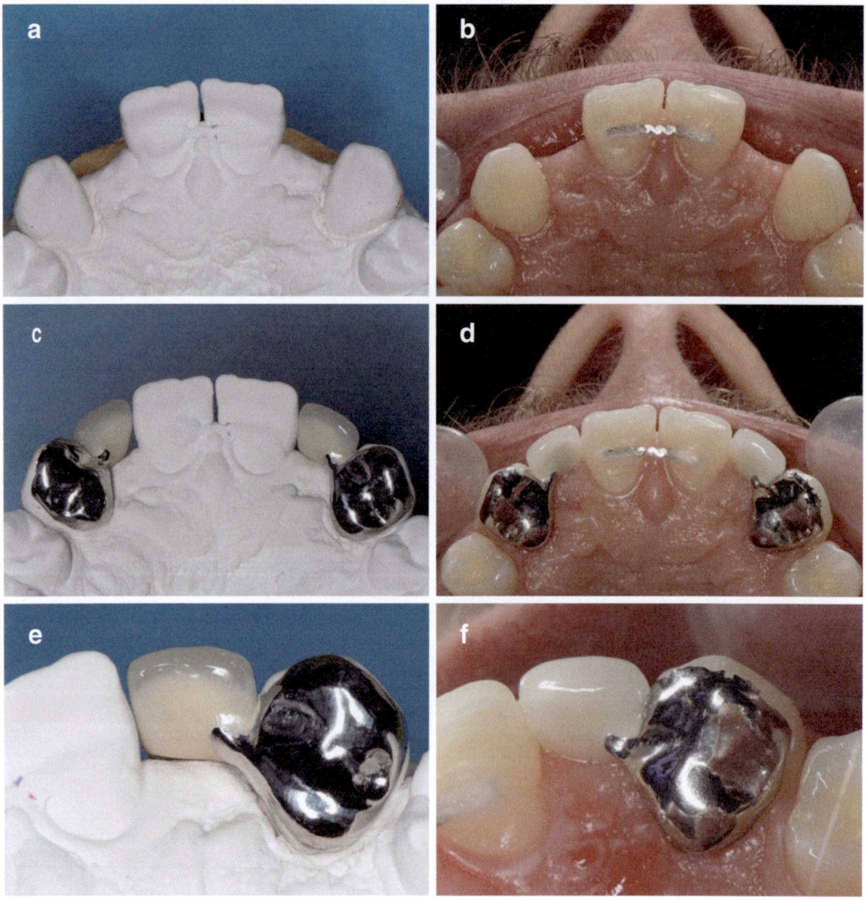

Fig. 9.12 (**a–f**) Cingulum enhanced occlusal platform of RBB retainer wings on maxillary canine teeth increasing thickness of restorations shown in a clinical case replacing missing maxillary lateral incisor teeth

clinician is faced with a decision to make. The two options in these circumstances may either be to intentionally increase the occlusal vertical dimension and load the abutment axially to accommodate a combination of intrusion and extrusion of the remaining units, or prepare the abutment tooth, prepare the opposing unit or a combination of both abutment and opposing tooth (Figs. 9.11 and 9.13). The former option requires the design of the contact surface to transmit occlusal force axially through the tooth and subsequently to the periodontium. This is largely achieved through an occlusal plane that is inclined to be perpendicular to the axial angulation of the tooth (Fig. 9.14). In contrast, the preparation of the abutment tooth removes the need for a change in the occlusion. The clinician needs to be wary that tooth preparation not only requires consideration for the intercuspal position and also dynamic movements, resulting in accommodating an even retainer wing thickness in all planes. If the canine is the abutment tooth, the clinician may be best advised to incorporate lateral movement guidance onto the retainer wing (Fig. 9.15).

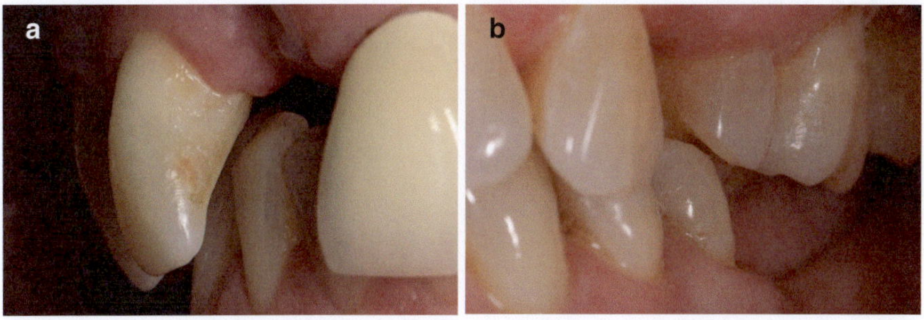

Fig. 9.13 (**a, b**) Preparation of the bridge abutment teeth and planned adjustment of the opposing teeth will allow sufficient interocclusal space to accommodate RBB retainer thickness without the need for altering the occlusal vertical dimension

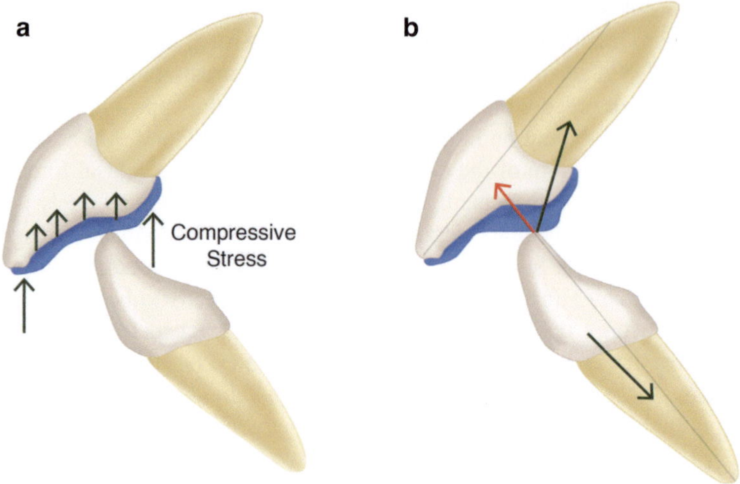

Fig. 9.14 RBB retainer wing design incorporating incisal edge coverage and cingulum enhanced occlusal platform allows favourable functional loading of: (**a**) the adhesive resin cement (compressive stress shown in green arrows) and (**b**) the abutment and opposing occluding teeth through their long axis (green arrows) with minimal off-axis loading (red arrow)

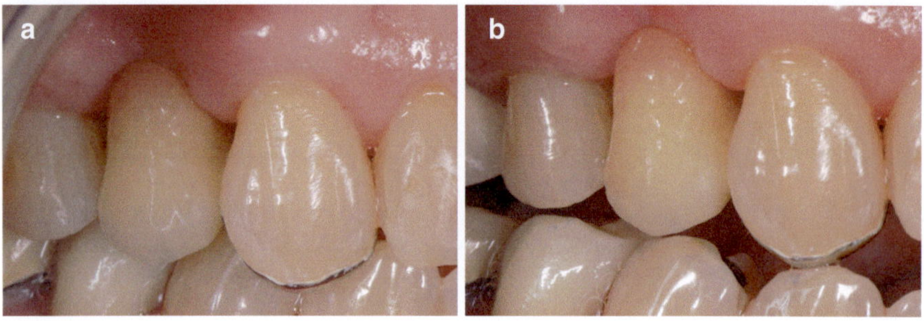

Fig. 9.15 (**a, b**) Canine guidance on RBB retainer wing allowing separation of the posterior teeth on lateral guidance

9.5 Tooth Preparation

Resistance and retention form, an improved path of insertion and increased connector height can be attained from minimal tooth preparation. One further advantage of tooth preparation is the greater ability to positively locate the bridge retainer onto the abutment. A cingulum rest, locating dimple or finish line (incisal or gingival) will aid the laboratory technician in the construction of the restoration, in addition to the clinician with the location of the restoration in the clinical scenario (Fig. 9.16).

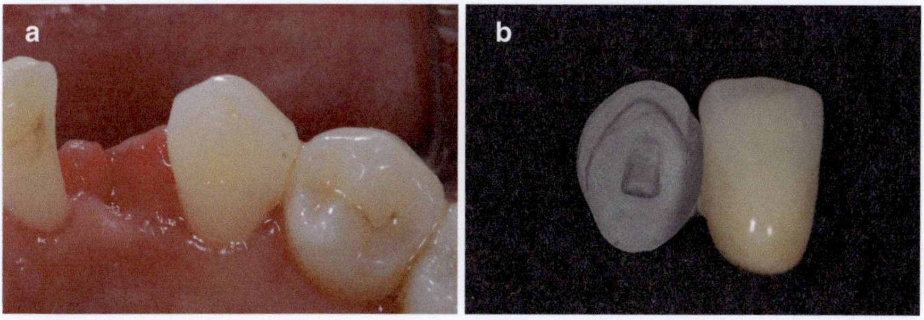

Fig. 9.16 (**a**) Incisal and cingulum rest preparation of tooth 43, (**b**) with reciprocal engagement features in the RBB wing retainer

Preparation guide planes on mesial or distal abutment surfaces, depending upon the position of the pontic, will limit the path of insertion and so minimise the potential for movement to cause restoration debond. Such guide planes modify the bulbosity of the tooth by altering the height of contour and will also result in a longer connector height between retainer and pontic, thus building further rigidity into the prosthesis framework (Figs. 9.7 and 9.11).

Other advantages of tooth preparation include the minimisation of metal work overlying maxillary palatal cusps and anterior incisal edges. When utilising occlusal coverage and respecting the need for adequate retainer wing thickness, metal work may become intrusive in the maxillary palatal area. This may also be more apparent in the patient's smile line. By reducing the palatal cusp, the restoration form is likely to be more tolerable and more aesthetic. Incisal edge coverage improves surface area, location and retention form but is unlikely to be tolerated from an aesthetic point of view. One preparation technique may be to provide a sub-incisal groove (Fig. 9.17).

If teeth are to be prepared, then the clinician has to incorporate a method to maintain the space; otherwise, axial movement of units may result in unwanted re-establishment of contact (Fig. 9.18).

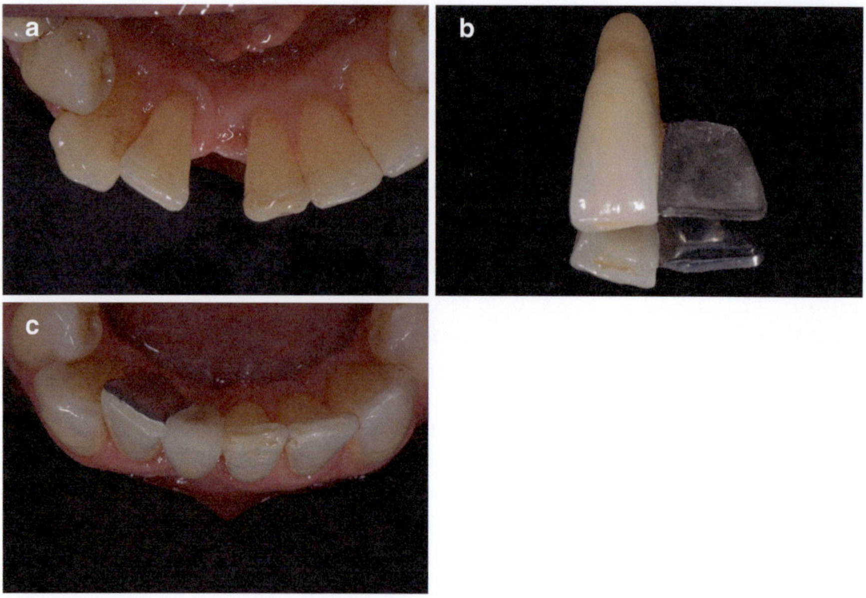

Fig. 9.17 (**a**) Subincisal groove preparation of abutment tooth 42 allows (**b, c**) partial coverage of the incisal edge, improving the functional engagement and aesthetic integration of the RBB restoration

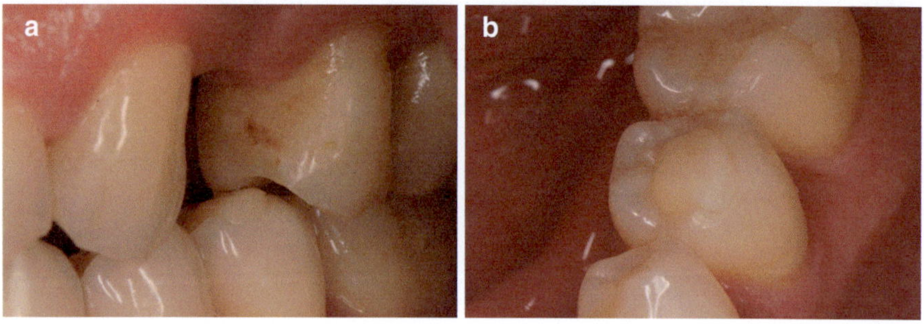

Fig. 9.18 (**a, b**) Glass-Ionomer cement occlusal space maintainer on occlusal surface of opposing tooth 35 to maintain prosthetic space during construction of the RBB restoration

9.6 Restoration Framework Design

The framework design is key to the restoration's success. The favoured material for the resin-bonded bridge prosthesis framework is a non-precious metal alloy of nickel chromium, largely due to its inherent rigidity, predictable bonding surface, ease in casting and its economic benefit. Cobalt chromium alloy, glass-matrix or polycrystalline high-strength ceramics (e.g. lithium disilicate and zirconia) may also be used as alternative aesthetic framework options and for those patients that present with a nickel allergy (Fig. 9.19).

Retainer wing design will inherently require considerations of the aesthetic and the functional component in addition to the adhesive aspects of retention.

With any choice of framework material, the retainer wing design should be unperforated and engage a maximum surface area across all available abutment tooth surfaces (mesial, distal, incisal/occlusal and cervical/lingual/palatal) to provide optimal retention. The greatest surface area contact provides the greatest engagement of the prosthesis. This is crucial in the ability of the technician and the clinician to locate the bridge prosthesis on the abutment that will aid compression of the bonding resin cement and favour axial directional loading of the supporting abutment tooth (Fig. 9.14). The minimal retainer wing thickness required for the nickel-chromium metal alloy is 0.7 mm (Fig. 9.20), and ceramic materials require a minimum of at least 1 mm. These requirements are to be detailed to the dental technician in the laboratory prescription. The design must be balanced against the aesthetic parameters in the aesthetic zone and the ability of the patient to access and cleanse the restoration margins. Incisal engagement of the retainer wing of an

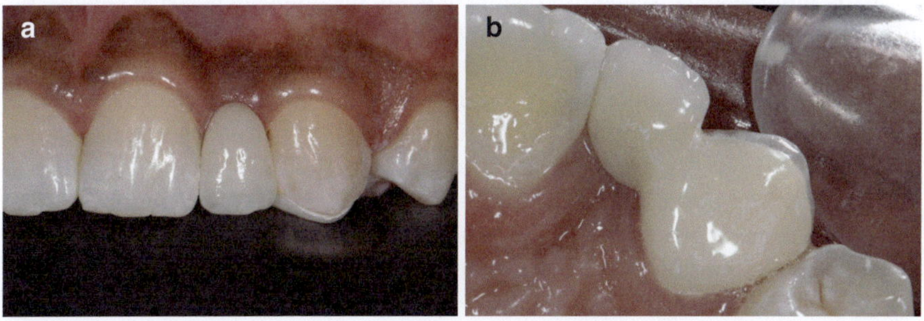

Fig. 9.19 (**a, b**) All-ceramic Zirconia two-unit cantilever RBB replacing tooth 22 from abutment tooth 23

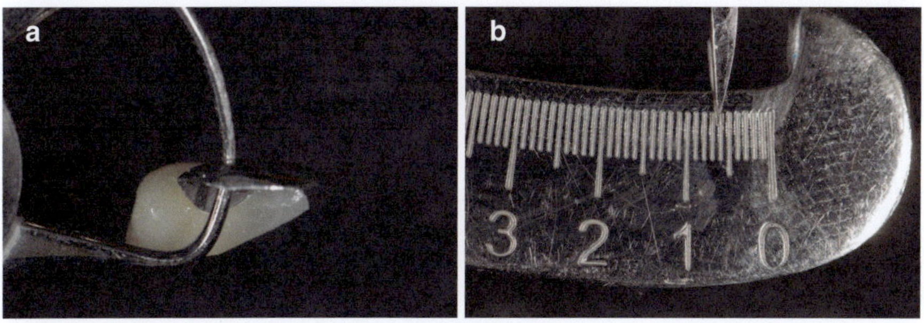

Fig. 9.20 (**a, b**) Measuring retainer wing thickness with an Iwansons Calliper to check the required thickness for the nickel–chromium metal alloy

anterior tooth will improve location of the prosthesis but may impede upon the ideal aesthetic outcome especially if a metal alloy framework is used. Cervical engagement of the retainer wing deep into the gingival crevice is likely to be counterproductive. Without adequate retraction, moisture control during the adhesive cementation phase is likely to be compromised. Where there is no preparation, the resin bridge is likely to create a positive margin; if this is situated at the cervical junction, the potential for gingival inflammation increases. To mitigate against these issues, the inferior margin of the retainer wing should be elevated 0.5–1 mm above the gingival margin, this will also be beneficial at the cementation stage where excess adhesive resin cement extrusion can be visualised and removed with relative ease.

Without the ease of retainer wing location on the abutment tooth, cementation of the prosthesis is significantly compromised and will result in a compromised outcome due to a lack of appropriate seating during the cementation process. Methods of mitigating such difficulties are numerous. One option that may introduce aesthetic compromise is overlapping the retainer wing over the incisal edge to ensure restoration. Once successfully located and cemented, the patient can return at a later date to have the overlapping portion adjusted to allow improved aesthetic integration of the restoration (Figs. 9.17 and 9.21).

In the same manner as anterior abutment teeth, the clinician needs to balance the advantages of tooth preparation versus no tooth preparation, although the nature of the abutment teeth posteriorly may influence the decision-making. Due to their pronounced occlusal platform, creating a surface that will be axially loaded is easier to achieve (Fig. 9.12). This change in occlusal vertical dimension needs to be tempered against how the remaining dentition and occlusal contacts will change. A 0.7 mm increase posteriorly will result, on average, in an approximate 2–3 mm space opening anteriorly. This may not be acceptable to the patient, especially if, in the long term, axial movements do not result in re-establishment of occlusal contacts. The junction between tooth and retainer wing is best kept remote from lateral movements of the opposing teeth and should also incorporate a portion overlaying the

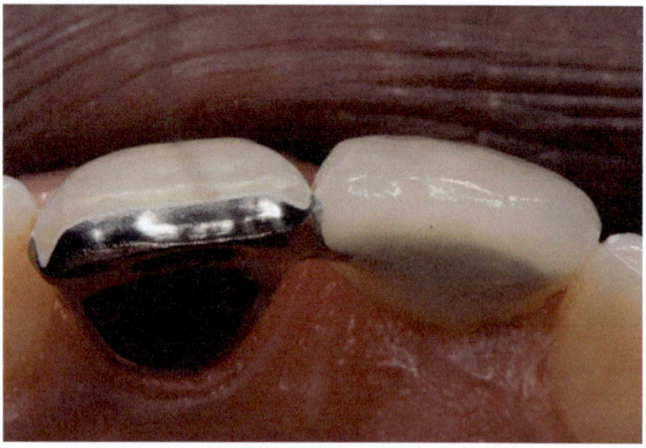

Fig. 9.21 Overlapping the retainer wing partially over the incisal edge to ensure restoration location and improved anterior aesthetics

occlusal surface. The extent of the coverage can vary. Retainer wings can either extend on the palatal and lingual cusp short of the central fissure, at the central fissure, past the central fissure or encompass the whole occlusal surface (Fig. 9.22). In areas where the likelihood that non-axial forces are not likely, the clinician may consider less extensive coverage. In contrast patients who parafunction greater coverage of the occlusal surface may be more beneficial. One aspect that is less crucial is the need to incorporate design features for location when compared to anterior abutments. Posterior teeth have occlusal fissure patterns which result in ease of location on the cast and intra-orally. If the fissure patterns are deep, the clinician may find it difficult for the bridge to seat. In these circumstances, technical colleagues could block out the fissure areas with a die spacer.

Other than improved adhesive potential, increased surface area coverage of the abutment tooth also plays a role in the manner in which the resin cement is loaded. Cements loaded in compression are less likely to result in failure than those exposed to shear or tensile forces. If the abutment tooth has an occlusal contact transition from retainer wing to tooth surface, this is likely to result in shear stresses being translated during lateral movement to this junction, and there is an increase in the risk of the restoration debonding via resin cement failure. To reduce these stresses, the greater the retainer wing extends in coverage across functional surfaces, the less risk there is of functional occlusal contact guidance moving across such a transition.

Metal alloys bend and flex due to their physical ductility, whereas the inherent brittle nature of ceramics allows them to catastrophically fracture through their weakest section (typically the connector). The degree to which this manifests depends on the dimensional size of the prosthesis framework itself. The longer and narrower the framework, the greater the potential for flexure and fracture. In contrast, thicker and shorter frameworks will have less potential for flexure and fracture due to the increase in stiffness. This phenomenon is relevant to the framework design of the prosthesis. The more flexure, the greater the risk of prosthesis debond or fracture as the prosthesis flexes away from the abutment tooth. To reduce this, the greater the thickness of the prosthesis framework and the shorter its length, the less flexure will occur. The parameters associated with this are directly related to the

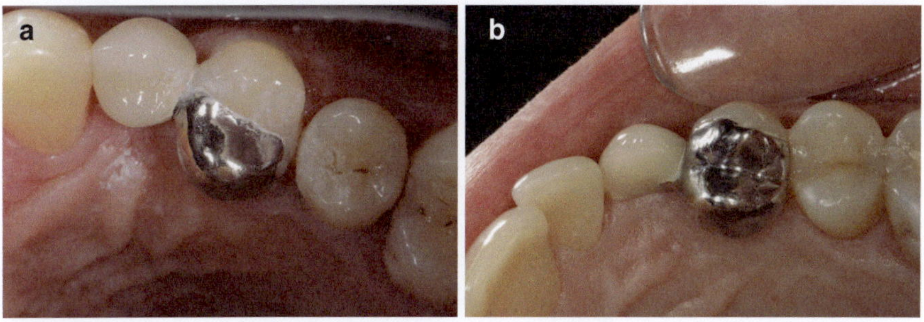

Fig. 9.22 (**a, b**) Retainer wing designs to engage a maximum surface area across the occlusal table, where possible, to provide optimal retention

number of abutments and the size of the pontic (span length), the framework thickness in cross-section and more specifically the connector width and length. For example, a resin-bonded bridge with multiple abutments and more than one pontic with short connector width and length will flex and bend more often than a single retainer single pontic framework. As such, the latter is less likely to debond or fracture.

The clinician has some scope of influence on the rigidity of the framework. In situations where the soft tissue profile is favourable in the vicinity of the prospective connector, gingival modification can increase the width and length of the connector to increase rigidity. In other circumstances, where teeth may be contoured, resulting in undercuts in mesial or distal surfaces, a guide plane preparation may also increase connector width and length.

9.7 Restoration Pontic Design

The shape, angulation and size of the pontic play a significant role in a number of aspects in bridge provision. The fit surface of the pontic influences the emergence profile and so the aesthetics. The pontic–edentulous ridge relationship plays a role in the emergence profile of the bridge, which in turn influences the ability to clean the embrasure space and the underlying mucosa.

The ovate pontic provides the most optimal emergence profile whilst also being the most cleansable pontic design (Figs. 9.23). The engagement of this pontic with the soft tissues gives the appearance of projection of the prosthetic tooth from the

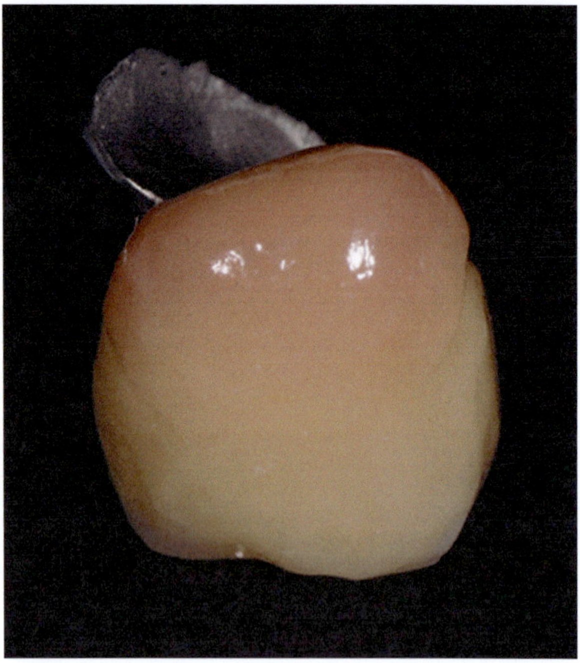

Fig. 9.23 Ovate ceramic pontic allows efficient cleansibility

edentulous ridge. The ovate nature of the fit surface allows cotton tufted floss (e.g. Superfloss) to be passed under and engage the surface fully, unlike the ridge lap or modified ridge lap pontic designs, which, due to their concave fit surface shape, may not be as easy.

The ability to provide an ovate pontic is heavily linked to the biotype and volume of the edentate site. If significant bone resorption has occurred, the scope for pontic development is limited, and a modified ridge-lap design may be the only option. Where oral hygiene in a thick biotype with good volume, the soft tissues can be engaged or even modified to the desired pontic shape (Figs. 9.4, 9.5 and 9.6). One option that can be considered is the utilisation of surgical techniques to either increase the pontic site volume or to remove tissues to make a gingival silhouette to later accommodate the pontic.

Other than the purpose of restoring the space aesthetically, the pontic design can have significant repercussions on the manner in which the bridge is loaded in function. In the intercuspal position, it is preferred that contact is present on the retainer wing, light or even absent occlusal contact on the pontic. More importantly, the absence of occlusal contact on the pontic is also preferred in the lateral movement of the mandible (Fig. 9.15). If contact is present on the pontic, this will serve to torque or twist the bridge away from the abutment, placing high tensile forces upon the adhesive cement and making debond of the restoration more likely. This aspect of design to avoid dynamic occlusal loading can only be reduced through mounting diagnostic and working casts on a semi-adjustable articulator and specific prescription relayed to technical colleagues (Table 9.1).

Table 9.1 Key features of RBB prosthesis design

Restoration component	Design feature	Biomechanical benefit
Framework material	Metal alloy—Nickel-Chromium Cobalt-Chromium Polycrystalline ceramic—Zirconia Glass-matrix ceramic—Lithium Disilicate	Strength Aesthetics Aesthetics
Framework retainer	Maximum surface area coverage Non-perforated 0.7–1+ mm thickness	Restoration engagement and compressive loading of resin cement Increased rigidity Reduction of flexure Increased surface area Increased rigidity Reduction of flexure Increased rigidity Reduction of flexure
Framework connector	Maximum connector width and length	Increased rigidity Reduction of flexure
Pontic	Ovate or Modified ridge-lap design	Aesthetic profile Cleansable

9.8 Adhesive Technique

The adhesive technique for resin-bonded bridge cementation does not vary a lot from direct resin bonding in that management of moisture in the operative area is key to restoration success. One other aspect of note is the plaque status of the abutment at fit. Commonly, plaque and biofilm may be present around the cervical margin of the tooth compromising the bond as this substrate area will not be adhesively prepared optimally. The abutment tooth should be cleaned with a prophylaxis and ultrasonic scaler prior to adhesive treatments to the recipient substrates. One may be hesitant to remove the surface contaminants in these areas just before adhesive bonding procedures, as gingival bleeding may prevent and potentially contaminate adhesive cementation at that visit. To avoid such circumstances, instilling appropriate oral hygiene measures in good time before bridge provision would be the best pathway.

Where challenges may arise is from the ability to successfully isolate the abutment to allow location of the retainer wing, which is likely to be in close proximity to the gingival margin and the pontic contact to the edentulous ridge, which can potentially make rubber dam isolation challenging. The importance of the bridge fitting passively onto the abutment at the diagnostic try-in stage, as well as the pontic onto the edentulous ridge site, should not be assumed but assured very early on in the treatment process (Fig. 9.24). Suboptimal rubber dam isolation will not only compromise moisture control but can also result in restoration misfit, where the

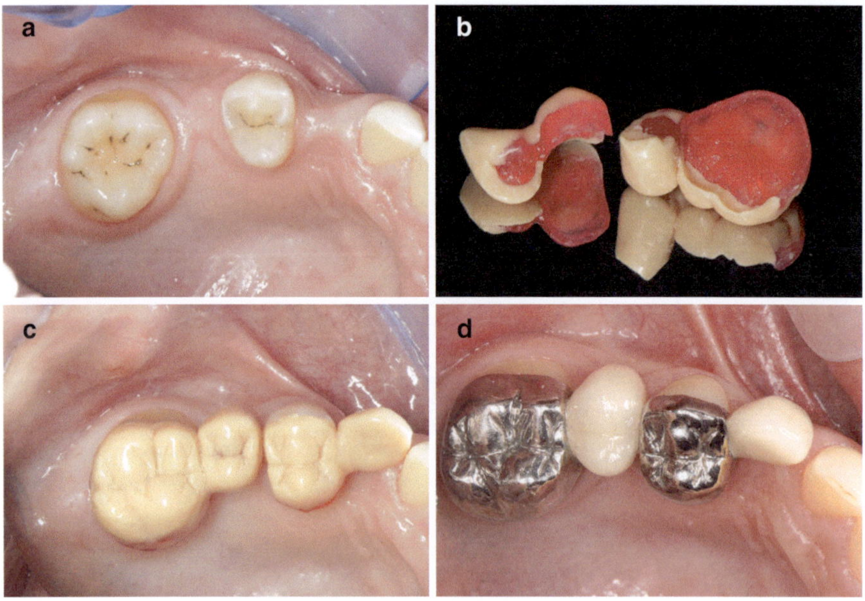

Fig. 9.24 (**a–d**) Diagnostic patterns (made of Duralay 2 burnout acrylic and wax) try-in stage of RBB restorations prior to their definitive fabrication and delivery

clamp or the rubber dam sheet prevents the restoration from fully seating, resulting in a misfit of the bridge restoration. Once isolated, the restoration is retried onto the abutment tooth. Both abutment and restoration surfaces to be bonded may also be alumina blasted with 50 micron alumina particles for surface roughening to improve upon micromechanical adhesion of the resin cement. The intaglio surface of the metal alloy retainer wing should be cleaned with alcohol to remove contaminant residue that may affect cementation. Ceramic retainer wings should be sandblasted or etched and cleaned with alcohol as indicated by the ceramic material used. The fit surface of the retainer wing bridge should then be treated as appropriate with the adhesive resin cement system primer and adhesive components. The optical properties of the resin cement are vitally important for success. Opaque coloured resin cements are advised in all circumstances where metal alloy framework alloys are used, as the metal shine through can be unsightly in the aesthetic zone. This is more crucial anteriorly, where the incisal edges of the teeth are thin and translucent, more likely to transmit the dark metallic colour of the retainer wing (Fig. 9.25).

Observing the manufacturers' guidance for the storage and mixing of the cement is paramount to the success of the adhesive procedure. The resin cement should be spatulated and loaded carefully onto the retainer wing with a microbrush to coat the cement into all areas of the surface. Both chemical-cure and dual-cure resin cements can be used.

On approximating the bridge restoration onto the abutment, cement will extrude from the restoration margins. This excess cement needs to be removed in a timely manner to avoid it being more challenging once fully polymerised. A microbrush or a cotton pledget can be effective at achieving this. The dual-cure cement may be light-cured initially to allow stability of the restoration and initiation of the chemical-cure of the cement. The full cure of the resin cement can be allowed to be undertaken with an oxygen-blocking agent to prevent the oxygen inhibition layer from forming. After full polymerisation has occurred, the excess cement may be removed by way of a No. 12 scalpel blade and careful use of an ultrasonic scaler. The area that is equally as important to manage is the embrasure space between the pontic and the abutment tooth. If cement is retained here, this can result in localised papilla/

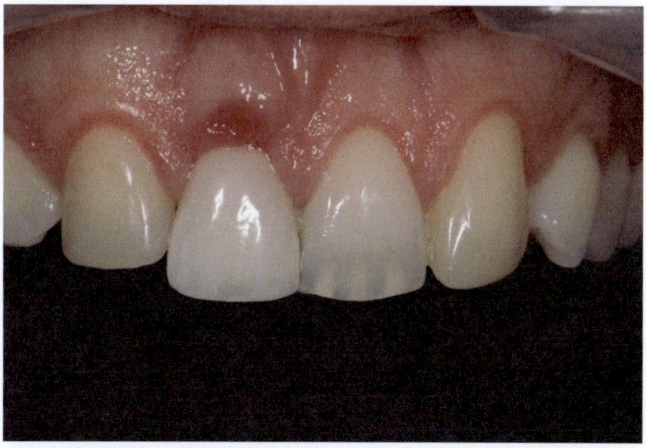

Fig. 9.25 Dark colour of RBB retainer wing showing through the supporting abutment tooth 21

gingival inflammation or periodontal attachment loss. A proficient way to manage this is the utilisation of suitably sized interproximal brushes (e.g. tepe brush) or cotton tuft floss (e.g. superfloss).

The summary of clinical stages for the adhesive cementation of a resin-bonded bridge restoration is listed in Table 9.2 and is shown in the three presented clinical cases (Figs. 9.26, 9.27, 9.28, 9.29, 9.30, 9.31, 9.32, 9.33, 9.34, 9.35, 9.36, 9.37, 9.38, 9.39 and 9.40).

Table 9.2 Summary of clinical stages of resin-bonded bridge restoration adhesive cementation

Clinical stages
1. Abutment tooth clean
2. Restoration try-in
3. Rubber dam isolation
4. Restoration re try-in
5. Abutment tooth sandblast/etch/bond
6. Retainer wing sandblast/etch/clean/prime/resin cement
7. Cement restoration
8. Excess cement clean-up
9. Oral hygiene instruction procedures

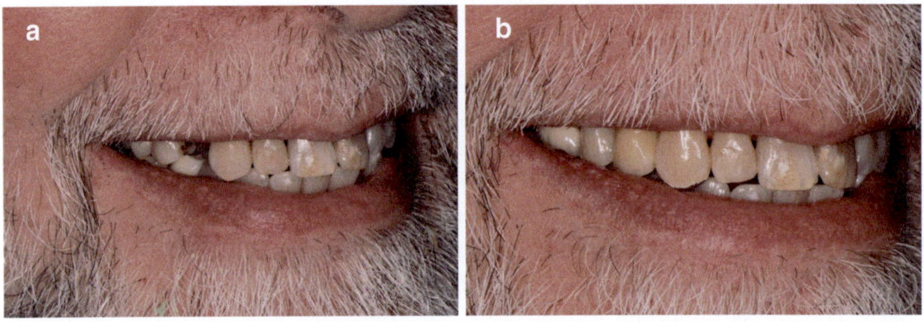

Fig. 9.26 (**a, b**) Clinical Case 1 showing before and after provision of 2-unit distal cantilever RBB from tooth 13 replacing tooth 14

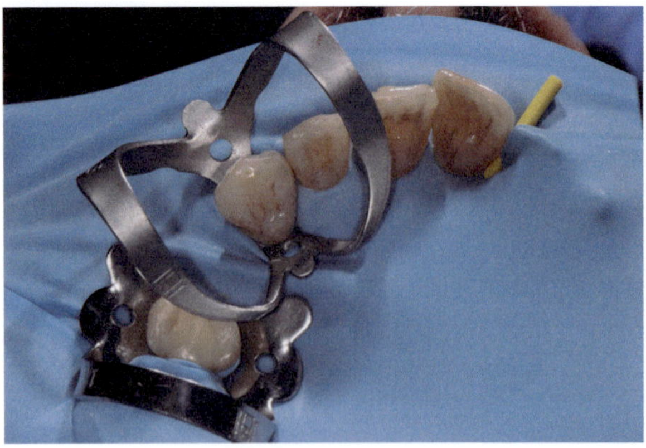

Fig. 9.27 Rubber dam isolation ensuring full exposure of abutment tooth 13 bonding surface

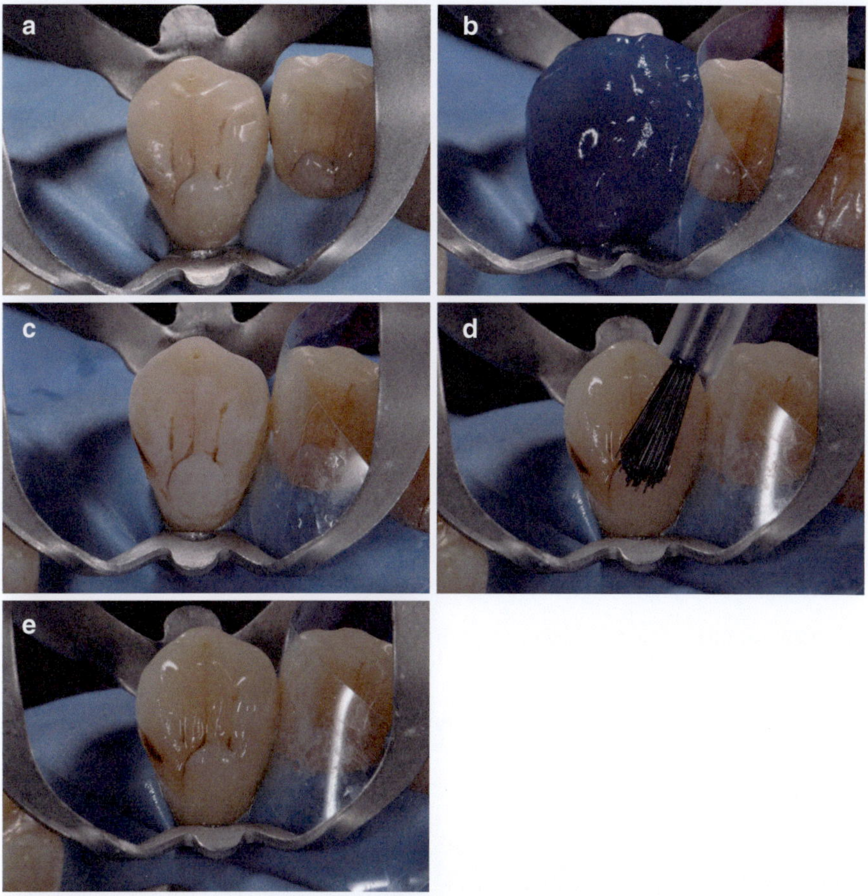

Fig. 9.28 Abutment tooth 13; (**a**) isolation, (**b, c**) etch and (**d, e**) bond

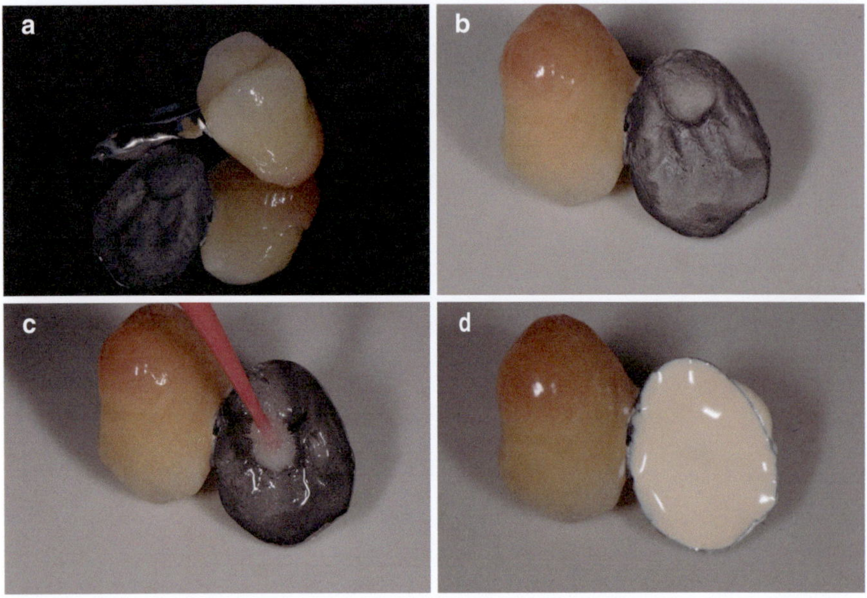

Fig. 9.29 (**a**) RBB restoration retainer wing; (**b**) sand blast, (**c**) prime and (**d**) resin cement

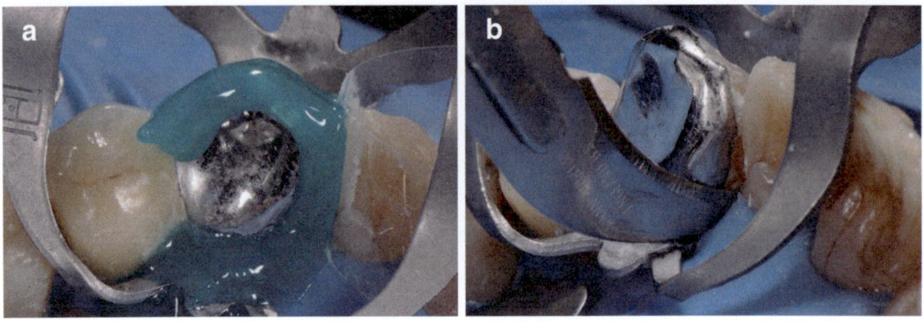

Fig. 9.30 (**a**) Cement RBB restoration (with oxygen inhibition paste Oxyguard) and (**b**) excess cement clean-up with scalpel blade no.12

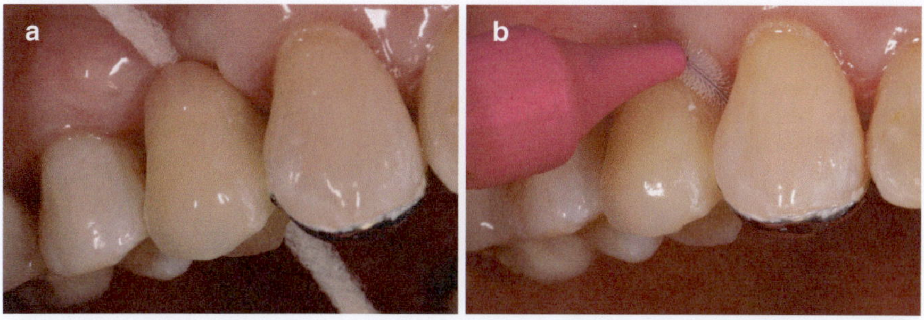

Fig. 9.31 Oral hygiene instruction procedures for RBB restoration using (**a**) cotton tuft floss and (**b**) interdental brushes

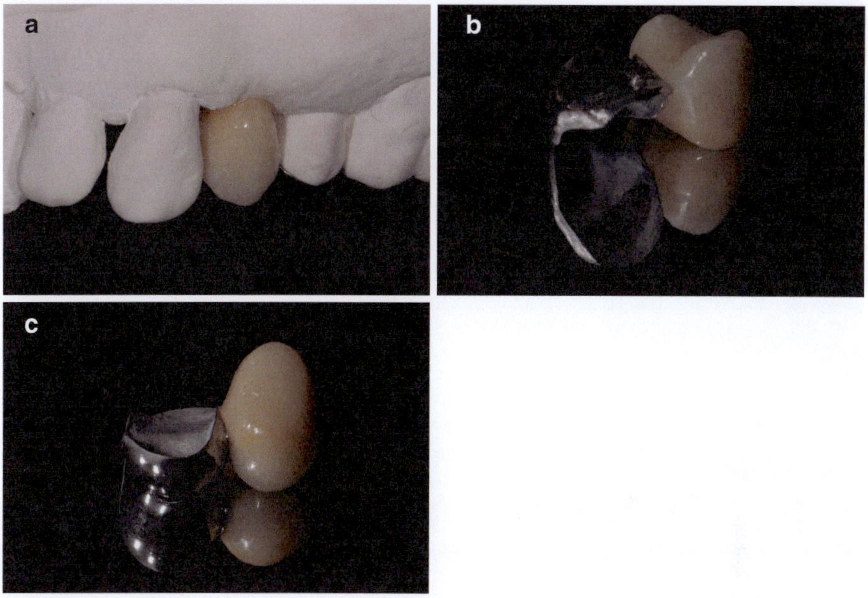

Fig. 9.32 (**a–c**) Clinical Case 2 showing planned provision of 2-unit cantilever RBB from tooth 24 replacing tooth 23

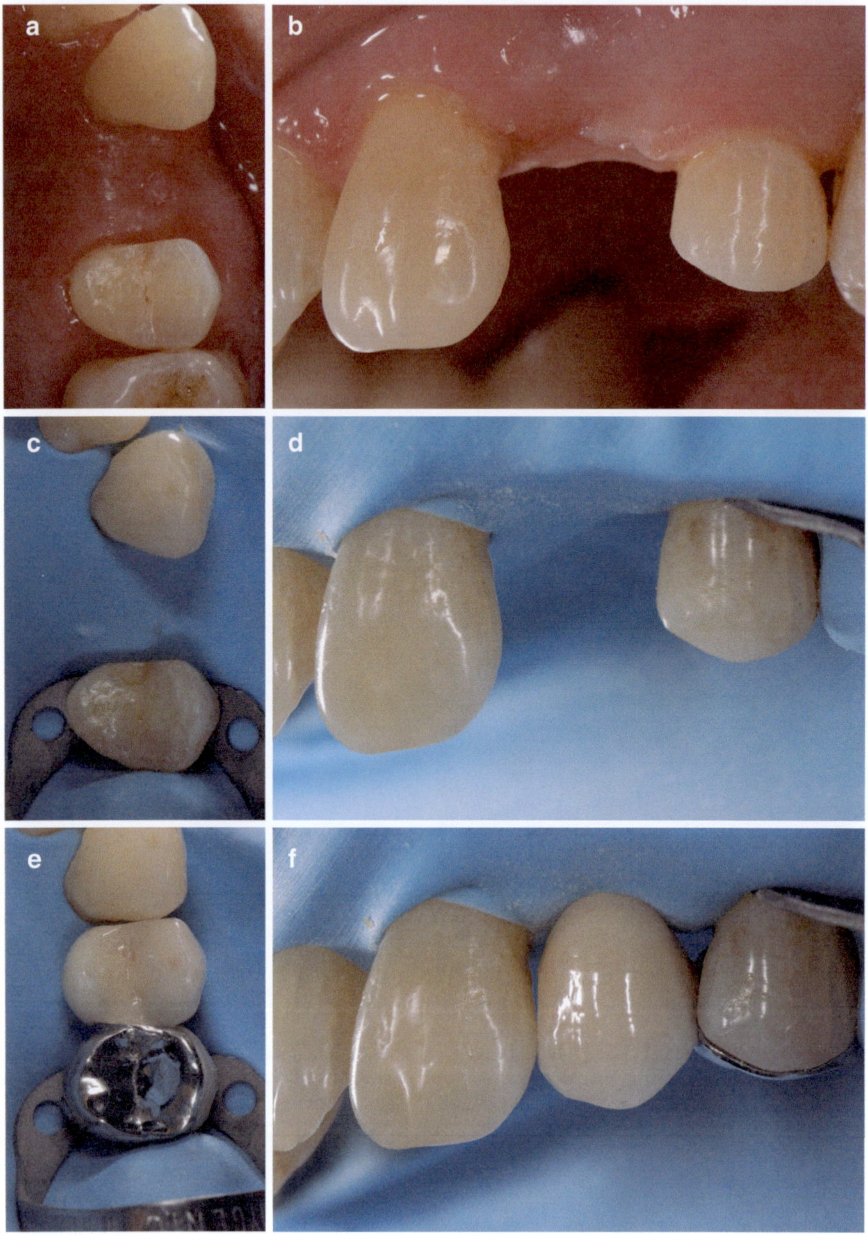

Fig. 9.33 (**a–d**) Rubber dam isolation and (**e, f**) restoration re try-in

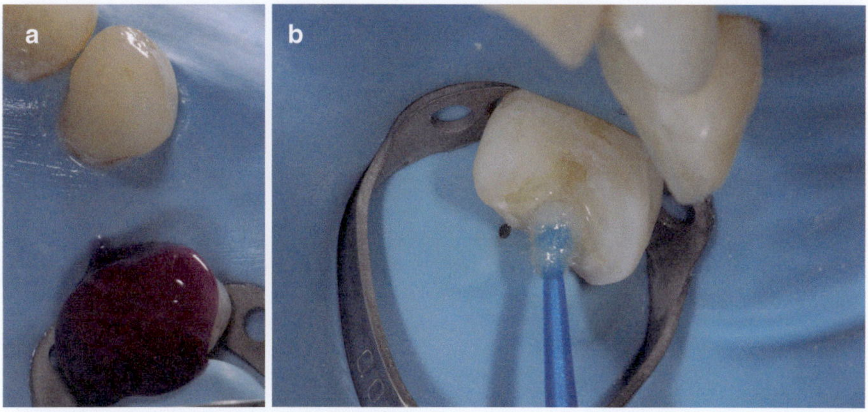

Fig. 9.34 Abutment tooth; (**a**) etch and (**b**) bond

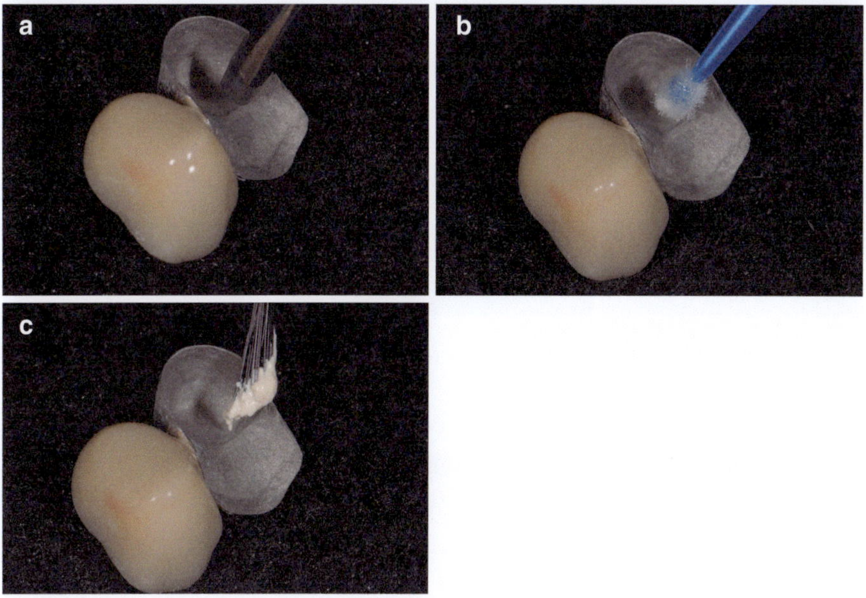

Fig. 9.35 RBB retainer wing; (**a**) sand blast, (**b**) prime and (**c**) resin cement

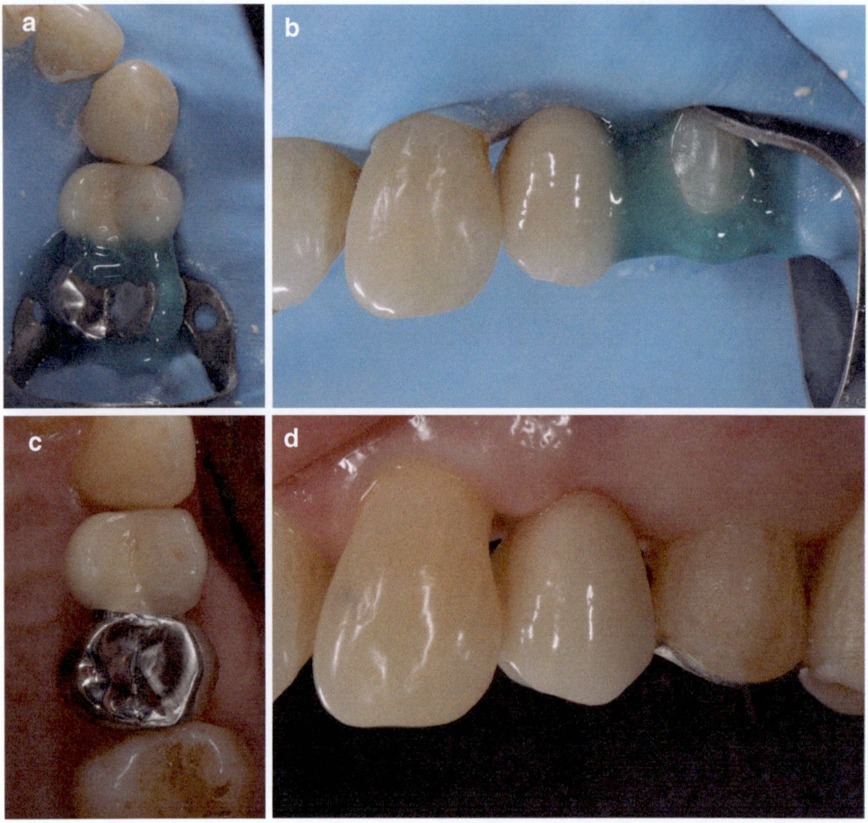

Fig. 9.36 RBB restoration; (**a, b**) cement (with oxygen inhibition paste Oxyguard) and (**c, d**) in situ

Fig. 9.37 Provision of 2-unit cantilever RBB from tooth 24 replacing tooth 23

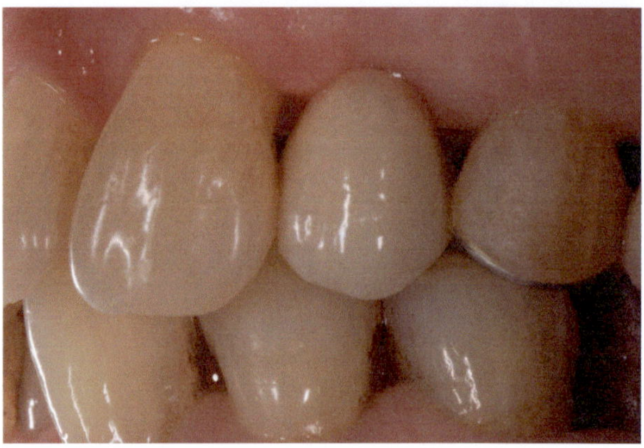

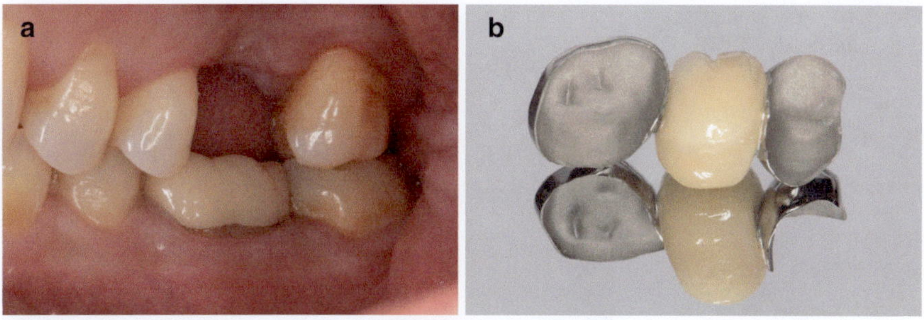

Fig. 9.38 (**a, b**) Clinical Case 3 showing planned provision of 3-unit fixed–fixed RBB from tooth 25 to 27 replacing tooth 26

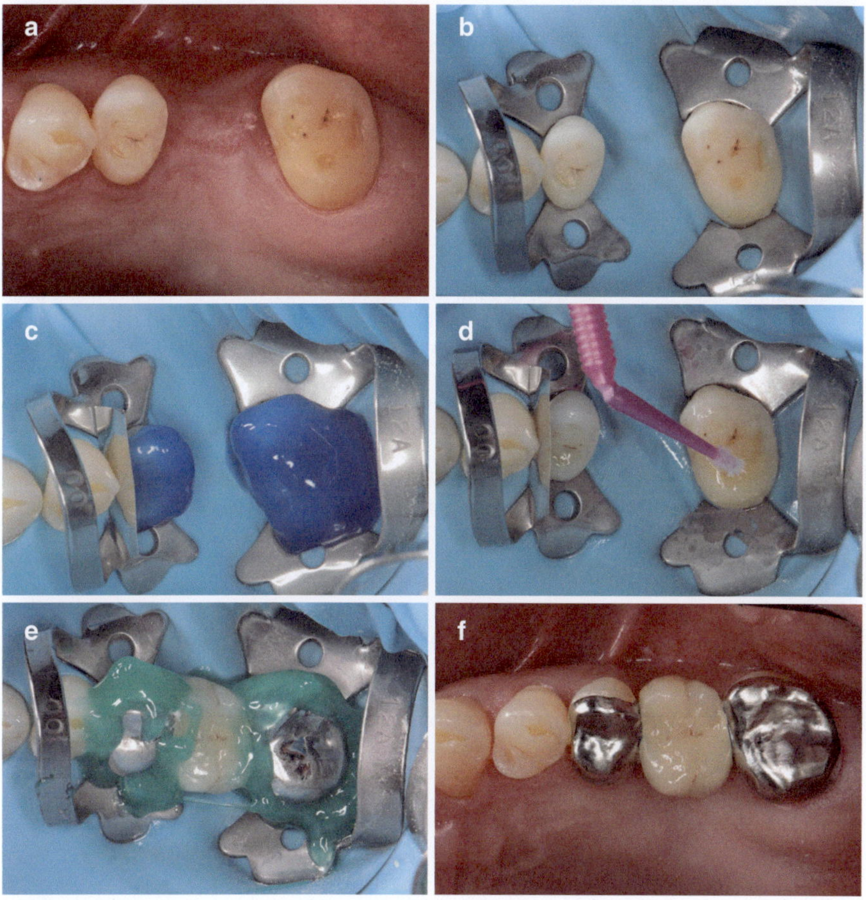

Fig. 9.39 (**a, b**) Rubber dam isolation; abutment teeth (**c**) etch, (**d**) bond, (**e**) cement (with oxygen inhibition paste Oxyguard) and (**f**) RBB restoration in situ

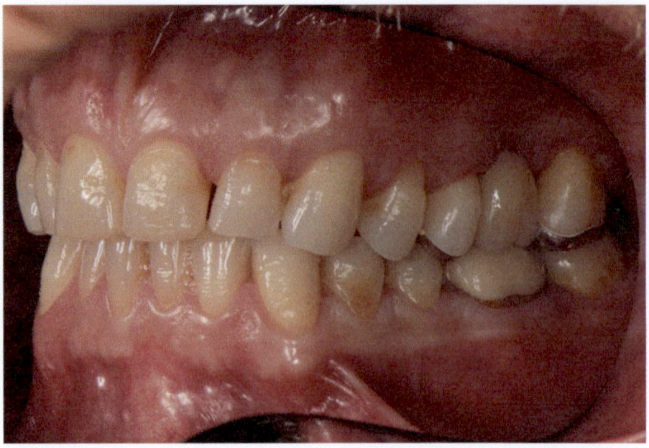

Fig. 9.40 Provision of 3-unit fixed–fixed RBB from tooth 25 to 27 replacing tooth 26

Further Reading

1. Djemal S, Setchell D, King P, Wickens J. Long-term survival characteristics of 832 resin-retained bridges and splints provided in a post-graduate teaching hospital between 1978 and 1993. J Oral Rehabil. 1999;26(4):302–20.
2. Garnett MJ, Wassell RW, Jepson NJ, Nohl FS. Survival of resin-bonded bridgework provided for post-orthodontic hypodontia patients with missing maxillary lateral incisors. Br Dent J. 2009;201(8):527.
3. Jagodin S, Sasse M, Freitag-Wolf S, Kern M. Influence of attachment design and material on the retention of resin-bonded attachments. Clin Oral Investig. 2019;23(3):1217–23.
4. Kern M, Knode H, Strub JR. The all-porcelain, resin-bonded bridge. Quintessence Int. 1991;22(4)
5. King PA, Foster LV, Yates RJ, Newcombe RG, Garrett MJ. Survival characteristics of 771 resin-retained bridges provided at a UK dental teaching hospital. Br Dent J. 2015;218(7):423.
6. Pjetursson BE, Tan WC, Tan K, Brägger U, Zwahlen M, Lang NP. A systematic review of the survival and complication rates of resin-bonded bridges after an observation period of at least 5 years. Clin Oral Implants Res. 2008;19(2):131–41.
7. Shah R, Laverty DP. The use of all-ceramic resin-bonded bridges in the anterior aesthetic zone. Dent Update. 2017;44(3):230–8.
8. Shahdad S, Cattell MJ, Cano-Ruiz J, Gamble E, Gambôa A. Clinical evaluation of all ceramic zirconia framework resin bonded bridges. Eur J Prosthodont Restor Dent. 2018;26(4):203–11.
9. Yoshida T, Kurosaki Y, Mine A, Kimura-Ono A, Mino T, Osaka S, Nakagawa S, Maekawa K, Kuboki T, Yatani H, Yamashita A. Fifteen-year survival of resin-bonded vs full-coverage fixed dental prostheses. J Prosthodont Res. 2019;63:374.
10. Zhang X, Li T, Wang X, Yang L, Wu J. Glass-ceramic resin-bonded fixed partial dentures for replacing a single premolar tooth: a prospective investigation with a 4-year follow-up. J Prosthet Dent. 2019;124(1):53–9.

Managing Occlusal Issues 10

Contents

Learning Outcomes

- Appreciate how adhesive dentistry techniques can aid in the management of occlusal issues.
- Recognise situations where adhesive restorations can be utilised to create or enhance anterior or lateral guidance.
- Be aware of the ability of adhesive techniques in reducing non-axial loading on vulnerable units.
- Appreciate how unfavourable axial movements into edentate sites can be managed through treatment which aims to induce intrusion and extrusion to accommodate prosthetic replacement.

10.1 Introduction

The traditional occlusal philosophy, the attainment of a cusp fossa relationship between opposing teeth statically and the ideal lateral and anterior guidance dynamically, may be a mantra that is unachievable for most patients outside of considering wholesale and destructive dentistry. Focus on attainment of the ideal for the dentition as a whole in this manner may distract away from situations where occlusal principles can be applied to individual tooth units or opportunities to prevent further

A. Alani, M. Patel, *Adhesive Techniques in Restorative Dentistry*, BDJ Clinician's Guides, https://doi.org/10.1007/978-3-032-07346-4_10

occlusally related pathology. Invariably, occlusal factors may contribute to the issues or tooth loss. Occlusal problems or developing pathology, such as non-working side interferences, are likely to be inconspicuous when compared to the more tangible signs of decay or periodontal disease. As such, recognising and treating occlusal problems from either a preventative or elective manner may not be as intuitive for practitioners.

The adhesive management of occlusal problems provides an avenue to optimise static and dynamic occlusal contacts to improve the dissipation of forces through the dentition to reduce forces that may either cause tooth surface loss or catastrophic fracturing or cracking of teeth.

10.2 Cracked Teeth

With the marked increase in parafunction and bruxism associated with more prevalent mental health issues and the desire by our patients to retain teeth, heavily restored or otherwise, occlusally related problems such as cracked teeth now have a greater incidence. Cracked teeth are difficult to diagnose and even more difficult to treat, as they have significant repercussions where cracks develop into a catastrophic fracture, rendering the tooth unrestorable. Where patients constantly parafunction and brux teeth undergo repeated cycles of axial and non-axial loading. Crack propagation results in pulpal symptoms where fluid, via the capillary effect, moves in and out of the crack and dentinal tubules as the tooth is loaded or exposed to temperature changes. As the crack widens, greater fluid exchange occurs, slowly increasing the painful stimulus. Once a crack becomes a fracture, the periodic nature of the pain can change to something more constant depending on the level at which the pulp is exposed or inflamed. Due to the nature of the fracture, teeth can become borderline restorable or even unrestorable. Steep angular fractures through the middle portion of teeth, mesio-distally or bucco-palatally, create defects difficult to retain either through direct or indirect restorations. The fractures tend to cleave through the passage of least resistance. This invariably puts teeth with mesio-occlusal or disto-occlusal or a combination of both at a greater risk, especially where the restorative material is amalgam alloy, large with an undercut cavity form. Teeth that may be more susceptible to fractures are molars and premolars due to the increased mastication forces imparted upon these teeth (Fig. 10.1). Unlike anterior teeth, posterior teeth are loaded axially, but non-axial occlusal forces can be detrimental, imparting stress and strain on the teeth that are involved in lateral or protrusive guidance on working and non-working sides. Maxillary premolar teeth are morphologically at a disadvantage due to their occlusal shape. The inherent deep valley of the central fissure from the mesial to the distal makes the wedging of cusps apart more likely during function. This observation needs to be borne in mind when looking at the cusp fossa relationship of any dentition. The greater the cusps engage into deep fissures the increased likelihood that during function, non-axial loads will occur. In essence, the depth of this relationship compounds

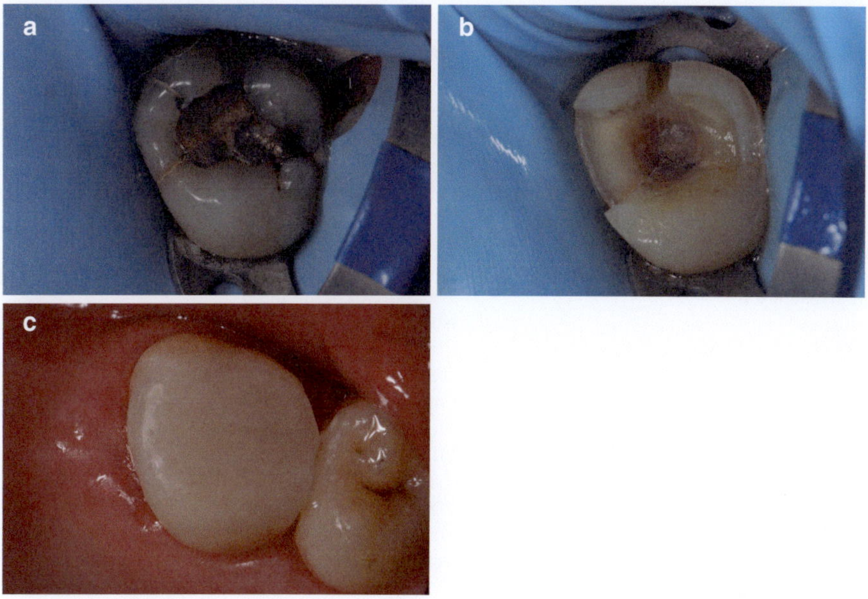

Fig. 10.1 (**a, b**) Extensive cracking within a maxillary second molar tooth 27 highlighted after removal of amalgam restoration. (**c**) Restoration with a full occlusal coverage direct composite onlay with shallow cuspal inclines and a flat basic occlusal anatomical profile to reduce functional stresses and help aid resolution of pulpal symptoms. This restoration will act as an adhesive bandage to help reduce further crack propagation. Indirect restoration is indicated as the long-term management strategy

occlusal loading, making unfavourable force distribution more likely. This issue is not exclusive to premolars. Teeth with restorations that are not optimally shaped can result in wedging forces. In this manner, the concept that the restoration is a tool or implement through which occlusal force is transmitted to the remaining tooth tissue needs to be recognised.

Prevention takes precedence over management, as it is likely to be too late once a crack has propagated. Preventive advice for parafunctional-related problems is underdeveloped and unlikely to be considered as important as that for plaque-related disease, despite both representing an equal threat to tooth vitality and survival. Early recognition of parafunction is likely to be difficult, but nonetheless, there are some signs and symptoms that patients and clinicians should be wary of (Table 10.1).

Once a tooth fractures as a result of occlusal forces, the patient and the dentist can be forgiven for focusing their efforts on this now severely injured tooth. What may be more intuitive once the problem is recognised is accepting the unfortunate fractured tooth as a compromised unit, but signalling a greater need to protect the remaining, otherwise intact units. What the clinician needs to be aware of is the constant or even ever-increasing masticatory or functional load the patient is applying to the teeth. If we say that on average a healthy patient has 28 teeth, one fracturing will result in the remaining 27 teeth managing the same

Table 10.1 Signs and symptoms of a pathogenic occlusion

Apparatus	Signs & symptoms
Temporomandibular joints	Pain Crepitus Clicking Locking
Musculature	Pain—acute/chronic Trismus Swelling Redness
Periodontium	Widening of periodontal ligament Isolated angular defects
Teeth	Cracks Wear Fracture Mobility/fremitus Migration
Restorations	Cracks Wear Fracture Decementation

occlusal loads, proportionally, the forces on these remaining teeth will increase and not decrease. Hence, the remaining units are now at a greater risk of fracture. Preventive devices such as stabilisation splints and bite raising appliances rely on compliance of the patient and, of course, cannot be worn all the time. These techniques could be considered to have their limitations in the prevention of further crack occurrences.

The purpose of a restoration, when faced with such extensive and catastrophic repercussions of non-axial loads, other than the widely accepted 'functional' and 'aesthetic' roles, should extend to the need for a 'protective' role. Restorations fill a void within a tooth but are also an apparatus that distributes occlusal force to the tooth, periodontal ligament and alveolus. A large amalgam alloy restoration, under- or over-contoured or with sharp line angles, is likely to concentrate forces internally in the tooth that increase the chances of fracture. Through a change in restoration design concept, a restoration can be engineered to be a tool through which force is dissipated more evenly through the trunk instead of focusing force down the aforementioned path of least resistance. Cuspal coverage through indirect full crown, partial crown or onlay restoration provision achieves this by bracing the remaining cusps and preventing flexure. An alternative method is the provision of a direct composite resin onlay restoration that would act in the same protective manner, but also evenly redistributes occlusal force and can change the nature of the static and dynamic contacts (Fig. 10.1).

10.3 Occlusal Redesign

The mechanical protection of teeth may occur through occlusal resign of the new restoration provided. The achievement of cuspal coverage has been more routinely achieved through the provision of an indirect crown, partial crown or onlay restoration. This can result in the removal of sound tooth tissue to achieve the occlusal aims to protect the remaining tooth tissue. In a situation where a molar tooth is heavily restored with an extensive three-surface amalgam alloy restoration, the treatment can take the form of simultaneous replacement of the restoration and reducing the risk of fracture. The first step would be to remove the restoration from the tooth and examine the floor of the cavity for signs of caries or fracture lines. At this point, if anything significant is observed, the patient should be made aware, as this may invariably signify a reduction in the prognosis of the tooth. Once the cavity has been restored with composite resin, attention may turn to the occlusal table. Rather than maintaining a deep cusp-fissure profile in the new restoration, an additive approach to cover both cusps with composite resin and flatten the occlusal table with a gentle cusp incline. This redesign results in the tooth and the restoration being loaded in compression with reduced wedging splitting forces (Fig. 10.1). To avoid localising occlusal contacts on this and other molar units in isolation, utilising this approach could be better suited in a direct adhesive rehabilitation where numerous teeth are restored and, as such, will share the occlusal load collectively in a different manner. This change in occlusal design can also be achieved through a resin-bonded bridge provision for the replacement of a maxillary canine cantilevered from the first premolar tooth. This change in occlusal design of the molar may be prudent for the pattern of tooth loss. The absence of a canine and its guidance, which aids in the reduction of lateral forces, results in a greater need to protect premolar and molar teeth in this manner.

The alternative to providing direct cuspal coverage is the provision of an indirect adhesive restoration. The crucial consideration in this respect is the reduction of tooth tissue to an adequate level to accommodate a restoration without compromising available enamel surface for bonding, the pulp and the thickness of material required for strength in compression. Where full coverage is required, tooth reduction should be minimised to accommodate the chosen material and ensure optimal fit. Knowledge of the requirements of the material should be borne in mind when examining the tooth and planning the preparation. Incorporation of residual restorations can be considered, but it may be more beneficial to remove any restoration, resulting in fewer interfaces and potential sources of failure.

10.4 Modifying Occlusal Guidance

Fortifying teeth, such as redesigning restorations and their occlusal loading, is one prophylactic measure to reduce cracks or fractures. A different approach may be to increase the likelihood of dis-occlusion of vulnerable units on anterior or lateral movements of the mandible. Anterior and canine guidance may be considered the gold standard for this role. Inevitably, over time, both may diminish as the teeth continually function and wear. In some patients, canine guidance may never have been present and can be created with the so-called 'canine riser' technique. This can be achieved through the direct provision of a composite restoration contoured to manage lateral loads to dis-occlude all other contacts on the working and non-working sides. The composite resin needs to be applied in a thick increment of at least 2 mm, which can be designed through diagnostic waxing on articulated study casts and then translated into the patient's mouth utilising a translucent silicone matrix technique (Fig. 10.2). Cases where aesthetic changes are proposed and require functional considerations may also be planned diagnostically and executed in this same manner, utilising matrix transfer techniques (Fig. 10.3).

Where the restoration is placed for this role is likely to be put under significant, and potentially constant occlusal loads, the clinician may consider an alternative material such as Type III gold alloy due to its superior wear characteristics and hardness (Figs. 10.4, 10.5 and 10.6). This would be retained utilising resin bonding in combination with a sandblasted intaglio surface. Other than ideal physical properties, this restoration modality can provide further advantages. The guidance surface can be designed on articulated models to ensure smooth transition from the intercuspal position laterally (Fig. 10.5). One disadvantage is that the metal alloy shows on the incisal and palatal surfaces, which are dependent on the smile line and tooth angulation, also (Fig. 10.6). Increasing parafunction and an ageing population are only likely to increase the instances where such restorations are indicated. Modification of functional occlusal guidance in this manner can be provided in isolation for patients with progressive wear of the canine tooth or incorporated into a treatment plan for either tooth replacement, such as implant provision, resin-bonded bridge provision or for tooth surface loss cases.

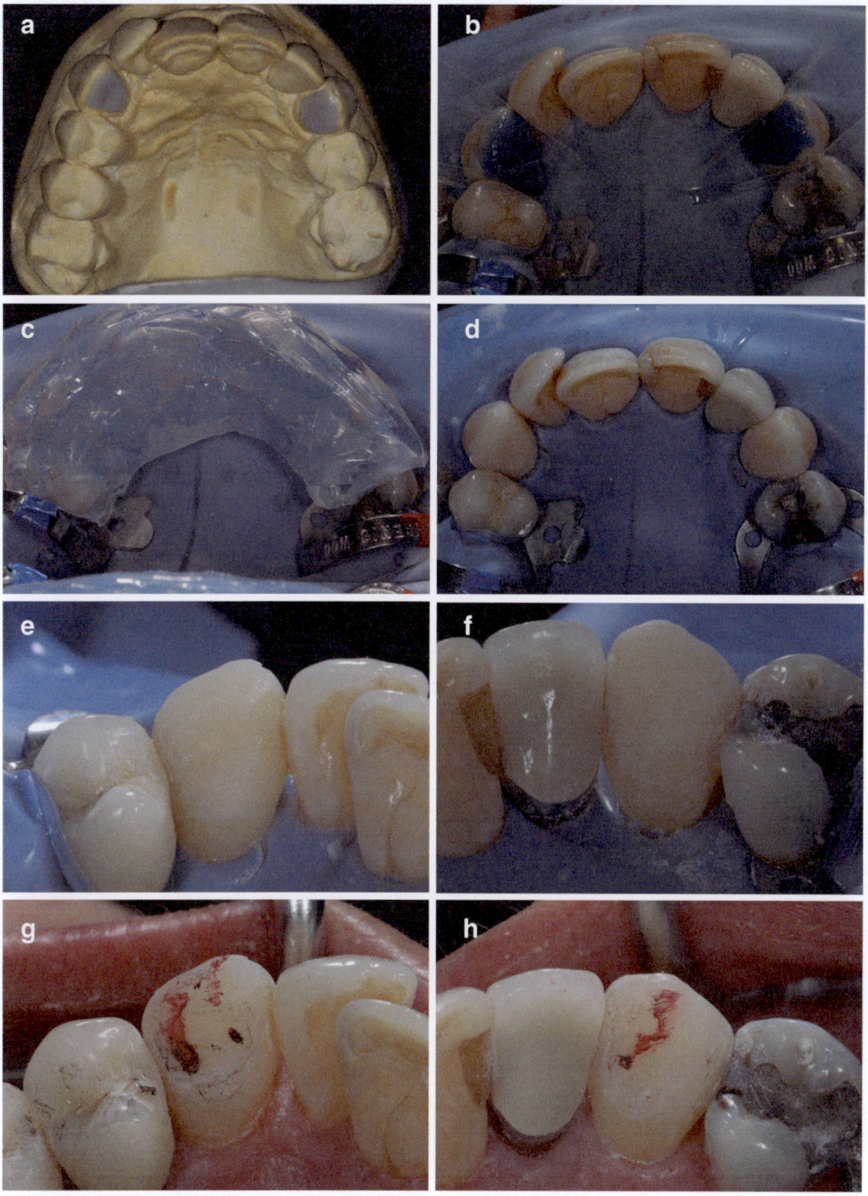

Fig. 10.2 (**a**) Diagnostic wax up of maxillary canine teeth 13 & 23 palatal surfaces to enhance canine guidance. (**b–f**) Subsequent isolation and adhesive technique utilising transparent matrix to deliver direct composite resin palatal veneers. (**g, h**) Static and dynamic occlusal markings on restorations verifying diagnostic planning

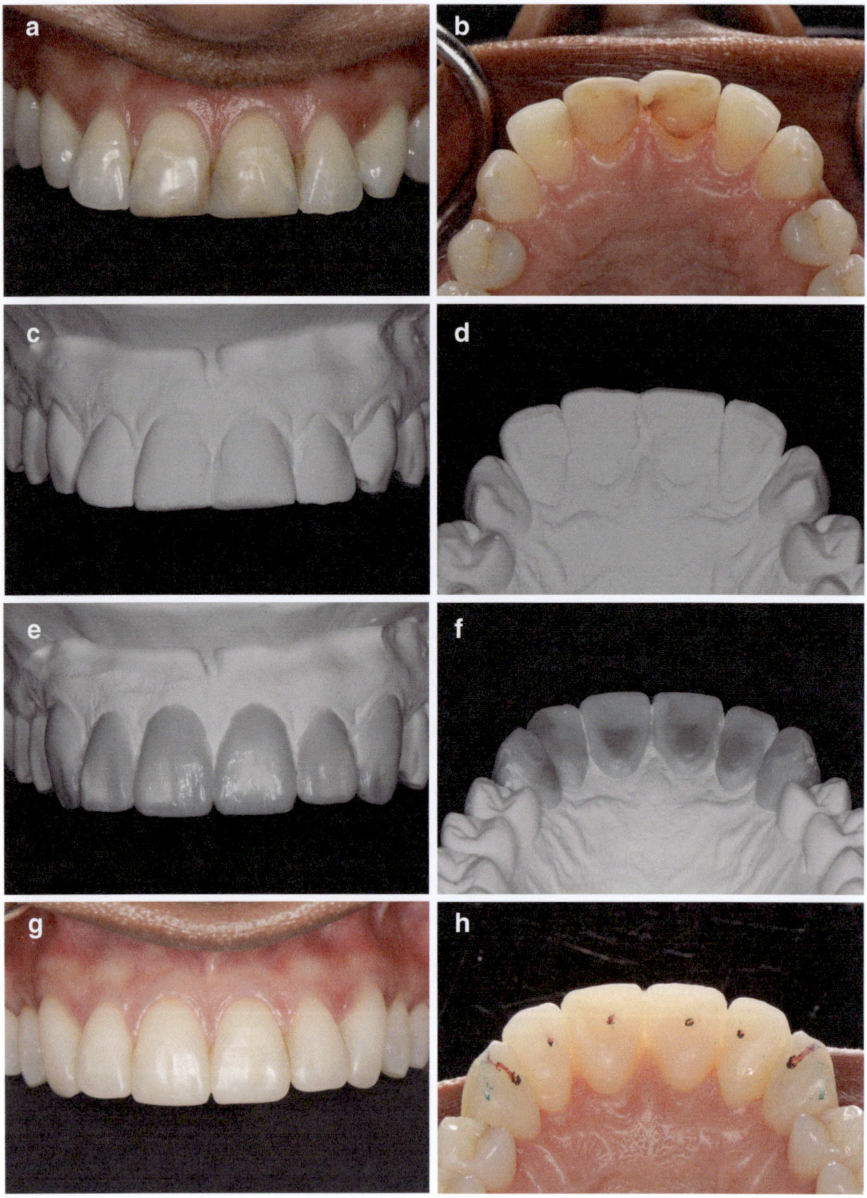

Fig. 10.3 Aesthetic and functional adhesive restoration of teeth 13–23 with composite resin restorations; (**a, b**) Pre-operative situation. (**c–f**) Diagnostic planning on articulated study casts with aesthetic and functional contour waxing. (**g, h**) Composite resin direct restorations of teeth 13–23 showing improved aesthetics with static and functional occlusal markings

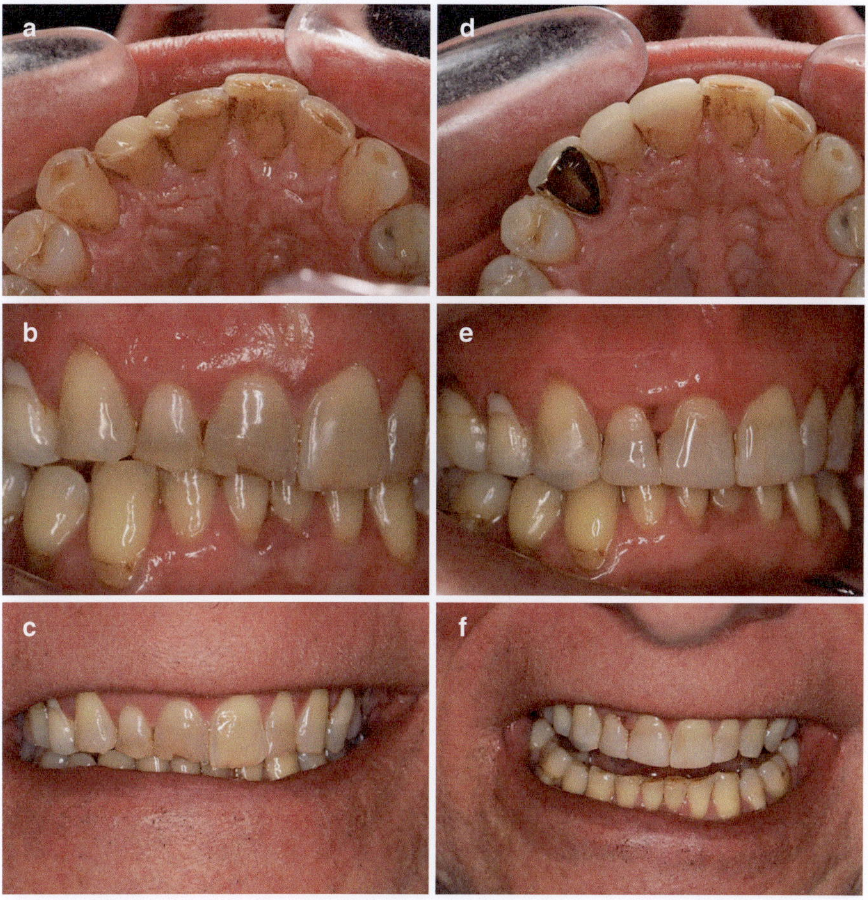

Fig. 10.4 Adhesive restoration of teeth 13, 12 and 11; (**a**–**c**) before and (**d**–**f**) after. A canine riser made from Type III gold adhesively bonded in place on tooth 13 re-established functional separation of anterior and posterior teeth to improve prognosis of composite resin restorations and aesthetic integration of teeth 12 and 11

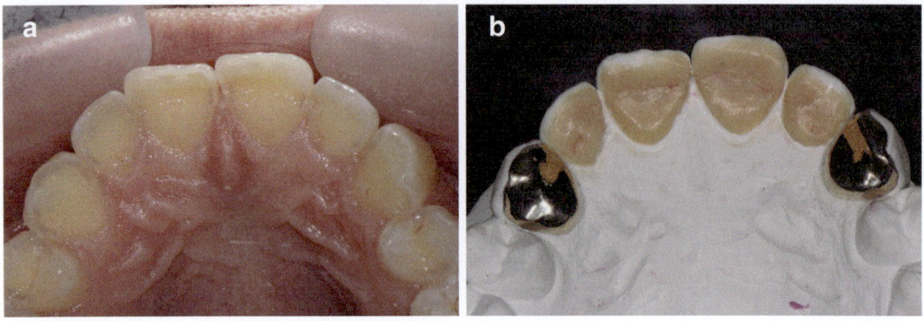

Fig. 10.5 Restoration of teeth 13–23; (**a**) Pre-operative situation. (**b**) Diagnostic wax up of teeth 12–22 and planned canine risers made from Type III gold on teeth 13 and 23 to allow functional separation of anterior and posterior teeth to improve the prognosis of planned composite resin restorations for teeth 12–22

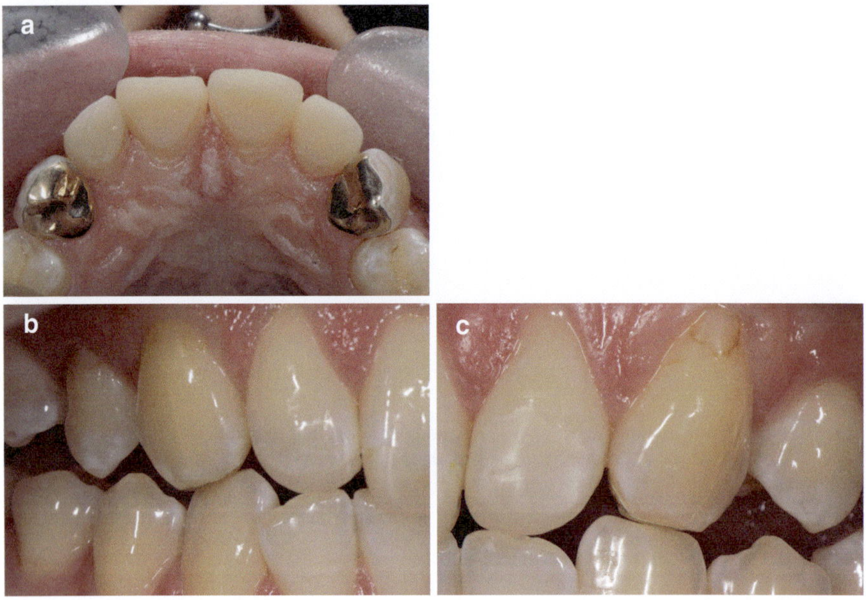

Fig. 10.6 Adhesive restoration of teeth 13–23; (**a**) Post-operative situation. (**b, c**) Type III gold alloy canine risers on teeth 13 and 23, allowing functional separation of anterior and posterior teeth to improve the prognosis of composite resin restorations of teeth 12–22

10.5 Tooth Over-Eruption

A variation on the presentation of localised occlusal changes is the overeruption of units into edentulous spaces. This situation can result in trauma to the opposing arch, an inability to restore the space with a prosthesis and restrictions on mandibular movements due to the 'locked-in' nature of the occlusion. This can be fairly frustrating and difficult to manage due to the extreme change in the occlusal plane. This almost classically occurs when a tooth is extracted and the missing unit is not prosthetically replaced, or in cases of tooth wear (localised or generalised), resulting in progressive dento-alveolar compensation. The loss or absence of an opposing tooth unit can result in the passive eruption of the tooth into that space. This situation can result in drastic measures to aide restoration of the space. Clinicians may consider extraction, severe occlusal adjustment or orthodontic intrusion of the aberrant over-erupted tooth. Full mouth rehabilitation to even out the occlusal plane and accommodate a prosthetic replacement may also be considered.

Occlusal situations where a tooth presents requires restoration without the requisite interocclusal space can be challenging to manage. This is compounded further where there is a lack of occluso-pulpal space, which makes any mode of preparation fraught with concern about maintaining pulpal integrity. The occlusal height in this situation is also likely to be compromised, hence reducing relative axial wall height for retention.

An occlusal intrusion device acts like an orthodontic appliance, and parallels can be drawn from the use of Dahl appliances. They can take many forms. Where a molar tooth has severe tooth surface loss, space for restoration is either gained from a change in the occlusal vertical dimension or by creating greater height through procedures such as crown lengthening. A direct restoration can be applied to the occlusal surface of the tooth, increasing its coronal height and localising contact on this unit in isolation. This, of course, results in a lack of contact on all remaining units in the intercuspal position. The design of the occlusal platform of the local intrusion device should be flat, lacking any occlusal morphology, to aid axial loading. Commonly, the device, due to its interim nature, can be provided in glass ionomer cement or composite resin. This change induces intrusion and extrusion movements to re-establish contacts on the adjacent teeth. Once the requisite movements are achieved, a more definitive restoration can be provided in composite resin, ceramic or gold alloy. This restoration, unlike the intrusion device, can have occlusal morphology incorporated with a more definitive cusp–fossa relationship (Figs. 10.7 and 10.8).

Where posterior teeth are over-erupted and occluding on the opposing edentate space, cementation of a prosthesis which occludes wholly on the over-erupted unit can also rectify what is an extreme change in the occlusal plane.

The 'local intrusion device' concept can be developed further by considering the placement of a resin-bonded bridge prosthesis, which restores the edentate space at an increased occlusal vertical dimension designed to create adequate pontic space through the occlusal changes provided by the contact on the retainer wing.

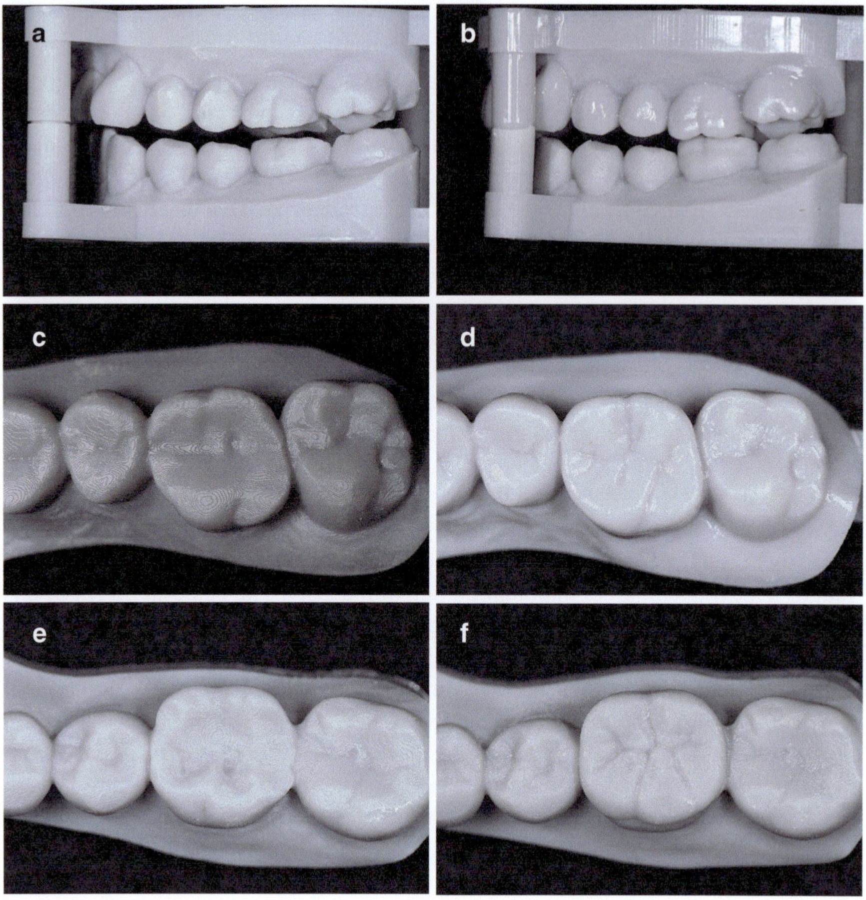

Fig. 10.7 (**a**) Diagnostic planning in centric relation. (**b**–**f**) Onlay Dahl appliances on first molar teeth 26 and 36 where localised tooth surface loss diminished restorative space for these teeth in maximum intercuspation. The opposing first molar teeth have been waxed into functional contact and will be the only contacting pairs of teeth

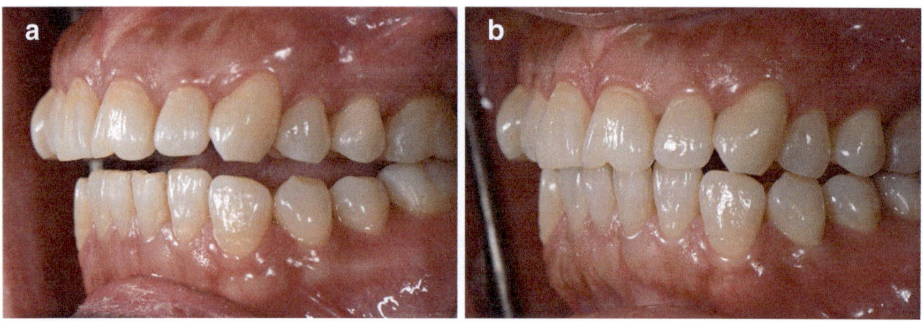

Fig. 10.8 (**a**) Direct composite resin onlay restorations on the first molar teeth utilised as the Dahl appliances; (**b**) after 6 months, re-establishment of all teeth occlusal contacts was obtained via dentoalveolar compensation

10.6 Open Bites

The presence or development of open bites (infra-occlusion) can be detrimental to both the function and aesthetics of the dentition. A lack of occlusal contact can be unsightly in the anterior dentition due to the spacing between the upper and lower teeth (Fig. 10.9). Similarly, a lateral posterior open bite may provide a further aesthetic issue where a unilateral difference between right and left can be just as unsightly for the patient due to asymmetry. These aspects of the smile may be worsened further in patients with high or wide smile arcs. From an occlusal perspective, the absence of posterior occlusal contacts from one or multiple units involved in open bites consequently means that the remaining functioning units are occlusally loaded more often or to a greater level (Fig. 10.10). Hence, establishing or re-establishing occlusal contact on such units has numerous benefits.

Due to the inherent space present between the teeth, the challenges in restoration provision are lessened. If direct or indirect adhesive restorations are to be provided, essentially making the teeth taller, the clinician needs to give attention to the new occlusal scheme design, the embrasure spaces, the interdental contact and the nature of the occlusal table. As the teeth are made taller, the crown–root ratio increases, and it may be prudent to consider a flatter occlusal anatomical plane to eliminate or minimise non-axial loading forces in dynamic function. When considering the restoration tooth margin interface, the clinician may consider creating a definitive preparation finish line if an indirect restoration is to be considered; however, a non-preparation approach may also be considered. Where direct restorations are provided, composite resin that is mechanically hard-wearing but also can be appropriately finished and polished is preferred for both functional and aesthetic reasons, where staining may develop. Ideally, the restoration should be confined to the occlusal table and have an identifiable, subtle margin for the purposes of future maintenance and/or replacement.

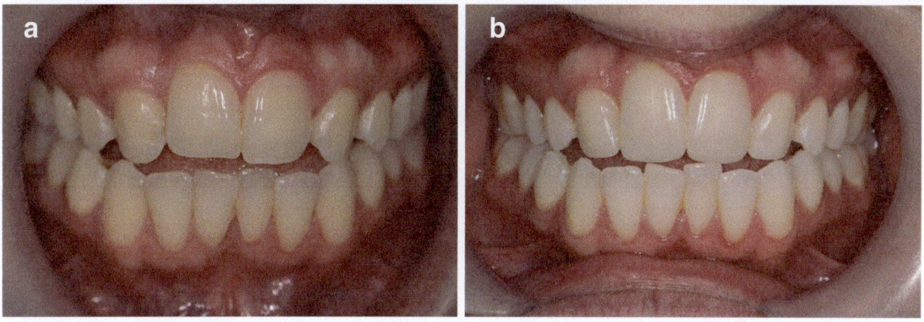

Fig. 10.9 (**a**) Anterior open bite and missing lateral incisor teeth. (**b**) Aesthetic improvement after vital tooth bleaching and restoration of canine and central incisor teeth with direct composite resin restorations

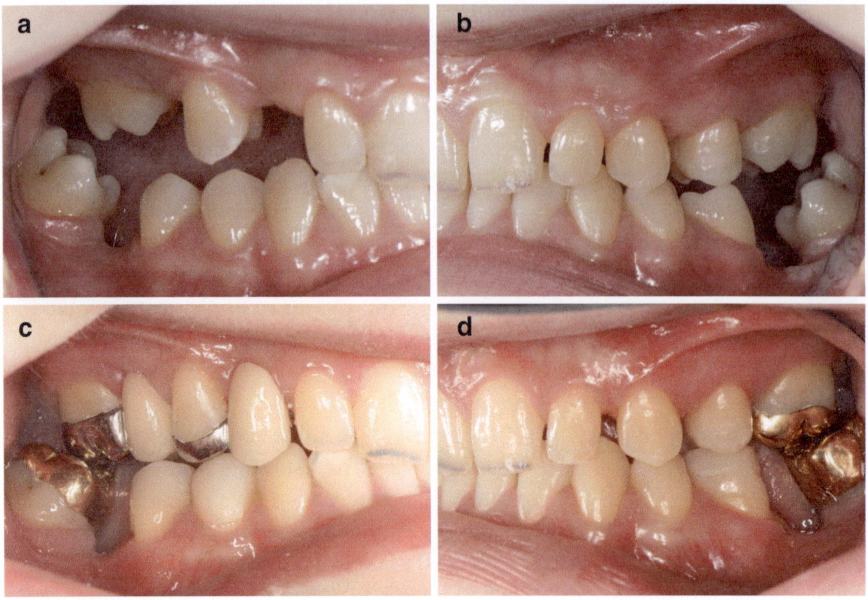

Fig. 10.10 (**a, b**) Bilateral posterior open bites and multiple missing teeth. (**c, d**) Functional improvement after provision of additive indirect adhesive Type III alloy and composite resin onlays, and resin-bonded bridge restorations

A variety of adhesive techniques previously discussed may be used to provide adhesive restorations in an additive manner to the abutment teeth to be built into occlusal contact in both anterior and posterior areas. Appropriate clinical examination, occlusal diagnosis and treatment planning would be prudent as part of the successful management of these unique cases.

Further Reading

1. Alani A, Patel M. Clinical issues in occlusion—part I. Singap Dent J. 2014;35:31–8.
2. Dahl BL, Krogstad O, Karlsen K. An alternative treatment of cases with advanced localized attrition. J Oral Rehabil. 1975;2:209–14.
3. Goldstein G, Campbell S. The Dahl concept: best evidence consensus statement. J Prosthodont. 2021;31:196–200.
4. Patel M. Treating tooth surface loss: adhesive restoration of the worn anterior dentition. Prim Dent J. 2016;5(3):43–57.
5. Patel M, Alani A. Clinical issues in occlusion—part II. Singap Dent J. 2015;36:2–11.
6. Poyser NJ, Porter RWJ, Briggs PFA, Chana HS, Kelleher MGD. The Dahl concept: past, present and future. Br Dent J. 2005;198:669–76.

Index

A. Alani, M. Patel, *Adhesive Techniques in Restorative Dentistry*, BDJ Clinician's Guides, https://doi.org/10.1007/978-3-032-07346-4

U

V

MIX
Papier aus verantwortungsvollen Quellen
Paper from responsible sources
FSC® C105338

If you have any concerns about our products,
you can contact us on
ProductSafety@springernature.com

In case Publisher is established outside the EU,
the EU authorized representative is:
Springer Nature Customer Service Center GmbH
Europaplatz 3, 69115 Heidelberg, Germany

Printed by Libri Plureos GmbH
in Hamburg, Germany